Locating the Medical

Locating the Medical

Explorations in South Asian History

Edited by

ROHAN DEB ROY

GUY N.A. ATTEWELL

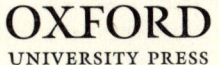

OXFORD

UNIVERSITY PRESS

OXFORD
UNIVERSITY PRESS

Oxford University Press is a department of the University of Oxford.
It furthers the University's objective of excellence in research, scholarship,
and education by publishing worldwide. Oxford is a registered trademark of
Oxford University Press in the UK and in certain other countries.

Published in India by
Oxford University Press
2/11 Ground Floor, Ansari Road, Daryaganj, New Delhi 110 002, India

ISBN-13: 978-0-19-948671-7
ISBN-10: 0-19-948671-9

Typeset in Trump Mediaeval LT Std 9.5/13
by Tranistics Data Technologies, Kolkata 700 091
Printed in India by Rakmo Press, New Delhi 110 020

CONTENTS

INTRODUCTION
Locating the Medical

ROHAN DEB ROY AND GUY N.A. ATTEWELL

Why should we 'locate the medical'? Because it pertains to an already established subfield of historical research, the call to 'locate' the medical may at first impression seem somewhat strange. Surely, locating the medical is what 'situated' studies in the 'social history of medicine', prominent since the 1970s and with a focus on the Indian subcontinent since the 1990s, have necessarily entailed? On one level this is certainly the case. But it is our contention that to focus analytical attention on the location of medicine is precisely to grapple with the common-sense understanding of medicine, to explore the different sites and ways of production of the category 'medicine', and to reveal the various objects of study, assemblages, and processes that are black-boxed by this capacious concept. Indeed, it could be suggested that the very establishment of the subfield of the history of medicine in South Asian studies—if this can be grasped by publications, congresses, institutional presence, and financing—carries with it the potential for the naturalization of the object of study. There is a risk in viewing 'medicine' as if it exists 'out there', waiting to be studied through what are often considered to be iconic sites, such as the hospital, the clinic, the pharmacy, and, typically for a historian, the places where its traces have been reposited into another kind of actual and potential existence, in the archives. This volume presents a challenge to the 'out there-ness' of medicine, and in the process aims to defamiliarize it. How is our understanding of the medical—its ontologies, modifying slightly the words of the political philosopher Johanna Oksala—achieved 'in social practices and networks of power rather being simply given?'[1]

The volume explores a variety of ways, sites, and nodes through which the category 'medical' has been consolidated and has been put to work. It does so through case studies from nineteenth- to twenty-first-century South Asia. Taken together, the chapters in this volume cover a wide spatio-temporal scope, ranging from colonial Bengal to contemporary Ladakh, from the Andaman Islands and British Burma to contemporary Maharashtra. It builds on the now extensive literature on the history of medicine in the Indian subcontinent, which has been instrumental in shaping our understanding of medicine during the period of colonial rule. The volume also showcases recent works that have focused on areas that were for long considered peripheral in mainstream South Asian historiography.

Even though the individual contributions make critical interventions, the volume as a whole is not intended as a critique of this or that perspective. Rather it seeks to add new perspectives by probing more explicitly, and in a more sustained fashion than has been attempted before, how the medical has been constituted by actors and agencies in specific times and places. As a collection of chapters, it complements several edited volumes on the history and sociology of medicine in India that have come out over recent years.[2] The strength of the contributions of this volume is to situate the enactments of the medical within the conditions of these enactments: sites, materials, instruments, documents, logics, experts, and their domains of expertise.

Locating the Medical builds on broader currents in the history of medicine. There is conscious overlap in the title with the 2004 collection of essays edited by Frank Huisman and John Harley Warner, *Locating Medical History*.[3] While Huisman and Harley Warner set out to explore the genesis and development of the history of medicine as a discipline in the United States and Europe, our volume is an appeal to unpack the multiple genealogies of the category 'medical' itself, with specific focus on modern and contemporary South Asia. However, certain reflections on the field in the Huisman and Harley Warner volume relate directly to our theme. In an obituary to the social in the 'social history of medicine', for example, Roger Cooter noted that the very idea of 'medicine' or the 'medical' had become destabilized, quoting Nikolas Rose: 'What we have come to call medicine is constituted by a series of associations between events distributed along a number of different dimensions, with different histories, different conditions of possibility, different surfaces of emergence. Its boundaries less clear and more porous than formerly thought, it consequently has become less sharp a category for analysis.'[4] Our contributions speak to these associations, events, dimensions, histories, conditions of possibility, and surfaces of emergence of the medical within the context of South Asian studies, in the history of law, technology, and mainstream history, with perspectives from anthropology. Although this is not the place for a systematic review of funding, publishing, and the institutional apparatus for the history of medicine in South Asia, we also open up the scope for greater intellectual reflection on the conditions under which the sub-discipline is gaining ground.

This volume calls attention to the notable successes in the subfield of medical history in South Asian studies. This success can be gauged by the growing institutional presence of the history of medicine in South Asian studies, by the rich variety of approaches adopted by historians, and in the number of publications and events within the field. At the same time, the volume confronts the potential pitfalls of this success—what Steven Shapin calls 'hyperprofessionalism'—in addressing the direction of the history of science.[5] This is, he writes, 'a disease whose symptoms include self-referentiality, self-absorption, and a narrowing of intellectual focus', carrying as its consequence the crisis of readership, which he observes in his own field. Clearly, the point Shapin is making is relevant to many domains of academic activity, including the history of medicine. Such a critique of self-referentiality, we feel, should inspire greater self-reflexivity among historians of medicine, who need to be more openly reflective about the ways in which their institutional locations, academic pedigree, and professional networks have shaped their own agendas. Although we are not positioning ourselves as diagnosticians, we are suggesting that this collection can throw into relief recurrent methods, resources, and archives that researchers are utilizing and mobilizing in the way they study the history of medicine, and this could serve as a useful corrective against disciplinary narrowing.

Therefore, this volume provides a platform for the traffic of ideas and approaches between the history of medicine as a sub-discipline and South Asian history, more generally. While conceiving the volume, the balance of the participants between those who would self-identify as historians of medicine, or whose work would be regarded as 'history of medicine', and those with other specialisms within history were considered, in order to generate systematic cross-disciplinary perspectives on the medical. As a result, various chapters in this volume connect the more conventional themes of medical history (illness, diseases, public health) with histories of material resources, bodies and organs, forensics, infrastructural and everyday technologies, legal codes and practices, protocols and regimes of governance, imperial prisons, and archival practices. The chapters are as attentive to the discourses and practices about the production of medicine in courts of law as among lineage healers and in the precincts of temple complexes, through cultures of translations in vernacular print, as well as the ethnographic framing of 'primitive' tribal cultures.

There is need for an interpretative axis, which, on the one hand, does not constrain the different approaches and analytical strategies adopted by the contributors, yet, on the other hand, helps to push, at a more abstract level, what they together achieve, an axis that they may rotate around. We call this axis 'historical ontologies of medicine'. While each chapter elaborates on its own position in relation to the relevant literature, in what follows, we proceed by setting out recent historiographical trajectories before we examine the theoretical purchase of historical ontologies for our project and provide a brief outline of chapters in this collection.

What Is Medical about Colonial Medicine?

The burgeoning of academic history of science, technology, and medicine in the subcontinent has its roots in the 1980s and early 1990s, first developing as an offshoot of imperial and colonial studies. There is now a rich literature, and it has become an indispensable field for understanding transformations in South Asian worlds over the last three centuries. The field has grown in conversation, even if sporadic and uneven, with sociological and anthropological approaches to health and medicine, as well as with histories of other regional, national, and transnational colonial and postcolonial situations. Several historiographical reviews have been written over the last twenty years that have grappled with its emerging forms.[6]

At a conference on histories of colonialism held in Birmingham in 1986, the historian Roy Porter posed a question that has proved to be remarkably enduring, and is now familiar to anyone working on the history of medicine in modern South Asia: 'What is colonial about colonial medicine?' The very same question was taken up a decade later by the then president of the Society for the Social History of Medicine, Shula Marks, and Waltraud Ernst addressed this question again another decade later.[7] It has become, as Ernst points out in her historiographical review of medicine in South Asia 'a hoary catchphrase' that has been used to frame a number of research directions in the field. The persistence of this question is an indication of the ways in which the history of medicine in modern South Asia has been shaped by the experiences and legacies of colonial rule. Following the tracks of 'new imperial histories', many studies have examined the extent to which modern medicine, more generally, emerged from intercultural encounters in colonial contact zones such as South Asia.[8] Medicine has also been seen as a 'tool of empire', which informed the ideological justifications as well as technologies of colonial control.[9] Colonial techniques of managing diseases, health, well-being, and populations, in turn, ended up redefining understandings about these categories themselves.[10] The question 'what is colonial in colonial medicine?' has further inspired analyses of the distinct historical trajectories witnessed in the colonial world vis-à-vis metropolitan Europe, by emphasizing the entanglements of medicine with histories of colonial governmentality and biopolitics,[11] race and gender,[12] marginality and cultural difference,[13] and epochs such as decolonization[14] and globalization.[15]

We draw attention to this question, 'what is colonial about colonial medicine?', not in order to launch another such investigation, but rather to use it as a convenient starting point for a different purpose—to point to what the many invocations of, and responses to, this question over the many intervening years seem to elide: what is medical about 'colonial medicine' or, for that matter, its conventional other, 'indigenous medicine'? To rephrase the question in a way that introduces process and contingency: how is the medical formed? How and in what conditions does an event, a substance, infrastructure, a technology of daily life, an actor, a body, a disposition, a socio-spatial configuration, or a particular situation of the body–mind become or cease to be 'medical' and according to whom (both the agents in prior times and the researcher of the present)?

Chapters in this volume examine numerous situations from colonial and postcolonial South Asia in which specific relationships, identities, as well as phenomena were designated as medical. We have aimed to capture situations that carry forward the task of the book to take seriously the question of difference (spatial–social–epistemological) in the constellations of medicine–sickness–health. Our 'map' is a patchwork. We have not set out to 'represent' each of the so-called medical systems, biomedical or other, or aspired to regional coverage. Commonplace narratives tend to universalize experiences encountered in the worlds of modern science, hospitals, laboratories, and so forth as exclusive manifestations of the 'medical'. Such narratives also either marginalize or exoticize practices that occur beyond these privileged sites. We argue that the emphasis on place and situation reveals the specific historical processes through which these distinctions between the medical and the non-medical were worked out. In so doing, we draw on recent interventions in the historiography of colonial medicine that have similarly adopted an expansive view of the medical by suggesting that the category needs to be opened up for analysis across multiple registers.[16]

Historical Ontologies of Medicine

The wide-angled perspective on the medical in this volume has the central aim of addressing how the medical is constituted (and in turn constitutes) in specific times and places. Our project charts a different course to several common theorizations of the making of medicine. Medicalization, and its twin de-medicalization, might appear at first impression a useful steering concept for our volume. They have been key concepts in theorizing extensions of the medical through insti-tutions and industrial concerns. John Burnham uses it as a cohering principle to structure his introduction to the field *What Is Medical History?* Each of his chapters can be read, Burnham asserts, 'in terms of the ways in which both historians and their subject were caught up in the tensions between medicalization and de-medicalization'.[17] One of the problems evident in such formulations, however, which our volume frontally addresses, is that the medical outlook is defined a priori. Not unlike a diffusionist model, such formulations suggest that medicine has an establishment and medicalization is the process by which medical authority is extended 'out' into 'society', where it may meet with resistance or accommodation. For almost similar reasons, we do not identify immediately with social constructivist approaches, which imagine the prior existence of a 'social' domain, waiting to engender (the shape and substance of) the world of medicine. In contrast to these potentially monochromatic renderings of medicine (and society) implied in social constructivist as well as medicalization theses, we propose to grasp the contingent co-constitutions of the medical and the social. Our approach is closely linked to what the philosopher of science Ian Hacking refers to as an exercise in 'ironic constructivism'. It is a perspective that would enable the recognition of the medical as 'highly contingent' and historically produced, and 'yet something we cannot, in our present lives, avoid treating as part of the universe in which we interact with other people, the material world and ourselves'.[18] This volume showcases various case studies where medical relationships figure both as historical artefacts and agents.

While grappling with these dynamics we need to search for the most appropriate vocabulary to describe our enquiry into locating the medical. We have already indicated that we call our approach 'historical ontologies of medicine' in South Asia. Our resort to it has been inspired by Hacking, who elsewhere compiled a collection of essays and lectures produced over a quarter of a century, which deployed the term 'historical ontology' as its title. Hacking's historical ontology seeks to map the emergence of possibilities in which beings and objects take shape and change in history.[19] Rather than reifying beings and objects as freestanding constants that exist on their own timelessly,[20] the project of historical ontology, according to Hacking, analyses 'the space of possibilities' in which they emerge, thrive, and evolve.[21] Hacking adopts a broad conception of beings and objects to include things, classifications, ideas, kinds of people, and institutions.[22] Similarly, Hacking proposes that historical ontology should study historical processes through which concepts are formed and sustained across time.[23]

However, at the same time, the project of historical ontology contests the impression that beings, objects, and concepts are passive historical artefacts. But rather, it also proposes to examine the ways in which these products of history, in turn, open up newer historical possibilities and opportunities.[24] 'The historical ontologist', argues Hacking, 'should be preoccupied by general and organizing concepts and the institutions and practices in which they are materialized.'[25] Therefore, drawing on examples from his case studies on child development and trauma, Hacking shows that while these concepts themselves were historically produced, they have also been used to organize an extensive range of activities.[26]

As an exercise in historical ontology, this volume situates medicine as an important organizing concept that is historically produced, and yet shapes discourses, practices, and subjectivities. Our project of historical ontologies of medicine is closely allied to what Hacking calls 'dynamic nominalism'. Through his thesis of dynamic nominalism, Hacking proposes to track the interactions between practices of naming and what is named.[27] Dynamic nominalism, Hacking elaborates further, reveals the 'historical dynamics of naming and the subsequent use of name'.[28] In this volume we trace some of the ways in which the historical circumstances that inform the designation of events, identities, people, and substances as medical are, in turn, reshaped by the designation.

Hacking is explicit that his conceptualization of historical ontology is derived from Michel Foucault's essay 'What Is Enlightenment?'[29] Foucault considered historical ontology as the study of how we constitute ourselves and are constituted as subjects according to three axes—knowledge, power, and ethics. In this essay Foucault proposed that 'historical ontology of ourselves' should be 'concerned with "truth through which we constitute ourselves as objects of knowledge," with "power through which we constitute ourselves as subjects acting on others," and with "ethics through which we constitute ourselves as moral agents"'.[30]

Compared to our purposes in this volume, Hacking's project, following Foucault's lead, is connected to a theoretically broader and more ambitious exploration of the 'historical ontology of ourselves'. Hacking's project is also overtly more philosophical in its orientation compared to our unambiguous engagement with disciplinary history in general and the histories of colonial and postcolonial medicine in particular.[31] Yet, we are inspired by the three 'cardinal axes' to explore various specific, locally situated, contingent histories from modern South Asia. We explore some of the ways in which the 'medical' was put together as an object of knowledge, as a subject impacting others, and as an ethico-moral organizing concept in specific moments in modern South Asian history.

In the following sections we indicate the ways in which historical ontology reveals itself in our project of locating the medical. We have accordingly grouped chapters into four themes, which are not self-contained but are rather intersecting and overlapping. We can begin to explore the historical ontologies of the medical in South Asian history by being simultaneously attentive to these interrelated questions: How do contingent political histories engender the medical? How does the medical, in turn, coalesce with, or reshape and sustain, political categories? Is the medical necessarily a stable, coherent, and continuous category? In what ways are the rigid boundaries between the medical and the non-medical blurred?

Production of the Medical

We argue that the medical is not a preordained designation. Rather the characterization of events or objects as medical emerges in specific historical conjunctures of time and place. Instead of aiming to propose a total history of the making of the medical as an overarching category in modern South Asia, case studies presented in this volume redefine the medical as a particular set of relationships between political authority, forms of corporeal knowledge, and objects of governance. The objects of governance examined in the various chapters in this volume include injuries, fingerprints, spleen, passengers, prisoners, primitives, private papers, intoxicants, road traffic, daily wage labourers, and factory workers. The medical is intimately tied to the specific entanglements of sociopolitical domains including law, governance, religion, domesticity, and literature, with material bodies, body parts, and landscapes. Three of the chapters in this volume draw upon examples from the constructions of the medical through efforts to classify bodies, culture, and society in South Asia. More specifically, they explore particular conjunctures of law and bodily intervention in nineteenth-century Bengal.

Durba Mitra analyses the intellectual and moral foundations of manuals on colonial medical jurisprudence in mid to late nineteenth-century Bengal, focusing in particular on cases of abortion. Physical investigations of women's bodies were imbricated with the histories of pathology, law, and sociological classification. Physical examination led to the production of new kinds of conceptions about 'deviant' females. These conceptions, in turn, shaped stereotypes about 'false' rape complainants, female criminality, and prostitution. Categories of deviance were created on the basis of physical evidence, understood as authoritative in contradistinction to oral testimony, and were used by a variety of actors (such as magistrates and other local authorities) to consolidate local hierarchies and prejudices (such as the exclusion of widows from property rights if they were sexually active). Mitra shows how manuals of medical jurisprudence were produced within a distinctive moral order, which intimately tied sexual activity to conceptions about social pathologies and crime.

Similarly, Chandak Sengoopta locates the medical at the intersection of the twin processes of colonial subject-making and bodily inter-ventions. The medical, both as a category and a set of practices, was sustained by regimes of colonial surveillance, governmentality, and asymmetrical interchanges of knowledge. Two late nineteenth-century colonial 'corporeal technologies', fingerprinting and mesmeric surgery, reveal how colonial relationships were not limited to political subju-gation, but, as we see also in Chapter 1, materialized in the bodies of the colonized. Fingerprinting techniques were developed in late nineteenth-century plantation economies in Bengal, first among indigo planters who used fingerprints as exteriorized material evidence in the making of contracts with their workers. As it became universalized as a technology of individual identification, applications of fingerprinting were increasingly restricted to criminal investigations. In the condi-tions of its colonial emergence, however, its applications were more wide-ranging, as they grew from within concerns of governance and surveillance. The second half of the chapter examines experiments in mesmeric surgery in mid nineteenth-century Bengal. It shows how various tropes of 'native' character traits were constructed in order to convince a primarily European audience about the effectiveness of a controversial method of removing pain during surgical intervention. These constructions enabled more extensive experimentation on native bodies of higher social position than was possible in Europe. The claim for the universal relevance of mesmeric surgery was founded ironically on the bureaucratic construction of cultural peculiarity of natives in a colonized province. Sengoopta re-emphasizes that medicine was both a product and a necessary ingredient of the twin colonial projects of asserting racial difference and violence.

Sudipta Sen's chapter on bodies (more particularly their parts) as icons of race, debility, social hierarchy, and surgical expertise pursues further the inseparable historical trajectories of the medical and the legal in South Asian history. It explores the location of the medical within the exercise of the law through the construction of the spleen as an organ of relative frailty in the bodies of poor Indians. This construction had a pivotal bearing on the legal handling of cases of violence meted out as 'corrections' by masters on their servants, a situation heightened in the late nineteenth century by the prospect of Indian magistrates sentencing European defendants. While analysing the 'notional divide between ideology and pathology', this chapter takes us through debates on legal controversies and traces a genealogy for the metonymic currency of the spleen in late nineteenth century. This genealogy embraces coroner's inquests, morbid anatomy, spleen theory, topography, and the classification of peoples, climates, and diseases of the tropics. Sen's chapter, much like the two preceding ones, situates the medical at the interstices of the histories of law, corporeal knowledge, colonial governance, and state violence.

Enactments of the Medical

The ascription of political meanings and authority to the category medical was not a story of rigid classifications and sterile constructions. We are particularly keen in tracing how medical relationships were lived, inhabited, internalized, contested, and, in the process, reconfigured. This volume argues that medical relationships in turn informed historical practices and discourses relating to various themes ranging from morality to criminality, from debility to normality, from primitivism to communication, from incomplete archives to religious beliefs, from spectacular events to the everyday. More specifically, two chapters in the volume urge us to reflect on the co-constitutive processes through which medicine and the state have shaped each other.

Jonathan Saha, for example, provides a detailed analysis of a devastating prison epidemic in late nineteenth-century British Burma and how prison officials attempted to manage it. While epidemics and prisons are established themes in the history of medicine, Saha draws on recent developments in state theory to argue against a common trope in the history of colonial medicine: that the British administrations 'deployed' medicine in order to secure its ambitions to govern populations in acquired territories. Rather than taking either the state or medicine to exist a priori, Saha's chapter is in tune with the constructivist–performative turn in the humanities and social sciences as it shows how the colonial state in British Burma was enacted into being, in this episode, through a spectrum of interventions. At the same time, the medical did not represent an already stabilized set of concerns amongst the British officials overseeing the prison. Rather, the medical was reconfigured among ostensibly 'non-medical' actors, as courts, the police, village headmen, and census workers took on roles that variously dealt with the collection and assessment of medical evidence, the propagation of sanitation, and the documentation of disease incidence. The medical, as an articulation of the state-in-the-making, itself appears as an emergent field, dispersed among an array of actors and practices, generated by specific concerns with governance and at the same time shaping the nature of governance. What we see is not straightforward 'medicalization' at the behest of the colonial state, but a firmer entrenchment of the medical domain inextricable from the practices of state formation.

Vishvajit Pandya and Madhumita Mazumdar take us to the post-Independence Andaman Islands through a close reading of a text by a Bengali doctor (Dr Kar), an 'agent of welfare' in the archipelago's tribal reserve forests. There they locate the 'medical' in the 'contingent yet pervasive presence of the state in the forest', drawing, like the previous chapter, on recent state theory, which argues that states are embodied forms, and not static entities. Kar's text can be read on two levels: as a realist ethnography of an Andamanese people, the Jarawas, and as a 'medical memoir' that narrates the state's presence in the forests as the 'custodian of its "primitive" population', positioned as 'an alterity that the state can only access, know and manage'. The Tribal Reserves are 'spaces of interaction and power' through which the state substantiates itself in the daily lives of communities. Through the partial vision into this 'distinct corporal habitus' of the state in the forest afforded by Kar's text, Pandya and Mazumdar draw attention to the co-constitutive dynamics of biomedicine, the state, and 'the primitive body'.

Rethinking Disconnections and Continuities

The agenda of locating the medical inspires various contributors in this volume to probe the assumption that the medical is a stable, coherent, and homogeneous category. The medical could be an ephemeral label, rather than a permanent and continuous property of objects and careers. Clare Anderson and Calum Blaikie argue in favour of exploring links between apparently disconnected worlds to examine the making of particular medical careers and genres. On the other hand, drawing on literature about 'biographies of objects', Jim Mills elaborates on the heterogeneous and multiple careers of an object usually considered as exclusively medical. Taken together, these authors resist essentialist conceptions of the medical.

In a historical anthropology of archives that straddle three continents, Anderson invites the reader to consider the ways in which archiving practices shape impressions about connection and disconnection between different worlds of medical genres and therapeutics. She explores the peripatetic life of J.P. Walker, who held a long career in British India as a medical officer and penal colony superintendent. Walker maintained a voluminous documentation on therapeutic themes, which he bequeathed to an American professor of eclectic medicine—a branch of medicine popular in North America from the mid-nineteenth century to the mid-twentieth century among physicians whose practices were pragmatically oriented around reports of beneficial actions of medicinal plants and formulations for patients, whatever their provenance. Walker's papers, now under the custody of a local repository in Cincinnati, are noted for their inclusion of remedies used by Native Americans and African Americans, and a relative elision of references to British India, where Walker carried out many medical and administrative experiments over many years as a ruthless colonial prison official. While analysing these elisions, this chapter draws attention to discrepancies between the archival holdings about Walker in South Asian, British, and North American repositories. By explaining and traversing the disconnections imposed by particular archival contexts, one can begin to assemble an analytical framework that is appropriate to make sense of the colonial and multiply connected medical worlds which men such as Walker shaped and inhabited. Walker's case is a reminder of the fact that political strategies shape particular archival collections, even when such repositories continue to be considered by many scholars as a transparent source for accessing objective historical pasts.

Blaikie takes us to the Indian Himalayan region of Ladakh to explore changes in the availability of materia medica since the 1960s, and to explain how they have transformed worlds of practice in Sowa Rigpa (a collectivization of forms of medical practice and tradition dispersed through the Indo-Tibetan highlands). These transformations were linked with apparently unconnected developments: the opening of roads to the region in the 1980s and the introduction of a cash economy. Previously rare materials, known through pharmacology texts in idealized formulations, became available in abundance, which have changed the nature of Sowa Rigpa pharmacy and therapeutic strategy, enabled new subjectivities through consumption, and motivated new modalities of exchange. Therefore, we can locate the contingencies of the medical by taking into account the ways in which material resources for medical practice have circulated. Although the author is careful not to erase the continuity of certain socially embedded practices within this time of great change, he highlights two crucial effects: the emergence of a distinctive medical realm itself as a professional space, marked by the presence of newer groups of producers, distributors, and consumers; and 'pharmaceuticalization', in which the consumption of powerful Sowa Rigpa drugs has become a symbolic social act. The unbecoming and becoming of therapeutic forms were connected with changing infrastructural–political–economic and material conditions. These changing conditions in turn can be explained in terms of an extensive socio-material network that included 'ever-shifting combinations of wild plants, their habitats and their collectors, farmers and their crops, traders and trade routes extending from Indonesia to Siberia and the Middle East, pilgrims, priests and tributary offerings, strangers, teachers and students, medical lineages, patients, kin and friends'.

Mills focuses on the multiple lives of a substance to argue that the medical was not necessarily a continuous or permanent label that could be imposed on objects. Contingencies of the medical can be revealed in the varied configurations of cannabis and its products during the nineteenth century: as therapeutic applications (as stimulants, painkillers, and anti-convulsives for a range of conditions including hydrophobia, cholera, and neuralgia), causes of ill health, as intoxicants, and significant excise articles for the British government in India. The credibility of its therapeutic, pathogenetic, as well as its commercial qualities was generated and circulated through various institutional apparatuses and mediations. Its multiple configurations existed in parallel until the rise to prominence of missionary networks and associated temperance movements. Mills examines both the labile nature of the medical, as also how the disparate histories of cannabis took shape.

Contours of the Medical

Indeed, the boundaries between the domains of the medical and the non-medical are more blurred and porous than it might appear. Contributions to this volume seek to defamiliarize the medical by reorienting attention on spaces such as police stations, courtrooms, coroner's chambers, forests, prisons, streets, or rice mills, while at the same time contesting the rigid distinctions between the world of the medical on the one hand, and the domains of the legal, the statistical, the literary, the religious, the superstitious, and well-being on the other.

Through an anthropological study of spirit-related suffering among daily wage labourers and factory workers, and their seeking relief at a temple complex in contemporary western India, Shubha Ranganathan calls for a re-imagining of what we mean by a 'healing system'. The conceptual differentiation between 'biomedical' and 'indigenous healing systems' does not square with the realities of people's everyday lived experiences. They are not two separate worlds that may be represented by biomedical/indigenous but rather they are forged together (practically and conceptually) and distinguished in various context-specific ways. Clear demarcations between the medical and the religious, between shrines and bureaucratic medical institutions should therefore be questioned. The multiple ways of making sense of, and intervening in, distress and suffering evinced in this study renders such demarcations implausible. Ranganathan speaks to the need for rethinking and refining the conceptual tools by which we can take into account the singularity of such therapeutic spaces and worlds.

In his chapter, Projit Bihari Mukharji extends further the agenda of rethinking the contours of the medical by focusing on a nineteenth-century fever epidemic, the 'Burdwan Fever' (after a locality in Bengal). Although various representations of the epidemic identified themselves as either fictional or factual accounts, they actually shared predomi-nant tropes and articulated similar concerns. Literary imaginations and literal descriptions of the event were not mutually exclusive processes. Mukharji provides a close and comparative reading of contemporary government reports, an essay (and its reviews), and a novel to examine how narratives about the epidemic were sustained, caricatured, and consolidated across genres. In so doing, this chapter evaluates the extent to which Bengali commentators in the 1870s domesticated early nineteenth-century Scottish and Irish notions about 'political medicine'. Bengali aetiological discussions about colonial illness and insanitation were entrenched within fledgling social commentaries and a wider political economic critique of British imperialism and the poverty and dearth it engendered.

David Arnold reinforces the need for historians of South Asia to examine disease with greater attention to occupation or lived circum-stances. Rather than focusing on the archetypal medical sites—the hospital, clinic, jail, asylum, and the pharmaceutical industry—this chapter analyses sites of the everyday, places where people live and work. It is an example of a 'doctor-less' approach to health/illness histories, which provides insights into the 'health–technology nexus' through three sites—the street, the home, and the factory. In each case the author describes the ways in which everyday technologies (the road, vehicular traffic, household stoves, and rice mills, among them) have been implicated in people's health and illness. Drawing on the wider histories and sociologies of health and well-being, this chapter poses questions about class- and occupation-specific conceptions of illness. It argues that responsibility for health might be 'shifted to new objects and agencies', and might extend to apparently non-medical professions such as the police, legal agencies, and factory inspectors.

Therefore, this volume showcases various trends in the histori-ography of medicine in South Asia. Taken together, the chapters in this volume reassert the material and metaphorical significance of the medical in shaping the histories of colonial and postcolonial South Asia. At the same time, the history of colonial and postcolonial

South Asia reveals various ways in which the medical, both as a category and a set of processes, was consolidated and domesticated. The different approaches towards locating the medical that have been adopted here should be relevant not only to the wider discipline of medical history more generally; these approaches should also be relevant to similar efforts to analyse various core discipline-defining concepts prevalent in other fields. While reflecting on these questions, the 'Afterword' by Mark Harrison provides a detailed meditation on the category medical in modern South Asian history. A distinct social and professional domain of the medical was carved out in colonial India, even when the boundaries between what could be considered medical and non-medical often appeared blurred and contentious in the nineteenth and twentieth centuries.

Notes

1. J. Oksala, 'Foucault's Politicization of Ontology', *Continental Philosophy Review* 43, no. 4 (2010): 447.
2. B. Pati and M. Harrison, eds, *Health, Medicine, and Empire: Perspectives on Colonial India* (New Delhi: Orient Longman, 2001); C. Palit and A.K. Dutta, eds, *History of Medicine in India: The Medical Encounter* (New Delhi: Kalpaz Publications, 2005); B. Pati and M. Harrison, eds, *The Social History of Health and Medicine in Colonial India* (London: Routledge, 2008); V. Sujatha and L. Abraham, eds, *Medical Pluralism in Contemporary India* (New Delhi: Orient BlackSwan, 2012); D. Kumar and R.S. Basu, eds, *Medical Encounters in British India* (New Delhi: Oxford University Press, 2013).
3. F. Huisman and J.H. Warner, eds, *Locating Medical History: The Stories and Their Meanings* (Baltimore: Johns Hopkins University Press, 2006).
4. N. Rose, 'Medicine, History and the Present,' in *Reassessing Foucault: Power, Medicine and the Body*, edited by Colin Jones and Roy Porter (London: Routledge, 1994), p. 50. Quoted in R. Cooter, '"Framing" the End of the Social History of Medicine', in Huisman and Warner, *Locating Medical History*, pp. 309–37.
5. S. Shapin, 'Hyperprofessionalism and the Crisis of Readership in the History of Science', *Isis* 96, no. 2 (2005): 238–43.
6. On the interface between the colonial state and medicine, see P. Chakrabarti, 'Introduction' to a special section on 'States of Healing: New Perspectives on the State in Histories of Medicine', *South Asian History and Culture* 4, no. 1 (2013): 1–8; on medical plurality, see W. Ernst,

'Beyond East and West: From the History of Colonial Medicine to a Social History of Medicine(s) in South Asia', *Social History of Medicine* 20, no. 3 (2007): 505–24; on histories of 'indigenous' medicine, see P.B. Mukharji, 'Symptoms of Dis-Ease: New Trends in the Histories of "Indigenous" South Asian Medicines', *History Compass* 9, no. 12 (2011): 887–99; D. Hardiman, 'Indian Medical Indigeneity: From Nationalist Assertion to the Global Market', *Social History* 34, no. 3 (2009): 263–83; on the need to critique the historiography of global connections, see S. Hodges, 'The Global Menace', *Social History of Medicine* 25, no. 3 (2012): 719–28.

7. S. Marks, 'What Is Colonial about Colonial Medicine?' *Social History of Medicine*, 10 (1997): 205–19; Ernst, 'Beyond East and West'.

8. M. Harrison, *Medicine in an Age of Commerce and Empire: Britain and Its Tropical Colonies* (New York: Oxford University Press, 2010); P. Chakrabarti, *Materials and Medicine: Trade, Conquest and Therapeutics in the Eighteenth Century* (Manchester: Manchester University Press, 2010); K. Raj, *Relocating Modern Science: Circulation and the Construction of Knowledge in South Asia and Europe, 1650–1900* (Basingstoke: Palgrave Macmillan, 2007).

9. On the modes of governance and logics of care, see R.M. MacLeod and M.J. Lewis, *Disease, Medicine, and Empire: Perspectives on Western Medicine and the Experience of European Expansion* (London: Routledge, 1988); D. Arnold, *Colonizing the Body: State Medicine and Epidemic Disease in Nineteenth-Century India* (Berkeley: University of California Press, 1993); M. Harrison, *Public Health and British India: Anglo-Indian Preventive Medicine, 1859–1914* (Cambridge: Cambridge University Press, 1994); A. Kumar, *Medicine and the Raj* (New Delhi: Sage Publications, 1998); M. Harrison, *Climates and Constitutions: Health, Race, Environment and British Imperialism in India* (Oxford: Oxford University Press, 2002); N. Bhattacharya, *Contagion and Enclaves: Tropical Medicine in Colonial India* (Liverpool: Liverpool University Press, 2012); S. Sehrawat, *Colonial Medical Care in North India: Gender, State, and Society, C. 1840–1920* (New Delhi: Oxford University Press, 2013); S. Mishra, *Pilgrimage, Politics and Pestilence: The Haj from the Indian Subcontinent, 1860–1920* (New Delhi: Oxford University Press, 2011). On animal health, see S. Mishra, 'Beasts, Murrains, and the British Raj: Reassessing Colonial Medicine in India from the Veterinary Perspective', *Bulletin of the History of Medicine* 85, no. 4 (2011): 587–619. On policy and strategies of control, see S. Bhattacharya, M. Harrison, and M. Worboys, *Fractured States: Smallpox, Public Health and Vaccination Policy in British India 1800–1947* (Hyderabad: Orient BlackSwan, 2005); S. Bhattacharya, *Expunging Variola: The Control and Eradication of Smallpox in India, 1947–1977*

(Hyderabad: Orient BlackSwan, 2006); C.W. McMillen and N. Brimnes, 'Medical Modernization and Medical Nationalism: Resistance to Mass Tuberculosis Vaccination in Postcolonial India, 1948–1955,' *Comparative Studies in Society and History* 52, no. 1 (2010): 180–209; M. Worboys, 'The Colonial World as Mission and Mandate: Leprosy and Empire, 1900–1940', *Osiris* 15 (2000): 207–18; J. Buckingham, *Leprosy in Colonial South India: Medicine and Confinement* (Basingstoke: Palgrave MacMillan, 2002). On ecological determinants of health, see I. Klein, 'Imperialism, Ecology and Disease: Cholera in India, 1850–1950', *Indian Economic and Social History Review* 31, no. 4 (1994): 491–518. On madness and psychiatry, see J.H. Mills, *Madness, Cannabis and Colonialism* (Basingstoke: Palgrave Macmillan, 2000); W. Ernst, 'Idioms of Madness and Colonial Boundaries: The Case of the European and "Native" Mentally Ill in Early Nineteenth-Century British India', *Comparative Studies in Society and History* 39, no. 1 (1997): 153–81; A.R. Basu, 'Emergence of a Marginal Science in a Colonial City: Reading Psychiatry in Bengali Periodicals', *Indian Economic and Social History Review* 41 (2004): 103–41.

10. For example on reproductive health and birth control, see P. Jeffery, R. Jeffery, and A. Lyon, *Labour Pains and Labour Power: Women and Childbearing in India* (London: Zed Books, 1989); S. Hodges, *Contraception, Colonialism and Commerce: Birth Control in South India, 1920–1940* (Aldershot: Ashgate Publishing Ltd, 2008). On the shaping of disease categories, see, for example, R. Deb Roy, 'Quinine, Mosquitoes and Empire: Reassembling Malaria in British India, 1890–1910', *South Asian History and Culture* 4 (2013): 65–86.

11. S. Legg, *Spaces of Colonialism: Delhi's Urban Governmentalities* (Chichester: Wiley-Blackwell, 2008); Hodges, *Contraception, Colonialism and Commerce*; I. Pande, *Medicine, Race and Liberalism in British Bengal: Symptoms of Empire* (Abingdon and New York: Routledge, 2010); R. Berger, *Ayurveda Made Modern: Political Histories of Indigenous Medicine in North India, 1900–1995* (Basingstoke: Palgrave Macmillan, 2013).

12. Pande, *Symptoms of Empire*; P. Levine, *Prostitution, Race, and Politics: Policing Venereal Disease in the British Empire* (London: Routledge, 2003); E. Wald, *Vice in the Barracks: Medicine, the Military, and the Making of Colonial India, 1780–1868* (London and New York: Palgrave Macmillan, 2014); A. Stoler, *Carnal Knowledge and Imperial Power: Race and the Intimate in Colonial Rule* (Berkeley: University of California Press, 2002).

13. See, for example, D. Hardiman and P.B. Mukharji, *Medical Marginality in South Asia: Situating Subaltern Therapeutics* (London: Routledge, 2013); P.B. Mukharji, *Nationalizing the Body: The Medical Market, Print, and Daktari Medicine* (London: Anthem Press, 2009); A.R. Basu, 'Historicizing

Indian Psychiatry', *Indian Journal of Psychiatry* 47, no. 2 (2005): 126–9; K. Sivaramakrishnan, *Old Potions, New Bottles: Recasting Indigenous Medicine in Colonial Punjab, 1850–1945* (New Delhi: Orient Longman, 2006); S. Alavi, *Islam and Healing: Loss and Recovery of an Indo-Muslim Medical Tradition, 1600–1900* (New Delhi: Permanent Black, 2007); G.N. Attewell, *Refiguring Unani Tibb: Plural Healing in Late Colonial India* (Hyderabad: Orient BlackSwan, 2007); M. Banerjee, *Power, Knowledge, Medicine: Ayurvedic Pharmaceuticals at Home and in the World* (New Delhi: Orient BlackSwan, 2009); Berger, *Ayurveda Made Modern*.

14. S. Amrith, *Decolonizing International Health: India and Southeast Asia, 1930–65* (Basingstoke: Palgrave Macmillan, 2006).

15. J.S. Alter, *Asian Medicine and Globalization* (Philadelphia: University of Pennsylvania Press, 2005).

16. For emphasis on spatiotemporal intersections behind the making of medicine in the colonial and postcolonial worlds, see, for example, Hodges, 'A Global Menace'; W. Anderson, 'Where Is the Postcolonial History of Medicine?' *Bulletin of the History of Medicine* 72, no. 3 (1998): 522–30; P. Chakrabarti, *Medicine and Empire* (Basingstoke: Palgrave Macmillan, 2014). See also, A. Digby, W. Ernst, and P.B. Mukharji, eds, *Crossing Colonial Historiographies: Histories of Colonial and Indigenous Medicines in Transnational Perspectives* (Newcastle: Cambridge Scholars Publishing, 2010).

17. J. Burnham, *What Is Medical History?* (Cambridge: Polity Press, 2005), p. 9.

18. I. Hacking, *The Social Construction of What?* (Cambridge, Massachusetts and London, England: Harvard University Press, 1999), p. 20.

19. I. Hacking, *Historical Ontology* (Cambridge, Massachusetts and London: Harvard University Press, 2002), pp. 4, 22, 23.

20. Hacking, *Historical Ontology*, p. 8.

21. Hacking, *Historical Ontology*, p. 23.

22. Hacking, *Historical Ontology*, pp. 2, 5.

23. Hacking, *Historical Ontology*, pp. 17, 25.

24. Hacking, *Historical Ontology*, pp. 4, 7, 17.

25. Hacking, *Historical Ontology*, p. 17.

26. Hacking, *Historical Ontology*, pp. 21–2.

27. Hacking, *Historical Ontology*, p. 2.

28. Hacking, *Historical Ontology*, p. 26.

29. M. Foucault, 'What Is Enlightenment?' in *The Foucault Reader*, edited by Paul Rabinow, translated by C. Porter (New York: Pantheon Books, 1984), pp. 32–50.

30. Cited in Hacking, *Historical Ontology*, p. 2.

31. Hacking, *Historical Ontology*, pp. 17, 23, 25.

I

PRODUCTION OF THE MEDICAL

I

SOCIOLOGICAL DESCRIPTION AND THE FORENSICS OF SEXUALITY

DURBA MITRA*

A Coroner's Inquest

Kally Bewah experienced many social deaths before she actually died in 1885, alone in a dilapidated house where she lay naked, bleeding profusely from an alleged abortion.

It is in the medical investigation of Kally Bewah's death that we learn scattered details of her life story.[1] She had belonged to a respectable Hindu family of colonial Calcutta, India. She married at the age of eleven, but three years into her marriage, her elderly husband died. In 1863, after her husband's death, Kally's brother-in-law forced her to leave her inherited property. Her own relatives rejected her as well, accusing Kally of having an illegitimate pregnancy. Thrown out by all of her kin, she would ask her sister Prosonno shortly before dying: 'How will I show my face among so many people?'[2] A few days later, Prosonno found Kally dead in a shack, yards away from the house in which she was born. Her nude body was decomposing, strewn across the floor, with bundles of bloody clothing under her head.

* My thanks to Rohan Deb Roy and Guy Attewell for inviting me to be part of the conference and the resulting volume on the 'medical' in South Asian history. My work has benefited from their wonderful editorial insights and feedback. Thanks also to the anonymous reviewers for their suggestions and to Manan Ahmed for his insightful critiques and suggestions.

Kally's death was recorded by E.W. Chambers, coroner of West Bengal in an official Coroner's Enquiry, narrated in a letter to the Jury of Inquest.[3] Chambers observed that the violent case before the Jury of Inquest was commonplace in colonial Bengal, as the 'evidence revealed ... facts which are ordinarily connected with the life of a Hindu widow'. He emphasized that Kally had led an 'unchaste life' and was therefore forcefully expelled by her family, prohibited from leading a respectable life. Her indiscretions increasingly visible to others through her pregnancy, Kally was 'literally hunted from house to house', never to return home again.[4]

In his medical report, the Coroner narrated Kally's social world. At stake for the coroner was the scientific truth behind the dead body, leading to a narration of Kally's life that anticipated the circumstances of her death. The purpose of the coroner's enquiry was to define the cause of death, and Kally's body betrayed the violence inflicted on her body. In describing his findings to the Jury of the Official Inquest, the coroner emphasized that the violence of Kally's physical death was only the end result of a life of shame and 'ill-fame', suggesting that the 'traditions' of Bengali society were culpable for her transgressions and subsequent social and physical degradation.

In the end, all that remained of Kally was her corpse, which became the domain of medical authority and the sole testimony to her life and death.

'This Essay Begins with a Transgression'[5]

In this chapter, I offer a few glimpses of women who emerge in colonial medico-legal descriptions as deviant bodies. As in Ranajit Guha's reading of the testimony of Chandra's death, I ask: how do such details of a woman's life, and death, come to appear in the archive? There are brief, constrained appearances of the precarious lives of women in official historical sources. I explore how experts claimed these lives for their own purposes. Multiple authorities lay claim to the narrative of Kally's death, including the Jury of Inquest, the law, and the colonial archive.[6] Yet, medical science endowed the coroner with the power to narrate Kally's death into an event. In his narrative, the coroner produced evidentiary truths premised on his claim to a specialized knowledge of the body. How are these bodies described in the language of medical science?

Using texts on medical jurisprudence and their use in colonial surveillance, I argue that medical jurisprudence, also known as forensic medicine, produced an ethno-scientific knowledge of the body that followed a recursive form of reasoning that linked sociological classifications of women to a forensic science of sex. I focus in particular on the medico-legal determination of abortion and its relationship to related forms of knowledge, including forensic knowledge of rape, virginity, and infanticide. This circular logic united scientific descriptions of anatomical attributes of women's bodies with sociological classifications that marked the sexual deviance of Indian women. As in Kally Bewah's report, narratives of forensic medicine travelled from the particularities of the physical body to broad and often fluid sociological categories like 'Hindu widow', 'unchaste woman', or 'prostitute'. These sociological typologies were subsequently invoked by the medical investigator to interpret the legal meaning of the physical features of the woman's body. Medico-legal texts on abortion extended beyond claims to legal veracity, constituting new authoritative forms of knowledge that united sociological and scientific methods to comprehend the potential dangers of women's sexuality.

How do we think of the 'medical' in an account such as the coroner's report? 'Medical' knowledge featured in medico-legal sources trafficked between women's anatomy, physiology, and law in the making of a robust colonial sociology of Indian women and society. Forensic medical writings from nineteenth century India on investigations of women's bodies, including cases of rape, abortion, and infanticide, deployed colonial discourses about the status of Indian women as a marker of civilizational difference.[7] I see the 'medical' as a unique site where claims of scientific objectivity, legal veracity, and social scientific authority silently converged. Colonial and medical authorities deployed this mode of sociological classification and scientific description to comprehend the nature of the Indian woman.

Forensic medicine—the use of medical science in the practice of law—described diverse circumstances in which medical evidence was used in the application of law. The science of medical jurisprudence for India began to appear in the early nineteenth century. By the middle of the nineteenth century, intersections between law and medicine were codified in the Indian Penal Code of 1860, the Criminal Procedure Code of 1861, and an emerging literature on the science of forensic medicine.[8] Medical evidence became crucial to legal proceedings through the Indian Evidence Act of 1872, which determined the types of evidence that were ascertained as 'facts', defined the role of evidence in demonstrating motive, and established the status of medical experts in legal proceedings.[9] The Indian Penal Code signalled a new approach to governance through criminal law in India. The Code sought to establish new kinds of governance in colonial India through the production of a standard set of rules and operating procedures. The Penal Code introduced an expansive set of laws that addressed women and their sexual and reproductive behaviour, including laws against foeticide, infanticide, and rape.[10] The Criminal Code thus set forth legal standards outlawing crimes that were often carried out in private and intimate spaces. According to colonial officials, forensic medicine could provide new forms of evidence to prove the criminal activity of Indian women hidden from the view of the colonial state.

With the circulation of new forms of scientific knowledge such as forensics in the nineteenth century, the gendered Indian body became visible in new and important ways. Perhaps the most cited example of medical writing on the female body in the colonial period is the medico-legal report concerning the child Phulmoni in debates over age of consent legislation in the late nineteenth century. Tanika Sarkar reads the in-depth medical description of Phulmoni's genitalia as representative of the horror of sexual violence and the complicity of the colonial state in child rape. Sarkar's careful reading of the Phulmoni case demonstrates how contentions about gender established both colonial and Bengali patriarchal authority. Yet questions about the status of medical knowledge in legal proceedings remain. Why did the genital examination come to have status as a key form of evidence in the colonial judiciary? What practices of knowledge linked claims of objectivity to the description of 'native' women's bodies?[11]

Feminist historiography has investigated important relationships between law, gender, and power in nineteenth-century colonial approaches to social reform.[12] I build on these histories by locating scientific knowledge as a foundational site in the making of not only new forms of gendered difference, but also new modes of sexual knowledge. The medico-legal science of sexuality established new forms of authority over women's bodies and produced new networks of social power and surveillance over women.[13] Thinking the 'medical' allows us to consider the formation of scientific knowledge alongside the formation of sexual norms. How do changing ideas of sexuality constitute new forms of medical knowledge? How were Indian women's bodies ordered and imagined in the nineteenth century? By addressing the construction of categories of sexuality through medico-legal textbooks and investigations, I suggest that nineteenth-century understandings of the 'medical' were constitutive of and constituted by a range of 'scientific' knowledge—anatomy and physiology, law, sociology, as well as history.

The Medico-legal Case as Sociological Study

In 1856 Norman Chevers, civil assistant surgeon in Calcutta, published an early textbook for forensic medicine for India, *A Manual of Medical Jurisprudence for Bengal and the North-Western Provinces* (1856). Chevers's influential text was the first in a growing field of treatises on Indian medical jurisprudence.[14] The medico-legal enterprise in India expanded following the publication of Chevers's influential textbooks, with widely circulating textbooks by colonial administrators I.B. Lyons and J.D.B. Gribble and the publication of a widely influential textbook by the Indian doctor and professor of medical jurisprudence in Agra, Jaising P. Modi, in 1920. Publications on Indian forensic medicine appeared in journals, textbooks, and administrative reports from the middle of the nineteenth century, and continued to gain prominence in the first decades of the twentieth century. Indian courts increasingly relied on the new forensic medicine to provide 'scientific' and 'objective' evidence of crimes.[15]

In chapters on crimes associated with women, treatises on forensic medicine produce detailed narratives of the physical bodies of women while invoking sociological categories of Indian custom to understand the significance of physical evidence of the female body. Chevers's 1856 edition of his *Manual on Medical Jurisprudence* outlined relevant applications of forensic medicine, categories that continue to be used in textbooks on medical jurisprudence and writings on forensic medicine today.[16] In his textbook, Norman Chevers emphasized the scientific need for the forced genital examination of women: 'The question of compulsory examination is beset with some difficulty. In cases with native women of questionable character, examination becomes a matter of legal necessity.'[17] In the narrative of the body's attributes, the medical expert blurred the boundaries between scientific and non-scientific forms of evidence.

Different manuals on forensic medicine for India arranged the sections on crimes involving women's genitalia in accordance with

Chevers's initial organization.[18] Textbooks included extensive discussions of the signs of virginity, 'rape', 'infanticide', and 'foeticide'. Often, these sequential chapters also include a section on 'Unnatural Offences' that describes crimes of sodomy and 'unnatural' crimes of sex between men. Publications addressed the range of sexual crimes committed on or by women that required genital examination and assessment.

While Chevers's textbook defined a field of enquiry, many genres of medico-legal writing emerged alongside that of the treatise of forensic medicine for India. From the 1870s, Robert Harvey, surgeon general for Bengal, published 'medico-legal' case studies in the widely read *Indian Medical Gazette* for the use of colonial administrators and medical authorities. His reports in the 1870s widely influenced Indian medico-legal science. In his report on medico-legal returns for Bengal for 1870–2, Harvey emphasized that alongside the mandatory examination of the body, non-medical observations were essential for determining women's criminality:

> Criminal Abortion is believed to be an exceedingly common practice in India, where the prohibition of widow marriage leads to much immorality, the discovery of which involves social ostracism and exclusion from caste, a punishment so severe, that all means are taken to avoid detection, even although death is risked. A thorough investigation into all the means used by the native Dhais and professed abortionists is still much needed, and although much valuable information has been collected by Dr. Chevers, it remains to be done before our knowledge of the crime, as it obtains in India, can be considered satisfactory. In these cases it is important to know the *whole history of the person*, and those in the returns treated purely in their medical aspect throw little new light on the subject.[19]

According to these texts, the questionable character and innate criminality of the promiscuous woman authorized the medical investigation of her body.[20] In narratives of the body, 'the whole history' of her sociological status was necessary to understand the anatomical facts of the case. Her physicality revealed her identity as a criminal subject while her identity defined the contours of her anatomy. The medico-legal case study used a narrative device that united the colonial sociological with the scientific: the extraordinary violence on the body was narrated alongside sociological terms and sub-clauses that detailed a woman's sexual 'character'.

Harvey's reports detailed cases with a primary focus on the forensics of women's bodies. In his reports of 1870–2, he offers detailed case studies of abortion. According to Harvey, these cases narrated how Indian women employed violent practices to induce abortion:

> In a case at Dinajpur a stick was thrust up the vagina of a prostitute aged 16, and caused her to abort. Mr. Webber found, 'the mucous membrane of the vagina entirely torn away and pushed upwards probably into the uterus' and gave it as his opinion that the woman would die. No post-mortem is recorded.[21]

In Robert Harvey's report in the *Indian Medical Gazette* from 1 December 1875, we again see sociological categories used in the narrative of the body's anatomy:

> INJURIES TO THE FEMALE GENITALS—25 cases are returned, where a stick or some hard substance has been thrust into the vagina, potentially to procure abortion. The motives of the crimes are seldom mentioned, but jealousy or desire to cover unchastity are the most common ones.
>
> Subject, *a Mussalmani widow*, aged 45... Entrance to the vagina contused and ruptured, upper part of the vagina and cavity of the cervix filled with blood, partly fluid, partly coagulated. Uterus was twice its normal size ... The woman, *a loose disreputable character*, charged three men with an assault ... Opinion—Death resulted from shock and hemorrhage consequent by the introduction of a blunt instrument. Only one of the accused was convicted. *The statements of the woman were considered wholly untrustworthy by the magistrate.*

In the next case, Harvey again invokes chastity in his scientific assessment:

> A girl, age 10, was found dead with a lacerated wound 1/4 of an inch long in the anterior wall of the vagina, with an inflamed uterus scraped of its contents. *Absence of the hymen showed that she had long been accustomed to intercourse.*[22]

The clinical writing of the anatomy of women is narrated seamlessly with an assessment of sexual behaviour. Each account united sociological descriptions of sexual behaviour with details of anatomical violence into a description that is sayable, knowable, and automatically medicalized in each case of child bride and widow. Here, as in Ranajit Guha's reading of the *ekrar* (statement or deposition) narrating Chandra's death, we see the entry of different colonized subjects into the official archive through a distillation of occurrences into the category of 'event' by the authority of a colonial official.[23] Social practices were entered into an archive of criminal evidence, with the evidence testifying to the event of the crime. In this event, the chastity, or lack thereof, of the prostitute girl, the widow, and the dead child-bride become significant to Harvey's assessment of the crime as well to his understanding of the body itself.

The juridico-medical abstractions produce a document that sets its own epistemological limits. Yet even as the 'event' of the crime of rape with foreign objects was reconstructed through evidence of medical knowledge, the violence itself seems to resist the medical language that codifies criminality through classifications of the injured body. Indeed, the medical descriptions of the crimes show a much more perverse concern for the sexual anatomy of the female body than it does for the crime itself. It is as if Harvey recognized the visceral effects of the narrative produced in the writing of these cases. Even as colonial authorities attempted to document these 'events' for their scientific value, Harvey recognized that medical description produces undesirable effects. He warns his readers that 'the cases [of rape and "unnatural crimes"] for the most part are of very little interest', cautioning against seeing these accounts beyond their objective value. He continues, noting, 'there is a general tendency to treat them with a reticence, which takes away all their medico-legal value—a reticence which savors of squeamishness in an enquiry which aims at the extirpation of the crime by making its detection easy'.[24]

In Harvey the use of anatomical detail alongside sociological categories in the account is essential in the 'detection' of crime. In order to reveal those hidden secrets, the medical enquiry was to map the body and character of the victim as deeply as possible to produce verifiable 'facts' in each case. Harvey's account travelled widely and shaped the understandings of cases of abortion. The widely read British medical journal *The Lancet* emphasized the 'admirable' work of Robert Harvey in his reports on medico-legal issues. According to the reviewer, from 'a section on criminal abortion we gather that the practice is exceedingly common in India, where the prohibition of widow marriage leads to much immorality'.[25] Early editions of Lyon's textbook, *Medical Jurisprudence for India* (1889), emphasized that Indians commonly employed the use of 'local violence', including the introduction of plant irritants and sticks.[26] With the circulation of Harvey's text, later editions of Isidore B. Lyon's textbook describe how Harvey's case studies demonstrate that Indians were 'prone' to use violence to hide their 'immorality' in cases of abortion: 'In India, cases of injury by thrusting a stick into the vagina are not uncommon. Harvey states that twenty-five such cases, ten of them fatal, were included in the Bengal, etc., returns for 1870–72.'[27] Harvey's reports circulated to create a general understanding that the crime of abortion was not only common in India, but also that its techniques were more violent.

In later editions of his textbook, Lyon offers case studies of supposed suicides, opining that women suspected of suicide more likely died from abortions. He describes these cases with extensive sociological details that surrounded each death:

(a) A widow seven months gone with child died rather suddenly; an inquest was held by the police, and a verdict returned of death from dysentery. Suspicion, however, being excited, a post-mortem examination was ordered, the result of which was the discovery of the pregnant condition of the woman (which had been concealed in the inquest report furnished by the police), and of the fact that the cause of death was arsenical poisoning. The district magistrate remarks, in reference to this case, that there is every reason to believe that all engaged in the inquest tried to conceal the true cause of death. Bo. Chem. An. Rep. for 1884, reported by the District Magistrate of Bassim, Hyderabad Assigned Districts.

(b) In this case, which occurred in the Surat district, as in above case, the cause of death was arsenical poisoning, and the deceased was a widow far gone in pregnancy. The brother and sister of the deceased confessed to having given her eight annas' worth of opium in order to procure abortion or to cause death, so as to avoid the disgrace arising out of her condition. No opium, however, could be discovered in the viscera of the deceased. *Ibid.*

(c) Case of poisoning by arsenic reported by medical officer, Tatta, Sind. Deceased was promised in marriage to a man of her caste (Mussulman), but before marriage she cohabited with him and became pregnant, and was advanced to above the fourth or fifth month, when her parents, to avoid disgrace, it is said, tried very much to procure abortion, but failed (much against her intended husband's will); so having failed to procure abortion, her parents, to save their reputation, it is suspected, gave her poison in her food. Bo. Chem. An. Bep., 1876–7.[28]

Even as these colonial medical manuals claimed only to be edifying and illuminating a *science* of the deviant body, the narrative effect extended far beyond self-imposed limits of scientific reason. The redundancies and exhaustive details of manuals of forensic medicine revealed the compulsive preoccupations that were claimed in the name of science, from the details of women's genitalia to the obsessive fascination with the pitiable characters that fell victim to Indian 'traditions'. A range of sociological types appear—promiscuous Hindu widows barred from the legitimate realm of marriage, young girls forced into child marriage, and women who engaged in sexual relationships outside of the confines of marriage. Indeed, as Harvey himself warned, medico-legal writing recounted the body and described the events of violence with such detail that they titillated and provoked a dramatic reaction in the reader.

These manuals described genital examination as a process where the investigator gradually closed in on the facts of the crime, starting with observations about the general appearance of the woman to a close and detailed reading of her physical parts, a description that moved from outside to inside. Textbooks of forensic medicine for India produce detailed instructions for conducting a genital examination in sections on rape, a procedure then referred to again in subsequent sections of textbooks on abortion and infanticide. For example, in Gribble's textbook, the investigation begins with broad observations on the appearance of the body. The most important outward observation was whether the suspect woman had the appearance of 'a person addicted to self-abuse or masturbation'.[29] The investigation then had to go further into the physical depth of the body. For virgins and women accusing rape, 'it is important to take note of whether the breasts are virginal, or show signs of having been manipulated'.[30] The doctor was to examine the external genital organs, which displayed evidence of sexual deviance and potential involvement in prostitution if there was the 'syphilitic sores'.[31] Finally, the examination culminated in the internal genital organs. The genital examination detailed whether the hymen was ruptured, the size and length of the vagina, and if there were any signs of disease.

Colonial desires for forensic, 'scientific' evidence reveal a preoccupation with graphic descriptions of violence, devices, and anatomies that portrayed the 'reality' of the crime through the body. These scientific investigations of native women's bodies read the character of the woman solely through an assessment of her genitalia.[32] At first glance, these manuals seem to do little except objectify the violence inflicted on the body, heightening the medical quantification of violence inflicted on women's genitalia to generalizations about 'native' sexuality. Yet it is *through* the modes of description that seamlessly unite sociological status and the effects of violence on Indian women's bodies that the medical investigation produced new and important associations between the sociology of women's sexuality, women's anatomical appearance, and the events of their death. The Indian woman's body was perceived as finite and legible, sanctioning a mode of inferential thinking that moved from visible indicators on the surface to invisible traits held inside the body.

Forensic Medicine and the Prostitute

The sexually deviant woman in particular was crucial to a powerful vision of modern society, testifying, through her physical appearance, to the depravity of the present condition of Indian society. The 'prostitute' emerges as a central concept in textbooks, a classification that tied Indian women's criminal behaviour to the inherently deviant sexuality of 'traditional' Indian society. In invoking concepts such as 'prostitute', medical authorities regularly cited Indian women's social and sexual deviance as the reason behind crimes of 'concealment'. For medical investigators, the hidden nature of crimes concealing sexual transgressions necessitated invasive investigative modes. By labelling those women who resided outside the regulated space of companionate marriage as 'prostitutes', forensic medical experts defined women outside of marriage as *inherently* sexual and criminal, simultaneously constructing the realm of female sexual desire exclusive of the 'legitimately' married woman.

The critique of widow remarriage and the inherent danger of unbridled widow sexuality are cited as the most important factors in chapters on abortion and infanticide. In Norman Chevers's depiction of widow remarriage, he explained the 'daily commission' of the crimes of abortion and infanticide: 'In a country like India, where true morality is almost unknown ... it is scarcely surprising that great crimes should be frequently practised to conceal the results of immorality, and that the procuring of Criminal Abortion should, especially, be an act of almost daily commission.'[33] It was so common that 'in the family of a single Koolin Brahmin, it was common for each daughter to destroy a child in the womb annually. The pundit who gave me this information supposed that 10,000 children were thus murdered in the province of Bengal, every month!'[34] In the second edition of his textbook, Chevers connected the crime of abortion to prostitution and emphasized the connection between Indian women's promiscuity and the Contagious Diseases Act of 1868. Chevers emphasized that perverse traditions fostered the existence of prostitutes in Bengal, 'a most striking illustration of the folly of the present system of preventing re-marriage of widows. Calcutta, with a population of 416,000, supports 12,419 women of ill-fame'. In depictions of women's crimes in forensic medicine textbooks, the dangers of abortion and prostitution were tied directly to the prevalence of deviant women who were unregulated by marriage.[35]

In Chevers, the prostitute emerged as the culprit in crimes conducted on the body of men as well. Chevers's *Manual on Medical Jurisprudence* featured a section entitled 'Rape by Females on Males', which detailed the marks of rape on men who manifested the signs of venereal disease. Chevers declared that prostitutes committed crimes that marked the bodies of young Indian boys in order to free themselves of the diseases acquired through prostitution. Explaining the appearance of syphilis and gonorrhoea in young boys, Chevers declared 'debauched women have an idea that they can rid themselves of venereal disease by having connexion with a child'.[36] The prostitute thus became responsible for many different crimes manifested in the private and hidden parts of the human body, from false accusations of rape to crimes of concealment like the abortion to the rape and infliction of disease on men.

Sexing and sexualizing the body were central to the investigation of crimes involving women. The chapters on virginity and rape of Indian girls feature extensive scientific discussions about the physical appearance and quality of the hymen of girls, especially those girls who accuse rape but showed evidence of being 'accustomed' to intercourse.[37] Lyon emphasized this point in his insistence that doctors investigate the presence of the hymen: 'Virginity. Is a certain female "*virgo intacta*" or not? The question arises in cases where women are falsely accusing rape, or an unmarried female is alleged to be a prostitute, a matter that is dealt with under the Contagious Diseases Act.'[38] It is through narratives that tied physical appearance to sociological categories that medical investigation authorized the assessment of the body.

Lyon's textbook describes 'Criminal Miscarriage' in much the same way it was described by Norman Chevers's text and Robert Harvey's reports. Abortion was 'especially common in India' because of the pro-clivity of Indian women to commit crimes in order to conceal their behaviour. As he describes, abortion was 'resorted to by both single and married women in order to get rid of the product of illicit inter-course. ... In India the custom of preventing the remarriage of widows tends directly to increase the prevalence of the offence'.[39] Indeed, the very investigation of crimes related to women required the medical investigator to understand the broad connections between the social phenomena of 'sexual crimes':

> Abortion and child-murder are most common amongst the unfortunate class of young Hindu widows, for whom re-marriage and social rights are denied by their religion. Amongst Mohammedans sexual crimes are much more frequent than amongst Hindus. Prostitution is much more extensively practised amongst the former, and sexual jealousy resulting in the murder of paramours and favoured rivals is probably the most frequent case of homicide amongst Mohammedans. In Bengal, for example, the greatest number of rape cases are reported from the Mohammedan districts of Mymensingh and Dacca. That fanatical form of homicidal insanity 'running amok' is more common amongst Mohammedan fanatics than Hindus.[40]

In this textbook on forensic medicine, we see a narrative technique that unites a disparate set of sociological types in the same epistemological field. For the medico-legal expert, abortion, prostitution, sexual trans-gression, and communalist depictions of Muslims and sexual violence were to be read as equivalent for the medical investigator.

Expanding Networks of Surveillance

Manuals of forensic medicine became significant as a form of knowl-edge because of their widespread use over the course of the nineteenth century, a crucial tool used to define legal understandings of women's sexuality. Forensic medicine was an essential tool in an expanding appa-ratus of colonial state surveillance and legal control. Nineteenth-century records from the colonial government of Bengal on the collection of evidence reflect a growing concern for the 'scientific' power of medical evidence in the detection and prosecution of crime. From the 1860s and until the 1890s, the government of India debated whether police in Bengal could legally conduct genital examinations on women who were accused of becoming pregnant and conducting either abortion or infanticide.[41] In these debates, local authorities emphasized that 'crimes of immorality' could only be detected through scientific fact. Police authorities continued to use the forced genital examination into the twentieth century, citing it as an essential tool in the collection of objective evidence in criminal cases of abortion and infanticide.

Following the enactment of a uniform set of criminal laws in the Indian Penal Code, new institutional apparatuses emerged to monitor and regulate women, and new types of experts were appointed by the state to decipher acts of crime. The Penal Code of 1860 was followed by the enactment of the new Indian Police Act of 1861, which established the Imperial Police and provided detailed guidelines that introduced a new system of policing in India.[42] The police emerged as a key actor in the detection of women's crimes as they were charged with the duty of investigating and discovering crime. Through the expansion of the authority of colonial police, the state began investing its agents with the power of direct regulation of women and their behaviour.

With the prohibition of abortion and infanticide in 1860, people across Bengal submitted petitions to the police that detailed suspicious activity of unmarried women suspected of pregnancy. These accusations often singled out young widows and suggested that they intended to abort or had already aborted unborn foetuses resulting from illegitimate sexual relationships.[43] An appeal to the state for official social regulation, these petitions from people within the community utilized new structures of colonial criminal law to reveal the daily practices of local women. Local authorities, such as village or neighbourhood elders, were to look after these potentially deviant women and to report any attempts at abortion to the subinspector of the police. Guardians of the suspect woman would then submit an ekrar assuring that there would be careful surveillance to ensure that no abortion took place and that they would report any suspicious activity to the police. In cases in which the accused woman denied the pregnancy, the sub-assistant surgeon examined the suspected woman regardless of her consent to collect evidence of her physical state and any signs of abortion or delivery to prove infanticide.[44]

According to police procedure, women were not to be genitally examined at the *thana* (police station) by the police, but, rather, were to be examined by the local medical authority, a state-designated surgeon. However, when women were suspected of crimes requiring a genital examination, police officers would often expose the woman to public shame, conducting the examination themselves: 'In some places where it is known or suspected that a widow is pregnant, she is summoned to the Thannah [police station] ... and that in cases in which the pregnancy is denied an examination takes place in order to ascertain the fact.'[45] In some instances the local *chowkidars* (reporters to the state) informed the police of the pregnancy of widows in their village in weekly reports. As a district magistrate suggests in an 1861 report on the medical examination of widows suspected of abortion, a suspected pregnancy out of wedlock was often a point of extortion and oppression by local neighbours and police. Upon learning that a widow had become pregnant, neighbours or the local police immediately accused the woman of intending to commit abortion or of perpetrating the crime, asking for hefty bribes to prevent a public accusation and forced genital examination at the local thana.[46] The forced genital examination of women, used to collect medico-legal evidence, became a crucial tool for governance over the most intimate aspects of everyday behaviour.

Complex networks of local and colonial authorities produced knowledge about women's deviance and their potential criminal behaviour. The police consistently cited the *dhobi* (washerman) as the primary informant on the sexual liaisons of women.[47] In Gribble and Heher's 1892 *Outlines of Medical Jurisprudence for India*, the text emphasized the significance of the dhobi for charges for a woman accused of abortion and infanticide:

> In this country, it is generally impossible to obtain evidence regarding the exact time of a woman's pregnancy, and it is only from an examination of the body that it can be decided whether it is that of a foetus or a viable child. If the former, the woman might be convicted of having caused an abortion, but it is only when the latter is proved that she could be convicted of infanticide or of concealment of birth. The statements made by the woman as to her condition are, for medico-legal purposes, untrustworthy. She may or may not willingly deceive, but she

may misinterpret her condition. ... The evidence generally produced to prove a woman's pregnancy is that of neighbours who have observed her figure, or that of a washerman who says that pregnancy for many months she has not menstruated [sic], judging from the clothes sent to him to be washed.[48]

Later the textbook describes a case where the dhobi played a pivotal role in bringing charges against a woman: 'A woman was arraigned on a charge of infanticide and also of having caused abortion. The evidence against her was that of the washerman to prove her pregnancy, a cloth stained with blood, and the finding of a decomposed body in a well.'[49] Because of his intimate knowledge of the daily goings on, the dhobi was designated as a key watch-guard to monitor the sexual lives of women.

As the state employed informal social networks in the formal surveillance of women's criminality, the local *samaj* (society) utilized state power to regulate social hierarchies and prevail in monetary and property disputes related to widow inheritance. Until 1873, families that brought civil property disputes to colonial courts could compel widows to forfeit their property rights on the basis of their 'unchastity', a requirement of forfeiture parallel to remarriage under conservative interpretations of Hindu law, where any relation with another man voided a widow's property rights.[50] In the 'Great Unchastity Case' of 1873, the Calcutta High Court decided, against the public opinion of outspoken Hindu elites, that a widow who had not remarried but was considered 'unchaste' or to have committed 'adultery' would retain her share of her husband's property regardless of her sexual indiscretions. With the decision that widows could inherit property despite 'unchastity', disputing families utilized colonial laws on abortion and infanticide to go beyond evidence of women's unchastity to identify the 'sexually deviant' widow as not only 'unchaste' but criminal, with the hope of recovering property from the widow. Petitions to the state demanding the investigation of women accused of abortion and infanticide continued through the end of the nineteenth century.[51]

According to local magistrates, women in India were prone to lie to cover up sexual relationships outside of marriage and, therefore, colonial surveillance of these intimate crimes depended on the collection of physical evidence. Without the compulsory genital examination of women, one magistrate insisted, 'false cases of rape and procuring abortion will largely increase, and we shall have scarcely any means of distinguishing between true and false cases'.[52] For another magistrate, requiring consent from women for genital examinations had the potential to 'cripple' the 'administration of justice'. Citing Norman Chevers's 1856 *Manual*,[53] the magistrate emphasized the untrustworthiness of Indians and the special significance of medical evidence in crimes hidden from the view of the state.

> In a country like India ... it is scarcely surprising that great crimes should be frequently practiced to conceal the result of immorality, and that the procuring of criminal abortion should especially be an act of almost daily commission ... it is necessary that every facility should be given to obtain evidence.[54]

Directly quoting Chevers's textbook on the frequency of abortion and widowhood in India in his argument for the necessity of the genital examination, the magistrate emphasized the frequency of concealed crimes committed by deviant women. He warned against policies that would require women's permission in their own genital examination, which he believed would render the colonial state powerless in a world of clandestine crime. Due to the suspect character of oral testimony in India, 'scientific and unerring material evidence' was more useful than any woman's testimony.[55]

Local authorities in Bengal insisted on the evidence of the 'truth' of women's bodies, asserting that local police had the right to assess a woman's genitalia, regardless of her consent. In response to calls by the government of India to end compulsory genital examinations of women, magistrates unanimously concluded that the examination was essential to substantiating crimes perpetrated by Indian women: 'When a charge of the commission of any of these offences [rape, abortion, or infanticide] is instituted, the Court must proceed with the examination *irrespective of the wishes of the women*.'[56] The medical examination of the accused woman's body was central to this intimate regulation of sexual relations, as it sanctioned the extension of authority over women and their bodies from the samaj to the state. Thus, for the practice of forensic medicine in relation to crimes of rape, abortion, and infanticide, the genital examination, as directed by authoritative textbooks, became a central site of medical investigation and an important form of governance over everyday behaviour.

A Forensics of Female Sexuality

In this chapter I have explored medico-legal narratives about Indian women. The 'medical' of forensic medicine was a site where scientific detail, legal authority, and sociological description converged to create new claims to authority. I have argued that forensic medical texts for India produced extensive knowledge about Indian women's sexuality that united anatomical science with modes of sociological description and the classification of Indian 'customs'. The widespread use of forensic medicine and examination by medical authorities as well as the police arm of the colonial state reveal the significance of forensic medicine to expanding institutions of colonial governance and surveillance over everyday practices and intimate social relationships in the late nineteenth century. Colonial officials described medical evidence of women's crimes to be more useful and factual than the testimony of Indian women, as it revealed the 'truth' behind a crime that was commonly hidden by social norms about sexual propriety and marriage. Forensic medicine extended beyond colonial practices of sociological data collection to become a foundational form of knowledge in the creation of new social scientific studies among Indians as well.[57] Narratives of medico-legal textbooks produced titillating details, which united social status with the physicality of a woman. These descriptions sought to reveal the depth of the character of crime through detailed narratives of violence and the inner recesses of the female body. Textbooks on forensic medicine sexualized the criminal behaviour of women, characterizing women who resided outside the domain of companionate marriage as socially deviant, unchaste, and potentially criminal.

Originating with these nineteenth-century manuals of forensic medicine for India, legal standards of medical evidence that unite corporeal observations and sociological categories continue to be significant today in the prosecution of rape and infanticide cases. Textbooks in contemporary India are fashioned after colonial manuals, and many reproduce nineteenth-century discussions of rape, virginity, abortion, and infanticide verbatim. Legal scholars of postcolonial India have suggested that courts perpetuate biases about women's sexual propriety through their dependence on conceptions of women's sexuality in medico-legal manuals.[58] Forensic medical textbooks continue to travel from the particular physical features of a woman's body to sociological prejudices about chastity, past sexual history, and the moral character of the woman. The continued significance of colonial medico-legal knowledge demonstrates the need for more historical investigations that focus on the relationship of sexuality to new forms of scientific authority, practices of governance, and sociological knowledge.

Notes

1. 'Letter from the Coroner of Calcutta to the Secretary to the Government of Bengal, Judicial Department, dated 14th December 1885', West Bengal State Archives (WBSA), Judicial Department, Judicial Branch, F.N.343, No. B 334 and 335, January 1886.

2. 'Letter from the Coroner of Calcutta to the Secretary to the Government of Bengal, 14 December 1885'.

3. In 1871, the Coroner's Act established the official position of the coroner and the Coroner's Inquest as an official judicial proceeding (Coroner's Act, Act 4 of 1871, 27 January 1871).

4. 'Letter from the Coroner of Calcutta to the Secretary to the Government of Bengal, 14 December 1885'.

5. Ranajit Guha, 'Chandra's Death', in *Subaltern Studies V*, edited by Ranajit Guha (New Delhi: Oxford University Press, 1985), p. 135.

6. Ranajit Guha, 'Chandra's Death', pp. 135–65.

7. For further discussion of medical jurisprudence, colonial difference, and gender in relation to the forensic investigation of rape, see Elizabeth Kolsky, *'The Body Evidencing the Crime': Gender, Law and Medicine in Colonial India* (PhD diss., Columbia University, 2005), pp. 278–347, 400–47 and Elizabeth Kolsky, '"The Body Evidencing the Crime": Rape on Trial in Colonial India, 1860–1947', *Gender and History* 22, no. 1 (2010): 109–30. Kolsky demonstrates how medico-legal understandings of rape shaped the establishment of the 'rule of law' in colonial India. See also Anjali Arondekar's discussion of same-sex archives, sodomy, and medical jurisprudence in her book, *For the Record: On Sexuality and the Colonial Archive in India* (Durham: Duke University Press, 2009), pp. 67–96.

8. See especially Norman Chevers, *A Manual on Medical Jurisprudence for Bengal and the Northwestern Provinces* (London: Carbery, 1856).

9. On the Evidence Act in relation to the implementation of the Indian Penal Code, see Wing-Cheong Chan, Barry Wright, and Stanley Yeo, *Codification, Macaulay and the Indian Penal Code: The Legacies and Modern Challenges of Criminal Law Reform* (London: Ashgate, 2013), pp. 34–8. On the

medico-legal expert, see Kolsky, *Gender, Law and Medicine in Colonial India*, p. 16. On the codification of the criminal code, see Elizabeth Kolsky, 'Codification and the Rule of Colonial Difference: Criminal Procedure in British India', *Law and History Review* 23, no. 3 (2005): 631–83.

10. See sections of the Code on foeticide (sections 315 and 316); infanticide (section 315), sentenced under the act of murder (section 302); the procurement of minor girls for illicit intercourse (section 366a); selling and buying of girls for prostitution (sections 372 and 373); and rape (section 376).

11. Tanika Sarkar, *Hindu Wife, Hindu Nation* (Bloomington: Indiana University Press, 2001), pp. 226–49. In her investigation of the significance of the Phulmoni case for the definition of the girl child under colonial law, Ishita Pande interrogates how colonial medico-legal discourse about Phulmoni constituted child marriage as a social and medical problem used to justify a 'humanitarian' intervention by the colonial state. Building on Pande's reading of the Phulmoni case, I would suggest that medico-legal narratives of Indian women's bodies constituted a range of crimes, including rape, abortion, and infanticide, as markers of the violent results of cultural difference. Beyond the question of authority, this chapter carefully interrogates medico-legal narratives to consider the power of the 'medical' in a sociology of sexual knowledge. See Ishita Pande, 'Phulmoni's Body: The Autopsy, the Inquest and the Humanitarian Narrative on Child Rape in Late Colonial India', *South Asian History and Culture* 4, no. 1 (2013): 9–30.

12. See Mrinalini Sinha, *Colonial Masculinity: The 'Manly Englishman' and the 'Effeminate Bengali' in the Late Nineteenth Century*, Studies in Imperialism (Machester: Manchester University Press, 1995); Janaki Nair, *Women and Law in Colonial India: A Social History* (New Delhi: Kali for Women, 1996); Lata Mani, *Contentious Traditions: The Debate on Sati in Colonial India* (Berkeley: University of California Press, 1998); Sarkar, *Hindu Wife, Hindu Nation*.

13. For more on the development of gynaecology and the sexing of the female body in Britain and the United States, see Ludmilla Jordanova, *Sexual Visions: Images of Gender in Science and Medicine between the Eighteenth and Twentieth Centuries* (New York: Harvester Wheatsheaf, 1989); Cynthia Eagle Russett, *Sexual Science: The Victorian Construction of Womanhood* (Boston: Harvard University Press, 1989); Ornella Moscucci, *The Science of Woman: Gynaecology and Gender in England, 1800–1929* (New York: Cambridge University Press, 1990); Alison Bashford, *Purity and Pollution: Gender, Embodiment and Victorian Medicine* (New York: Palgrave Macmillan, 1998). For important inquiries into the question of sexuality and sexual

difference in science in India, see Supriya Guha, 'The Nature of Woman: Medical Ideas in Colonial Bengal', *Indian Journal of Gender Studies* 3, no. 23 (1996): 23–38, her 'The Unwanted Pregnancy in Colonial Bengal', *The Indian Economic and Social History Review* 33, no. 4 (1996): 403–35, and her unpublished dissertation, 'A Science of Woman' (University of Calcutta, 1996); also see an important discussion of gender in relation to liberalism in Bengal in Ishita Pande, *Medicine, Race and Liberalism in British Bengal: Symptoms of Empire* (London: Routledge, 2009). For important and influential studies of colonial discourses of colonized women's female sexuality in other contexts, see, for example, Luise White, *Comforts of Home: Prostitution in Colonial Nairobi* (Chicago, IL: University of Chicago Press, 1990); Anne McClintock, *Imperial Leather: Race, Gender, and Sexuality in the Colonial Context* (New York: Routledge, 1995); Ann Laura Stoler, *Race and the Education of Desire: Foucault's History of Sexuality and the Colonial Order of Things* (Durham, NC: Duke University Press, 1995); Nancy Rose Hunt, *A Colonial Lexicon: Of Birth Ritual, Medicalization, and Mobility in the Congo* (Durham, NC: Duke University Press, 1999).

14. *A Manual of Medical Jurisprudence for Bengal and the North-Western Provinces* (1856) was published after Norman Chevers's initial report on medical jurisprudence from 1854. Chevers modified his manual for all of India based on case law in Bengal. This modified edition became *A Manual of Medical Jurisprudence for India* (1870). On the development of these textbooks from early colonial courts and the role of these textbooks in colonial discourses of difference, see Elizabeth Kolsky, *Gender, Law and Medicine in Colonial India*, pp. 278–347.

15. The second manual on medical jurisprudence in India, J.D.B. Gribble's *Outline of Medical Jurisprudence for India*, was published in 1885. In 1888 Isidore B. Lyon published his *Medical Jurisprudence for India with Illustrative Cases*. Lyon's book continues to be published today, with more than eleven editions. Following Lyon's manual, an Indian doctor and professor of medical jurisprudence in Agra, Jaising P. Modi, published *A Textbook of Medical Jurisprudence and Toxicology* in 1920. Since its publication, Modi's textbook, which reproduced many of Chevers's ideas about crimes of 'Chastity, Infanticide, and Foeticide', has been crucial to the jurisprudence of rape, abortion (until its legalization), and infanticide. It is the reference most often cited for determinations of medical fact in criminal cases involving women in postcolonial India and continues to be used in Indian courts today, with the most recent edition published in 2016 and separate editions published for use in present-day Pakistan and Bangladesh.

16. Flavia Agnes, 'To Whom Do Experts Testify? Ideological Challenges of Feminist Jurisprudence', *Economic and Political Weekly* 40, no. 18 (30 April–6 May, 2005): 1859–66.

17. Norman Chevers, *A Manual of Medical Jurisprudence for India* (Calcutta: Thacker, Spink & Co., 1870), p. 746.

18. Chevers, *A Manual of Medical Jurisprudence for Bengal and the Northwest Provinces*, pp. 460–532.

19. Robert Harvey, *Report on the Medico-legal Returns Received from the Civil Surgeons in the Bengal Presidency during the Years of 1870, 1871, and 1872* (Calcutta: Calcutta Central Press Co., 1876), p. 295. Emphasis added.

20. The medical investigation was scientific, contrary to the 'suspect' practices of the dhai or midwife. On the colonial marginalization of midwifery, see Geraldine Forbes, 'Managing Midwifery in India', in *Contesting Colonial Hegemony: State and Society in Africa and India*, edited by Dagmar Engels and Shula Marks (London: German Historical Institute, 1994), pp. 152–72.

21. Harvey, *Report on the Medico-legal Returns*, p. 305. Emphasis added.

22. Robert Harvey, 'Report on Medico-Legal Returns', *Indian Medical Gazette* (1 December 1875), pp. 309–10. Emphasis added.

23. Guha, 'Chandra's Death', pp. 135–65.

24. Harvey, 'Report on Medico-Legal Returns', p. 309.

25. 'Review of Robert Harvey's Reports', *The Lancet* (8 July 1876), p. 63.

26. Isidore B. Lyons, *Medical Jurisprudence for India, with Illustrative Cases* (Calcutta: Thacker, Spink, & Co., 1889), pp. 376–7.

27. Isidore B. Lyons, *Medical Jurisprudence for India, with Illustrative Cases* (Calcutta: Thacker, Spink, & Co., 1921), p. 139.

28. Lyon, *Medical Jurisprudence for India* (1921), pp. 275–6.

29. Gribble, *Outlines of Medical Jurisprudence for Indian Courts* (Madras, 1885), pp. 239–40.

30. Gribble, *Outlines of Medical Jurisprudence*, p. 274.

31. Gribble, *Outlines of Medical Jurisprudence*, p. 243.

32. This dependence on the Indian woman's genitalia stands in contrast to important studies of prostitutes in the nineteenth century that looked to different 'truth apparatuses' to decipher the nature of the deviant woman. The most influential physiognomic description of prostitutes in the nineteenth century was A.B. Parent-Duchatelet's 1836 anthropological study of prostitutes in Paris, *De la prostitution dans la ville de Paris* (Paris: J.B. Baillier, 1836). For a discussion of physiognomic texts in relation to perceptions of black sexuality, see Sander Gilman, *Difference and Pathology: Stereotypes of Sexuality, Race, and Madness* (Ithaca, NY: Cornell University Press, 1985). Italian physician and criminologist Cesare Lombroso's criminal

types widely shaped the modern field of 'criminology', a comprehensive science of criminal types that could be used in the creation of theories of crime and detection. See, in particular, Cesare Lombroso and Guglielmo Ferrero, *Criminal Woman, the Prostitute, and the Normal Woman*, translated by Nicole Hahn Rafter and Mary Gibson (Durham: Duke University Press, 2003).

33. Chevers, *Manual on Medical Jurisprudence for India*, p. 712.

34. Chevers, *Manual on Medical Jurisprudence for Bengal*, p. 491.

35. Chevers, *Manual on Medical Jurisprudence for India*, p. 712fn.

36. Chevers, *Manual on Medical Jurisprudence for Bengal*, p. 705.

37. 'Signs of defloration, ie, of loss of virginity—Just as the presence of an intact hymen is the most reliable sign of virginity, so rupture or laceration of this membrane is the chief sign of defloration or promiscuity available' (Lyon, *Medical Jurisprudence* [1889], p. 324). See further discussion of the connection and conflation of chapters on virginity and rape in Durba Mitra and Mrinal Satish, 'Testing Chastity, Evidencing Rape: The Impact of Medical Jurisprudence on Rape Adjudication in India', *Economic and Political Weekly* 49, no. 41 (2014): 51.

38. Lyon, *Medical Jurisprudence for India* (1889), p. 324.

39. Lyon, *Medical Jurisprudence for India* (1921), p. 317.

40. Lyon, *Medical Jurisprudence for India* (1921), p. 33.

41. 'Measures for Putting a Stop to the Practice of Police Officers Making Enquiries into the Pregnancy of Widows', Judicial Proceedings of the Government of Bengal, Proceedings 76–78, February 1861, and 326, April 1861 (WBSA); 'Interference of Police with Cases of Illegitimate Pregnancy with a View to Prevent Miscarriage', Judicial File 232, Proceedings 87–89, March 1881 (WBSA); 'Examination of Women in Criminal Cases', Judicial File 830, Proceedings 19–25, December 1888 (WBSA).

42. M.B. Chande, *The Police In India* (New Delhi: Atlantic Publishers and Distributers, 1997), pp. 72–88.

43. 'Measures for Putting a Stop'.

44. 'Measures for Putting a Stop'.

45. 'Interference of Police'.

46. 'Measures for Putting a Stop'.

47. The role of the *dhobi* in this intimate form of surveillance assumes the presence of menstrual blood on clothing encountered by the dhobi, and the absence of such clothing from suspect women. See Guha, 'The Unwanted Pregnancy in Colonial Bengal': 403–35.

48. J.D.B. Gribble and Patrick Heher, *Outlines of Medical Jurisprudence for India* (Calcutta: Thacker, Spink & Co., 1892), pp. 364–5.

49. Gribble and Heher, *Outlines of Medical Jurisprudence*, p. 367.

50. Dolores Chew, 'The Case of the "Unchaste" Widow: Constructing Gender in 19th-Century Bengal', *Colonialism, Imperialism, and Gender* 22, nos 3 and 4 (fall/winter 1993): 33–43.

51. 'Examination of Women in Criminal Cases', Judicial File 830, Proceedings 19–25, December 1888 (WBSA).

52. 'Examination of Women in Criminal Cases'.

53. 'Criminal Abortion', in Chevers, *Manual of Medical Jurisprudence for Bengal*, p. 489.

54. Chevers, *Manual of Medical Jurisprudence for Bengal*, p. 489.

55. Chevers, *Manual of Medical Jurisprudence for Bengal*, p. 489.

56. Chevers, *Manual of Medical Jurisprudence for Bengal*, p. 489. Emphasis added.

57. See, for example, a manual on women's medicine, *Gurbini Bandhab* (A Companion Guide to Pregnancy) (Calcutta: 1875), which details the causes of abortion and the detection of criminal abortion as well as the symptoms of pregnancy.[57] In a section on *papasrido gorbhosrab* (the criminal disposal of the womb), the author, Harinarayan Bandhyopadhyay, explains the reasons for unnatural abortion in colonial Bengal and the instruments and poisons used to induce abortion among Bengali women. He cites Chevers's textbook as well as the Contagious Diseases Act of 1868.

58. See for example, Agnes, 'To Whom Do Experts Testify?': 1859–66; Pratiksha Baxi, 'The Medicalisation of Consent and Falsity: The Figure of the Habitué in Indian Rape Law', in *The Violence of Normal Times: Essays on Women's Lived Realities*, edited by Kalpana Kannabiran (Delhi: Women Unlimited, 2005) and her book, *Public Secrets of Law: Rape Trials in India* (New Delhi: Oxford University Press, 2014); Durba Mitra and Mrinal Satish, 'Testing Chastity, Evidencing Rape: The Impact of Medical Jurisprudence on Rape Adjudication in India', *Economic and Political Weekly* 41 (2014): 51–8.

2

TREACHEROUS MINDS, SUBMISSIVE BODIES
Corporeal Technologies and Human Experimentation in Colonial India

CHANDAK SENGOOPTA

Analysing the 'style of thinking' of colonial states, Benedict Anderson has remarked that their aim was 'total surveyability' of the colonial domain. This transparency was sought through the construction of 'a totalizing classificatory grid' that could be used to order 'peoples, regions, religions, languages, products, monuments'. The grid ensured that one could identify and situate people and things in definitive ways—'that', to quote Anderson again, 'it was this, not that; it belonged here, not there'.[1] In this chapter I explore how projects for the definitive identification of individuals as well as human experimentation of dubious kinds were not shaped solely by an abstract drive for total classification but also by cultural convictions about the bodies and minds of the colonized. The vast literature on the history of colonial medicine has taught us much about the ways in which the management of epidemics, the institutionalization of laboratory research, or the treatment of 'lunatics', to varying extents, drew upon and shaped ideas of racial difference. We know rather less, however, about the role of colonial conceptions of 'native' bodies and minds in the emergence of such 'scientific' and universally applicable technologies as fingerprinting in British India or, at the other extreme, in the brief second life that 'mesmeric surgery', out of favour in the metropole, experienced in colonial Bengal. Although their Indian roots have been explored in earlier studies, their relevance to the history of colonial medicine as well as colonial governmentality has not been fully assessed.[2]

The Submissive and Duplicitous Native

One recurrent theme in British discourse on Indians concerned the duplicity of natives. John Strachey, in his authoritative and influential handbook *India* (first published in 1888) observed that 'if lying be the test of dishonesty, it would be hard to equal the dishonesty that you meet with in India'.[3] In 1899 Sir Edwin Arnold, translator of the *Bhagvad Gita*, warned that an 'atmosphere of lies' clung 'like an evil mist' to legal proceedings in India.[4] As late as in 1914, an authoritative textbook of forensic medicine lamented that virtually in every case involving Indians 'more or less false evidence is given, whether it be from fear, stupidity, apathy, malice or innate deceit', and that evidence was 'generally supported by marvellously minute direct and circumstantial details'.[5] Bengalis had the worst image of all. 'It is not too much to assert', George Otto Trevelyan (1838–1928) had observed in the 1860s, 'that the mass of Bengalees have no notion of truth and falsehood.'[6] More than two decades before Trevelyan, his uncle and old India hand Thomas Babington Macaulay (1800–1859) had put it far more floridly and famously: 'What horns are to the buffalo, what the paw is to the tiger, what the sting is to the bee, what beauty, according to the old Greek song, is to woman, deceit is to the Bengalee.'[7]

But malice and dishonesty were not all there was to the Bengali character. The race was also quite astoundingly passive and indolent. The Bengali, remarked Macaulay, 'shrinks from bodily exertion; and, though voluble in dispute … seldom engages in a personal conflict. … There never, perhaps, existed a people so thoroughly fitted by nature and by habit for a foreign yoke'.[8] Praising north Indians for their near-European 'manliness and vigour', John Strachey averred: 'But for the presence of our power, Bengal would inevitably and immediately become the prey of the hardier races of other Indian countries. … Englishmen who know Bengal, and the extraordinary effeminacy of its people, find it difficult to treat seriously many of the political declamations in which the English-speaking Bengalis are often fond of indulging.'[9] Although ideas on the duplicity and passivity of Bengalis were primarily used, as in the statement by Strachey, to justify the (benevolent) despotism of the British, they also generated and enabled techniques and initiatives targeting the native body. Although some excellent research has been done on colonial interventions on criminal bodies, the reach of colonial corporeal technologies was wider and far more diverse.[10] I shall establish that contention in this paper by examining the development of two techniques that were apparently very different in their nature, purpose, and impact. Nevertheless, their histories were rooted in their perceptions about the psychological, moral, and racial characteristics of Indians (and more specifically, of Bengalis), and show how the colonial relationship was not simply limited to political or cultural subjugation but inscribed on the very bodies of the colonized.

Lying Natives, Truthful Bodies

As long ago as in 1684, the British physician and pioneer botanist Nehemiah Grew (1641–1712) had pointed out in the *Philosophical Transactions of the Royal Society* that the human fingertips were covered by 'innumerable little ridges', and the British engraver Thomas Bewick (1753–1828) had used his fingermarks in 1804 and 1818 to 'sign' his books on birds. In 1823 the Czech physician and physiologist Jan Evangelista Purkyne (1787–1869) had even classified fingerprints into nine different types. None of these observations led, however, to the creation of a system of identification by fingerprinting.[11] If necessity is the mother of invention, then the necessity to invent a scheme to identify individuals by some simple, indisputable marker was not acute at the time of Grew's, or even Purkyne's observations. Not acute, that is, in Europe. It was a different story in India. European anxieties about habitual criminals and other marginal people, to be sure, heightened over the nineteenth century, but they were almost negligible in comparison to the problems of identity and identification confronting colonial administrators.[12] It is scarcely surprising, therefore, that a viable system for the identification of individuals by fingerprints was first developed in British India, and not by a scientist, or even a policeman, but by a civil servant: William James Herschel (1833–1917), grandson of the astronomer who discovered the planet Uranus and son of the celebrated Victorian scientist John Herschel.[13]

Unlike his illustrious ancestors, William James Herschel had chosen a career in the Indian Civil Service and was posted in administrative positions in various parts of Bengal. In 1858, while negotiating with a Bengali contractor named Rajyadhar Konai for the supply of construction material, Herschel was worried that the man might later disown the contract. In the hope of frightening 'Konai out of all thought of repudiating his signature thereafter', Herschel, on a sudden whim, asked him to stamp the contract with a print of his right palm. After obtaining the print, he later recalled, 'We studied it together, with a good deal of chaff about palmistry, comparing his palm to mine on another impression.'[14] The use of the entire palm being inconvenient, Herschel wondered whether it might be better to use the fingertips for the purpose. He does not seem to have imagined, as yet, that the ridge-patterns of the fingertips were so distinctive and so enduring that disowning them might lead to conviction for perjury. All he sought at this point was a device to frighten Indians into truthfulness. 'My executive and magisterial experience had', Herschel explained, 'forced on me that distrust of all evidence tendered in Court which did so much to cloud our faith in the people around us.'[15]

The real power of Herschel's discovery became evident to him only after much experimentation with his own fingers and those of friends and visitors. Herschel was indefatigable in collecting specimens from friends and colleagues and his 'fad' became well known wherever he was posted. He never encountered a duplicate pattern, and as far as he could see from prints taken repeatedly from the same person across time, each individual's ridge patterns persisted unaltered through time.[16] Purely by chance, he seemed to have stumbled upon a foolproof way of identifying individuals, and he would realize how administratively useful such a tool could be when he was posted to Nadia as magistrate. That was in 1860, when Nadia was the nerve centre of the so-called Indigo Rebellion.[17] From the late eighteenth century, the East India Company had supported the cultivation of indigo in India, and especially in Bengal, by providing advances to European planters.[18]

The planters, in turn, entered into contracts with peasants (*rayats*), who had come to hate the meticulousness required in cultivating indigo and to resent the low profits.[19] The indigo planters, however, were a powerful group and ran almost a parallel colonial regime of their own, there being few Europeans in rural regions except magistrates, many of whom were ready to turn a blind eye to the doings of other white people. The bullying of peasants, destruction of food crops, forging contracts, the forcible sowing of indigo, and countless other acts of petty despotism were only too frequent.[20] When peasants in village after village began to rebel against the planters, the government of Bengal ordered investigations of complaints of coercion. It was only after the government appointed a commission of enquiry into the indigo trade that the disturbances began to subside—the report was highly critical of the planters and the majority of magistrates.[21]

Violence and bullying were not all there was to the indigo business, however. Since the cultivation of indigo was done on contract, one easy way of compelling a peasant to grow the crop was to forge a contract. Likewise, for a peasant, an easy way of denying the obligation to grow indigo was to repudiate a genuine contract, alleging it to be a forgery. 'The Indigo disturbances in the district', Herschel wrote, 'had given rise to a great deal of violence, litigation, and fraud; forgery and perjury were rampant.'[22] Documents submitted in court, he recalled, 'were frequently worth no more than the paper on which they were written. ... Things were so bad in this and other ways that the administration of Civil Justice had unusual difficulty in preserving its dignity'.[23] There just was no simple way of determining whether a contract was real or forged, and as the magistrate in charge of pronouncing on such matters, Herschel came to appreciate the practical significance of his 'hobby'.[24] In his testimony to the Indigo Commission, Herschel declared:

> If personification at the time of signature, or false pleas of personification afterwards, were rendered impossible by any peculiar mode of signature, nine-tenths of the difficulty of forming a decision would disappear, and with it nine-tenths of the process necessary to bring the trial to an issue. I can suggest a signature of exceeding simplicity, which it is all but impossible to deny or to forge. The impression of a man's finger on paper cannot be denied by him afterwards.[25]

The enquiry commission ignored this suggestion completely and Herschel failed to convince the government of Bengal to enforce the use of 'fingerprints' on contracts.[26]

When appointed the magistrate and collector of the Hooghly district in 1877, Herschel finally had enough authority to go it alone. He demanded fingerprint signatures from those collecting pensions (because he suspected that many of the genuine pensioners had long died and been replaced by impersonators), and then instituted the use of fingerprints in registration of deeds for sale of land or property.[27] Finally, he began to use it in the jail to ensure that a convict could not get somebody to serve out his sentence 'for a consideration', which, apparently, was common practice. In all of these areas, the technique worked exceedingly well. Fingerprinting, Herschel exclaimed in a letter to his wife, was 'a miracle, a miracle from on High!'[28] Herschel failed again, however, to persuade the government to use his technique and his work was not widely known when he retired in 1877. After he retired from the civil service and left India, fingerprinting was discontinued even in Hooghly.[29] Back in England, Herschel continued collecting fingerprints but published nothing on his work in India.[30]

The importance of Herschel's work was first appreciated by Francis Galton (1822–1911). In the 1890s, Galton was working on techniques for identifying individuals by their bodily features.[31] The editor of *Nature* introduced him to Herschel, who was delighted to share his collection of prints with Galton. Having examined them, a stunned Galton declared: 'There seems no persistence in the visible parts of the body, except in these minute and hitherto too much disregarded ridges. ... They existed before birth, and they persist after death, until effaced by decomposition.'[32] Here, obviously, was an ideal means of permanently identifying each individual. Although such identification was essential in the East—'While the natives of India and of Egypt have beautiful traits of character and some virtues in an exceptional degree, their warmest admirers would not rank veracity among them', wrote Galton—it was far from inapplicable in Britain itself.[33] People saving money at the post-office savings bank, Galton suggested, should be asked to record their finger impressions in the deposit book 'and that these should be used as a means of identification, when the depositor sought to draw money from a post-office where he was not known'. It was so easy to learn the rudiments of matching fingerprints that 'it might well be part of the training of many minor civil servants, postmasters, Public Trustee employees, War Office and Admiralty pension-officers, and many other similar officials'.[34] Despite Galton's persistent pleas, however, none of those 'civil' uses of fingerprinting were ever seriously considered in Britain. It was only the Home Office that showed interest in fingerprints.

From the mid-nineteenth century, administrators, policemen, and politicians in Britain had been much concerned with identifying so-called habitual criminals, who, it was widely believed, constituted a distinct class and should be punished more severely than first-time offenders.[35] To achieve that, however, the police needed a foolproof system whereby a *specific* prisoner could be identified as having committed other crimes before the present one; but there was, as yet, no simple, reliable, and inexpensive method to do so.[36] Fingerprinting was cheap as well as reliable but to use fingerprinting in routine police work, one needed a reliable and easily searchable system whereby a fingerprint, whether one found at a scene of crime or one taken from an individual suspect, could be compared with prints (with identities) on record. But an easily searchable database of fingerprints seemed impossible to create. The infinite diversity that made the ridge patterns unparalleled as identifiers also made it impossible to order them systematically.

That problem, too, was to be solved in Bengal by the inspector general of the Bengal police, Edward Richard Henry, with considerable assistance from two Indian subinspectors, Azizul Haque and Hem Chandra Bose, but it would take us far beyond the remit of this paper to explore its technicalities here.[37] The availability of a classificatory scheme, as one might expect, led to the immediate introduction of fingerprinting in police work in India. Rather more surprising was the mighty resurgence in its 'Herschelian' applications. All military and civil pensioners were now fingerprinted, as were all executants of deeds.[38] Even more reminiscent of Herschel's experience during the Indigo Revolts was the use of fingerprinting in the opium department. As with indigo, opium was cultivated by rayats, who were not particularly fond of the crop and contracts with whom were often forged by middlemen. This had finally come to an end because 'the finger impression of the payee is now required to authenticate acknowledgment of receipt'.[39] Similar problems with contracts for indentured labourers were also resolved by fingerprinting.[40] Huge organizations such as the Survey of India or the post office maintained registers of their employees' thumb impressions and 'if a particular man is dismissed for misbehaviour, a photo-zincograph of his impression is sent to all the working parties, which ensures that he cannot again get taken on, even by assuming a false name'. From 1895, illiterate people were required to sign for money orders and postal savings accounts with their thumbprints.[41] The medical department of the Bengal Presidency stopped issuing medical certificates without recording the thumb impression of the patient.[42] The potential applications of fingerprinting in colonial administration seemed as unlimited as the mendaciousness and duplicity of Queen Victoria's Indian subjects.

Once fingerprinting had been established in India, it was adopted in Britain itself, but at first *only* for the identification of criminal recidivists. Although the police would secure permission to use fingerprinting for other kinds of offenders, the technique would never be allowed out into the 'civil' sphere. Henry himself was appointed assistant commissioner of the Metropolitan Police and charged with supervising the transplantation of the imperial sapling on home soil. Scotland Yard's fingerprint bureau was founded in 1901 and the first conviction on fingerprint evidence occurred the very next year. What was a universal technique for identification in India came to be reserved in Britain for criminals, and only for those regarded as the most incorrigible. No less a figure than Francis Galton regretted this restriction. His student and biographer Karl Pearson emphasized that Galton 'did not think finger-prints were useful solely as a matter of criminal identification' and it was 'almost a catastrophe that the process of finger-printing should have become tainted in the popular mind by a criminal atmosphere'.[43] Galton's laments and other pleas notwithstanding, the bodies of law-abiding British subjects were left inviolate and the numerous 'Herschelian' applications, developed to combat Indian mendacity, were never welcomed into the metropole.

Mesmerism in Hooghly: Animal Magnetism and the Brutish Bengali

Let us now turn to what is apparently a completely different kind of corporeal intervention—invasive surgery or, more precisely, anaesthesia in preparation for such surgery. Reliable chemical anaesthetics came into use in the West in the late 1840s but that was preceded by a brief but controversial period of experimentation with anaesthesia by mesmeric influence. Few topics in the history of European medicine and psychology are more intriguing than mesmerism and its offshoots, the most enduring of which has, of course, been hypnotism.[44] The originator of mesmerism, Franz Anton Mesmer (1734–1815), claimed to have discovered that all living beings possessed an intangible magnetic fluid, which could be influenced by a healer through 'magnetic passes' (slow and sweeping hand movements that came very close to the patient's skin but did not touch it).[45] Eventually, the subject being mesmerized would fall into a trance and could manifest many strange phenomena ranging from loss of sensation to clairvoyance. From the late 1830s, there was keen medical as well as popular interest in mesmerism in Britain. John Elliotson (1791–1868), professor of practical medicine at University College London, performed many spectacular public demonstrations of mesmeric techniques on his hospital patients. Although Elliotson had to resign from his university post after the credibility of one of his subjects was challenged, he remained an enthusiast and published extensive reports on the applications of mesmerism in *The Zoist*, a journal he co-founded in 1843.[46]

Mesmerism was known to produce insensibility but it was only after the 1842 amputation of the leg of a mesmerized labourer in Nottinghamshire that the anaesthetic utility of mesmerism began to be discussed widely.[47] Although anaesthetic gases like nitrous oxide had been known for many years, there had been no serious effort by surgeons to use them for anaesthesia, and surgical anaesthesia by ether came to be used only in the mid-1840s.[48] For a few years before the introduction of ether, mesmeric anaesthesia came to be well known, and was very controversial.[49] In the history of those controversies, the Scottish surgeon James Esdaile (1808–1859), working in distant Bengal, was to play a role that was arguably more significant than that of any European practitioner.

Esdaile was born in Scotland and trained in medicine at the University of Edinburgh. In 1830 he joined the East India Company, arriving in Bengal in 1831. From 1839 to 1846, he was in charge of a hospital at Hooghly—the same Hooghly where, more than three decades later, William Herschel would launch the official use of fingerprinting. Esdaile's success with mesmeric surgery there led to his transfer to Calcutta, where he was put in charge of a new mesmeric hospital. His work received much praise from the governor general, Lord Dalhousie, who made Esdaile a presidency surgeon in 1848. Esdaile left India in 1851 and retired from the East India Company's service in 1853. He became the vice president of the London Mesmeric Infirmary, but his research on mesmerism never seriously advanced beyond his Indian experiments and he died in relative obscurity in 1859.[50]

Esdaile had become aware of mesmeric phenomena from the early reports of John Elliotson.[51] Shortly before his first experiment, he wrote to a friend in England,

> What think you of this new mystery, Mesmerism? For my part, I am thinking seriously about it, and cannot help suspecting that we have hit upon one of Nature's great secrets. I keep myself perfectly neutral, and hear the *pro* and the *con*. If it turns out to be a delusion, I shall be happy to assist in digging its grave.[52]

Whether or not one takes this statement at face value, there is no reason to assume that Esdaile was a zealot on the subject. His first venture into mesmeric research was, he claimed, entirely fortuitous.[53] A prisoner named Madhab Kaura, with a double hydrocele, had been brought into his hospital and treated, as was routine at the time, by tapping of the fluid and injection of a corrosive substance into the scrotal sac. The latter, expectedly, was severely painful and Esdaile thought of using mesmerism to abate the pain. Placing the patient's knees between his own, Esdaile made mesmeric passes but it was only after an hour that they had a significant effect: 'All appearance of pain now disappeared; his hands were crossed on his breast, instead of being pressed on the groins, and his countenance showed the most perfect repose. He now took no notice of our questions, and I called loudly on him by name without attracting any notice.'[54]

To test the genuineness of the trance, the patient was pricked repeatedly with a pin, then 'fire was ... applied to his knee, without his shrinking in the least' and finally, he was given a strong solution of ammonia to inhale, which 'seemed to have revived him a little'. Offering him a drink, Esdaile 'took the opportunity to give, slowly, a mixture of ammonia so strong that I could not bear to taste it; this he drank like milk, and gaped for more'.[55] All of this was done in the presence of a local judge and the collector since it was essential to have the testimony of 'intelligent witnesses'. The witnesses were suitably impressed and signed a statement declaring that they were 'thoroughly convinced that there was a complete suspension of sensibility to external impressions of the most painful kind'.[56] Esdaile was now confident enough to perform actual surgery under mesmeric anaesthesia.

Since the other side of the same patient's hydrocele remained to be treated, he was again mesmerized a few days later. A group of European witnesses was brought in, including the governor of the French colony of Chandannagar (Chandernagore). The operation went ahead without any sign of the patient feeling the slightest pain. When he woke up, he was in some pain but not in agony and there was an unexpected bonus—his chronic diarrhoea seemed to have been relieved. 'What a blessed prospect this opens to sufferers who may be sensible to the Mesmeric influence', gushed Esdaile. 'Although I should never succeed again, I will in future think, speak, and write of Mesmerism as being as much a reality as the principle of gravitation, or the properties of opium.'[57]

He did not deny that mesmeric influence might have a mental dimension, but no such mental influence could have acted in the present case, 'for the individual is only one (?) degree above the brutes, and if his mind can be acted upon, I suspect it must be by some one who has more sympathy with his mental constitution'.[58] Many other patients followed Madhab Kaura and most were operated on for hydroceles or scrotal tumours.[59] Virtually all the early patients were Indians, almost all of them belonging to the poorest classes, and mesmerism, Esdaile discovered, was also of use in a variety of non-surgical conditions from retention of urine and rheumatism to nervous headaches and hiccups.[60] After the first few cases, he stopped inducing the trance himself and left that tedious task to his native assistants. 'I never mesmerise now', he wrote to John Elliotson in 1846, 'for others do the work just as effectually, and it was killing me. I wonder that you do not keep a mesmeric corps too; but I have a great advantage in the docility and patience of my agents and patients.'[61] 'The mesmeric power', he observed, 'is a far more general gift of nature than has hitherto been supposed.'[62] As his clientele grew, Esdaile also began to use water that had been mesmerized by him and which, when given orally, produced mesmeric effects.[63]

The government of Bengal appointed a seven-member committee to assess the worth of Esdaile's work. Although the committee's report was not unanimous, a majority found mesmeric surgery to be deserving of support.[64] Esdaile was transferred to Calcutta to head an 'experimental mesmeric hospital', where he could establish 'the applicability of this alleged agency to all descriptions of cases, medical as well as surgical, and all classes of patients, European as well as native'.[65] His work would be open to scrutiny by visitors appointed by the government. The hospital was funded only for a year and during his time there, Esdaile continued to perform the usual scrotal operations on Indians under mesmeric anaesthesia. He also used mesmerism to treat patients with nervous and psychiatric disorders and many of these latter patients were European. The results were reportedly good, but there was much criticism too. One medical observer declared that all the effects were faked by the patients and the time and attention required to mesmerize each patient was considered by many observers to be exorbitant.[66]

The hospital closed after a year, as originally scheduled. Influential people, including Governor General Lord Dalhousie, considered it to have been successful and Esdaile was promoted to the post of Presidency surgeon in recognition of his achievements. The recognition did not in fact help Esdaile to continue his work, since there was now no hospital where he could practise mesmerism. There were many demands from the indigenous elite of Calcutta for a mesmeric hospital, but the government was unwilling to fund it.[67] Eventually, a group of Indian and British residents of Calcutta raised the funds to open a new mesmeric hospital as part of a charity dispensary. Esdaile was appointed as its superintendent, but this institution does not seem to have been as active as its predecessor, and it definitely lost status by being associated with a charity dispensary. After Esdaile left India in 1851, he was succeeded by Alan Webb, who taught anatomy at the Calcutta Medical College. The fortunes of the hospital showed little improvement, however, and it closed towards the end of the decade.[68] The introduction of ether and then chloroform by the end of the 1840s, in any case, had undermined mesmeric anaesthesia more effectively than any of its medical critics ever could.[69]

Much has been written on Esdaile, the enduring value of his work, and on what the strange career of mesmerism in colonial India reveals about the relationship of science with magic, superstition, and Eastern exotica.[70] It is not the aim of this chapter to rehearse those discussions or to question their conclusions. Instead, I would like to emphasize how Esdaile's work was grounded in particular conceptions of the psychological, moral, and cultural nature of Indians. Esdaile always claimed that different races responded differently to mesmerism. 'Men', he asserted, 'are nearly the same all the world over: an universal vital law reduces all to the same level of animal, and the cooly, therefore, may be able to mesmerise the philosopher.'[71] He even went out of his way to interact with local magicians and healers, arguing that their techniques often worked because they were fundamentally mesmeric in nature.[72] The effects of mesmerism, Esdaile declared, were the same 'on the banks of the Thames, and the Seine, the Rhine, and the Hooghly'.[73]

There was considerable strategic justification for such Enlightenment-style assertions. If Esdaile's reports were to be deployed in defending the interests of mesmerism in Europe, as was done, for instance, by John Elliotson in issue after issue of *The Zoist*, then it was imperative to avoid the impression that mesmerism worked only on the 'lower' races. In one of his editorials Elliotson wrote,

> Dr Esdaile relates a few interesting facts which presented themselves unexpectedly to him in his Asiatic patients and are *precisely the same as astonished us in England on their first occurrence*—proving that they occurred *according to the laws of nature*, and that the human beings who manifested themselves were *not impostors, as the uninformed foes of mesmerism clamorously declared.*[74]

Esdaile and Elliotson remained consistent in their universalism, although an occasional unguarded admission can be found in their reports.[75]

At the same time, however, Esdaile insisted that Indians were ideal experimental subjects because of their *difference* from Europeans. First of all, mesmerism was unknown there under its modern name and it was inconceivable that 'some clever rogue' would know enough to feign to be mesmerized.[76] More importantly, the low mental and moral status of poorer Indians ensured that there could be no question of collusion with a European doctor. It went almost without saying that 'the difference in *morale* [between doctor and patient] is so great … as to preclude all sympathy, and to often amount to actual antipathy, and mutual repulsion'.[77] The reality of mesmerism could never be adequately proved by experiments upon 'some highly sensitive female of a nervous temperament, and excitable imagination, who desired to submit to the supposed influence'. What was special about his own studies was that they began with a man like Madhab Kaura, 'the very worst specimen of humanity ... a Hindu felon of the hangman cast'.[78] Successful inductions of mesmeric trance in such individuals meant that imagination and 'mental sympathy' did not play any role in mesmerism—animal magnetism was purely a *physical* force like electricity or magnetism, exactly as its champions in the West had been suggesting.[79] 'My patients and I', Esdaile declared, 'have probably too little in common to admit of mental sympathy between us.'[80]

The other great advantage of working with poor Indian patients was the range of experimentation that was permissible. One could test insensibility by burning the patient with fire or acid or sticking pins into him without any hesitation. One could also afford to ignore the shock experienced by many patients on 'coming out' of the trance. The first few moments after the end of the trance was a 'trial of the nerves, to which it would be very imprudent, and unsafe, to subject any but such singularly impassive beings as my patients ... *I would not dare to take such liberties with European temperaments*'.[81] The best thing about working with the people of Bengal, however, was that 'the people of this part of the world seem to be peculiarly sensitive to the mesmeric power'. It was obvious why Bengalis were more impressionable than Europeans since it was an established fact that 'a depressed state of the nervous system' facilitated the exertion of mesmeric influence. And nobody had a more depressed nervous system than Bengalis. 'Taking the population of Bengal generally,' Esdaile explained, 'they are a feeble, ill-nourished race, remarkably deficient in nervous energy; and natural debility of constitution being still further lowered by disease, will probably account for their being so readily subdued by the Mesmerist.' The mesmerist found his task much easier with such a primitive and passive people:

> We have none of the morbid irritability of nerves, and the mental impatience of civilised man, to contend against.... The success I have met with is mainly to be attributed, I believe, to my patients being the simple, unsophisticated children of nature; *neither thinking, questioning, nor remonstrating, but passively submitting to my pleasure*, without in the smallest degree understanding my object or intentions.[82]

Colonial India and its 'natives', in short, provided the optimal conditions for establishing the truth of the doctrine of animal magnetism—'*passive obedience* in the patient, and a sustained attention and patience on the part of the operator'.[83]

* * *

Many historians have remarked that colonial India represented a huge laboratory where social, administrative, and corporeal interventions, often of dramatically novel kinds, could be tried out far more freely than in the metropole.[84] In that metaphorical laboratory, indigenous Indians, of course, served as guinea pigs, but their role has yet to be extensively analysed. In this chapter, I have explored how two colonial experiments invaded, in very different ways, the bodies of the colonized and did so on the basis of specific, racialized concepts of the psychology and character of a subset of Indians. The reason why fingerprint identification was developed by a colonial administrator in Hooghly was not because William James Herschel knew more than Grew or Purkyne about the individuality of ridge patterns, but because the British in India urgently needed a weapon to combat what they regarded as the *innate* duplicity of Bengalis. Although fingerprinting was found to be universally valid, its colonial applications were to remain far more numerous and they were usually driven by the perceived need to combat the dishonesty of 'natives'.

With mesmeric surgery, the brutish nature of Indians was a vital presupposition but the venerable trope of native mendacity was entirely absent. The reasons for that absence are not difficult to identify. Unlike fingerprinting, mesmeric surgery was not only known in Europe but very controversial; one major aim of Esdaile's experiments was to provide valuable supportive evidence to metropolitan defenders of mesmerism who, because of the controversies surrounding the practice, no longer had the opportunity to conduct much human experimentation. Esdaile argued that if mesmerism worked on a race as ignorant, passive, and mindless as the Bengalis, then mesmerism could not be based, as metropolitan sceptics alleged, on mental suggestibility. But it was also essential to rule out conscious imposture and that explains the absence of any reference to the fabled dishonesty of Bengalis in Esdaile's writings.

For Macaulay, the duplicity and passivity of Bengalis had represented two sides of the same coin. When we juxtapose the history of Herschel's work on fingerprinting and Esdaile's mesmeric operations, however, we can appreciate that the two themes were not necessarily inseparable in conceptual terms. One useful way of appreciating the diversity of British ideas of Indians and their material significance, this chapter suggests, is to investigate how specific ideas of 'native' character governed particular uses of 'native' bodies. Needless to say, much has been written on colonial ideologies and racial stereotypes, and the literature on colonial medicine is no less voluminous. What this chapter argues is that the two approaches can be fruitfully combined by broadening the idea of the 'medical' to include all bodily interventions, regardless of their professional provenance, goals, and current scientific status.

Notes

1. Anderson does not address specific technologies of identification, although he does mention postcolonial Indonesia's compulsory photo IDs as an example of a residue of the colonial dream of total surveyability. See Benedict Anderson, *Imagined Communities: Reflections on the Origin and Spread of Nationalism* (London: Verso, 1991), pp. 184, 185.

2. See, for instance, Waltraud Ernst, 'Esdaile, James (1808–1859)', in *Oxford Dictionary of National Biography*, available at http://www.oxforddnb.com/view/article/8882, accessed 29 January 2006. For the broader contexts of Esdaile's work, see Waltraud Ernst, '"Under the Influence" in British India: James Esdaile's Mesmeric Hospital in Calcutta and Its Critics', *Psychological Medicine* 25, no. 6 (1995): 1113–23; W. Ernst, 'Colonial Psychiatry, Magic and Religion: The Case of Mesmerism in British India', *History of Psychiatry* 15, no. 1 (2004): 57–71; and Chandak Sengoopta, *Imprint of the Raj: How Fingerprinting Was Born in Colonial India* (London: Macmillan, 2003).

3. John Strachey, *India* (London: Kegan Paul, 1888), p. 286. On the importance of Strachey's book in building British opinion on India for decades, see Eric Stokes, *The English Utilitarians and India* (Oxford: Clarendon Press, 1959; reprint, Delhi: Oxford University Press, 1982), pp. 137, 305.

4. Quoted in Vinay Lal, 'Everyday Crime, Native Mendacity and the Cultural Psychology of Justice in Colonial India', *Studies in History* 15, no. 1 (1999): 145–66, 155. Lal's illuminating article cites countless other examples of British observations on the same theme.

5. See L.A. Waddell, *Lyon's Medical Jurisprudence for India with Illustrative Cases*, 5th ed. (Calcutta: Thacker, Spink & Co., 1914), p. 19, and for an even later elaboration of the same theme, see William Willcox's contribution to

the discussion on Lancelot Sanderson, 'Law and Order and Medicine in India in the Future', *The Medico-Legal and Criminological Review* 2 (1934): 129–40, at 137.

6. George Otto Trevelyan, 'Letter from a Competition Wallah: Letter VIII – About the Hindoo Character', *Macmillan's Magazine* 9 (1863–4): 198–211, 205 and 207. Trevelyan's letters were later published in book form: see G.O. Trevelyan, *The Competition Wallah* (London: Macmillan, 1864).

7. T.B. Macaulay, 'Warren Hastings' (1841), in Macaulay, *Critical and Historical Essays*, available at http://www.columbia.edu/itc/mealac/pritchett/00generallinks/macaulay/hastings/txt_complete.html, sec. 4, accessed 9 June 2013. Macaulay served in India from 1834 to 1838. On his contributions to British ideas and representations of India, see Balachandra Rajan, *Under Western Eyes: India from Milton to Macaulay* (Durham, North Carolina: Duke University Press, 1999), pp. 174–96.

8. T.B. Macaulay, 'Lord Clive' (1840), in his *Critical and Historical Essays*, available at http://www.columbia.edu/itc/mealac/pritchett/00generallinks/macaulay/clive/clive08.html, accessed 9 June 2013.

9. Strachey, *India*, pp. 4, 336. The charge of Bengali effeminacy, interestingly, was partly endorsed by Bengali nationalists and inspired many initiatives to overcome it. See John Rosselli, 'The Self-Image of Effeteness: Physical Education and Nationalism in Nineteenth-Century Bengal', *Past and Present* 86, no. 1 (February 1980): 121–48; Mrinalini Sinha, *Colonial Masculinity: The 'Manly Englishman' and the 'Effeminate Bengali' in the Late Nineteenth Century* (Manchester: Manchester University Press, 1995); and Indira Chowdhury, *The Frail Hero and Virile History: Gender and the Politics of Culture in Colonial Bengal* (Delhi: Oxford University Press, 1998).

10. On the colonial interest in 'criminal bodies', see Clare Anderson, *Legible Bodies: Race, Criminality and Colonialism in South Asia* (Oxford: Berg, 2004); and Mark Brown, 'Ethnology and Colonial Administration in Nineteenth-Century British India: The Question of Native Crime and Criminality', *British Journal of the History of Science* 36, no. 2 (2003): 201–19. See also Radhika Singha, 'Settle, Mobilize, Verify: Identification Practices in Colonial India', *Studies in History* 16, new series (2000): 151–98; and Sengoopta, *Imprint of the Raj*.

11. See Simon Cole, *Suspect Identities: A History of Fingerprinting and Criminal Identification* (Cambridge, Massachusetts: Harvard University Press, 2001).

12. On European concerns with identification, see Alain Corbin's essay 'Backstage', in *A History of Private Life*, vol. 4, edited by Michelle Perrot (Cambridge, Massachusetts: Harvard University Press, 1990), pp. 451–667.

13. The basic biography is well summarized in A. Spokes Symonds, 'Herschel, Sir William James, second baronet (1833–1917)', in *Oxford Dictionary of National Biography*, rev. Katherine Prior (Oxford: Oxford University Press, 2004), available at http://www.oxforddnb.com/view/article/37539, accessed 10 June 2013. See also Eileen Shorland, 'Sir William James Herschel and the Birth of Fingerprint Identification', *Library Chronicle, University of Texas*14, new series (1980): 25–33.

14. William James Herschel, *The Origin of Finger-Printing* (London: Oxford University Press, 1916), pp. 7–9. Many have wondered just why Herschel thought of this particular procedure. Herschel himself observed dismissively that there was nothing very original about it: instances had long been known of the hand, or the nail or even the teeth being used to 'certify a man's act, or a woman's'. As a boy, he recalled, he had loved Thomas Bewick's work on birds, although, by the time he had asked Konai for his handprint on the contract, he had forgotten all about Bewick's habit of affixing his thumb mark to his books. He also acknowledged that illiterate Indians used finger-dabs as signatures (*tip-soi*) but since those dabs were mere smudges without any identifying attributes, they did not, he asserted, inspire him to study the individuality of fingerprints. But even if he was wrong or dishonest about this and it *was* the supposedly unidentifiable tip-soi that had induced him to explore whether more carefully taken fingermarks might serve to record a person's identity, his use of the whole palm remains a mystery.

15. Herschel, *Origin of Finger-Printing*, 7.

16. See H.J.S. Cotton, *Indian and Home Memories* (London: Unwin, 1911), p. 68.

17. On the indigo revolts, see Blair B. Kling, *The Blue Mutiny: The Indigo Disturbances in Bengal, 1859–1862* (Philadelphia: University of Pennsylvania Press, 1966); and Amiya Rao and B.G. Rao, *The Blue Devil: Indigo and Colonial Bengal* (Delhi: Oxford University Press, 1992).

18. In the late eighteenth century, Joseph Banks, the president of the Royal Society and Scientific Advisor to the East India Company had urged its directors to cultivate sugar, cotton, coffee and indigo—none of which could be grown in Europe—in India. See David Arnold, *Science, Technology and Medicine in Colonial India* (Cambridge: Cambridge University Press, 2000), p. 52.

19. See *Report of the Indigo Commission Appointed under Act XI. of 1860, with the Minutes of Evidence*, available most conveniently in *House of Commons Parliamentary Papers*, 44 (1861), pp. 335 et seq., on p. xviii.

20. The *Report of the Indigo Commission* is full of examples; for independent confirmation, see John Beames, *Memoirs of a Bengal Civilian* (London: Eland, 1984).

21. This account relies on Kling, *The Blue Mutiny*.

22. Herschel, *Origin of Finger-Printing*, p. 11.

23. Herschel, *Origin of Finger-Printing*, p. 11.

24. Herschel was in favour of summary punishment for anybody infringing a contract and never hesitated to rule against *rayats*, when he considered them to be in breach of contract. He repeatedly warned the peasants that he would enforce contracts impartially and, if necessary, call in the military police to aid him. But he was equally strict with planters and was greatly disliked by them. See Kling, *Blue Mutiny*, pp. 150–1.

25. *Report of the Indigo Commission*, p. 573.

26. Many years later, however, Herschel heard from a senior civil servant that the inaction had been motivated by the fear that the introduction of fingerprinting might well trigger a new controversy just when the indigo situation was improving. See Herschel, *Origin of Finger-Printing*, pp. 14, 15.

27. See Herschel, *Origin of Finger-Printing*, pp. 18–21.

28. See Shorland, 'Sir William James Herschel and the Birth of Fingerprint Identification': 30.

29. See note from F.W. Duke dated 6 January 1893, Galton Papers, 172/5B, University College London Library Services.

30. See 'Sir William Herschel', *The Times*, 27 October 1917, p. 9.

31. See Francis Galton, *Finger Prints* (London: Macmillan, 1892); Paul Rabinow, 'Galton's Regret: Of Types and Individuals', in *DNA On Trial: Genetic Identification and Criminal Justice*, edited by Paul R. Billings (Plainview, New York: Cold Spring Harbor Laboratory Press, 1992), pp. 5–18; and Cole, *Suspect Identities*, pp. 99–113.

32. Galton, *Finger Prints*, 98, 10.

33. Francis Galton, 'Identification Offices in India and Egypt', *Nineteenth Century* 48 (1900): 118–26, 119.

34. Karl Pearson, *Life, Letters and Labours of Francis Galton*, 3 vols in 4 parts (Cambridge: Cambridge University Press, 1914), 3A, pp. 156–7.

35. See Leon Radzinowicz and Roger Hood, 'Incapacitating the Habitual Criminal: The English Experience', *Michigan Law Review* 78 (1980): 1305–89; and 'Papers Relating to the Bill for the More Effective Surveillance and Control of Habitual Offenders in India and Certain Connected Purposes', in *Selections from the Records of the Government of India (Home Department)* (Calcutta, 1893), p. 300, British Library Asia, Pacific and Africa Collections, MF 1/530–534.

36. On identification procedures in British police forces in the late nineteenth century, see C.E. Troup, A. Griffiths, M.L. Macnaghten, *Report of a Committee Appointed by the Secretary of State to Inquire into the Best Means*

Available for Identifying Habitual Criminals (Command Paper C-7263), 1894, in the *House of Commons Parliamentary Papers*, 72 (1893–4), pp. 209–91.

37. See E.R. Henry, *Classification and Uses of Finger Prints* (London: HMSO, 1901). Generally on Henry, see F.E.C. Gregory, 'Henry, Sir Edward Richard, baronet (1850–1931)', *Oxford Dictionary of National Biography*, available at http://www.oxforddnb.com/view/article/33822, accessed 14 February 2006; and Maurice Garvie, 'The Life and Times of Sir Edward Henry', *International Criminal Police Review*, no. 480 (2000): 24–31. On the role of the two Indian subinspectors, Azizul Haque and Hem Chandra Bose, in developing the so-called Henry classification, see Singha, 'Settle, Mobilize, Verify'; and Shreenivas and Saradindu Narayan Sinha, 'Personal Identification by the Dermatoglyphic and the E-V Methods', *Patna Journal of Medicine* 31 (1957): 97–108.

38. Henry, *Classification and Uses of Finger Prints*, pp. 6–7. Since the introduction of the technique, Henry claimed in his annual report for 1896, 'Cases have been instituted in twenty districts for false personation and convictions obtained in twenty-five cases, in which sentences varying from seven years to six months have been inflicted.' See E.R. Henry, *Report on the Administration of the Police of the Lower Provinces, Bengal Presidency for the year 1896*, British Library, Asia, Pacific and African Collections V/24/3202.

39. Henry, *Classification and Uses of Finger Prints*, p. 7.

40. Henry, *Classification and Uses of Finger Prints*, p. 8. Recruiters of indentured labourers (that is, those agreeing to serve abroad for a fixed number of years, usually in plantations in far-flung parts of the British empire from the British Caribbean to Natal) frequently resorted to ruses to entice illiterate villagers into signing such bonds. Fraudulent contracts were common and so were repudiations of contract by labourers who discovered too late the falsity of the stories of untold riches and wonderful lives in foreign climes. On the history of indentured labour, see Hugh Tinker, *A New System of Slavery: The Export of Indian Labour Overseas* (London: Oxford University Press, 1974) and Madhavi Kale, *Fragments of Empire: Capital, Slavery and Indian Indentured Labor Migration in the British Caribbean* (Philadelphia: University of Pennsylvania Press, 1998).

41. Henry, *Classification and Uses of Finger Prints*, p. 8.

42. Henry, *Classification and Uses of Finger Prints*, pp. 7–8.

43. See Pearson, *Life, Letters and Labours of Francis Galton*, 3A, pp. 156–7.

44. On the relationship between mesmerism and hypnotism, see Alison Winter, *Mesmerized: Powers of Mind in Victorian Britain* (Chicago: University of Chicago Press, 1997), pp. 184–5.

45. There is a vast literature on the general history of mesmerism. For comprehensive overviews, see Henri F. Ellenberger, *The Discovery of the Unconscious: The History and Evolution of Dynamic Psychiatry* (New York: Basic Books, 1970), esp. pp. 53–109; and Alan Gauld, *A History of Hypnotism* (Cambridge: Cambridge University Press, 1992). Winter's *Mesmerized* is the most comprehensive study of mesmerism in Victorian Britain, but see also Roy Porter, 'Under the Influence: Mesmerism in England', *History Today* 35 (September 1985): 22–9; and Fred Kaplan, '"The Mesmeric Mania": The Early Victorians and Animal Magnetism', *Journal of the History of Ideas* 35 (1974): 691–702.

46. On Elliotson, see Elizabeth S. Ridgway, 'John Elliotson (1791–1868): A Bitter Enemy of Legitimate Medicine?', parts 1 and 2, *Journal of Medical Biography* 1 (1993): 191–8; 2 (1994): 1–7.

47. See Winter, *Mesmerized*, p. 42.

48. See A.J. Youngson, *The Scientific Revolution in Victorian Medicine* (London: Croom Helm, 1979), pp. 42–72.

49. Winter argues that ether, the administration of which was by no means as simple then as it was to become later, was endorsed by powerful sections of the medical profession in order to keep mesmerism out of orthodox practice. See Winter, *Mesmerized*, pp. 178–83. For examples of contemporary reports, debates and controversies, see *The Zoist: A Journal of Cerebral Physiology and Mesmerism* 3 (1845–6): 207–16, 380–9, 490–7; *The Zoist: A Journal of Cerebral Physiology and Mesmerism* 4 (1846–7): 1–8.

50. On Esdaile, see Ernst, 'Esdaile, James (1808–1859)'; Ernst, '"Under the Influence" in British India"'; Ernst, 'Colonial Psychiatry, Magic and Religion'; and Winter, *Mesmerized*, pp. 187–212.

51. Esdaile was so keen to establish his complete lack of bias that he sometimes appeared to contradict his own admission that he had grown interested in mesmerism after reading Elliotson's writings on the subject. 'I had never read a Mesmeric book, when I made my first experiment', he claimed at one point, 'and having succeeded in getting nature to speak, I determined to listen only to her for some time ... all that I know about Mesmerism has been acquired by reading the book of nature, without guide or interpreter.' See James Esdaile, *Mesmerism in India and Its Practical Application in Surgery and Medicine* (London: Longman, 1846; reprint, New York: AMS Press, 1976), p. 73.

52. Esdaile, *Mesmerism in India*, p. 35.

53. There is some evidence suggesting that Esdaile had already been practising mesmeric techniques on prisoners and others. For details, see Ernst, 'Esdaile, James (1808–1859)'.

54. Esdaile, *Mesmerism in India*, pp. 44–5.

55. Esdaile, *Mesmerism in India*, pp. 45–6. Later, the patient complained of pain in the sites 'tested' for insensibility and Esdaile declares that he immediately decided never 'to put a patient to the "question" in this way again. It is only excusable for the first time, when we can hardly believe the evidence of our senses'. See Esdaile, *Mesmerism in India*, p. 54. Such 'tests' were also criticized by John Elliotson, but he blamed them not on Esdaile himself but on the unreasonable demands of sceptics. See Elliotson's remark inserted into a report by Esdaile in *The Zoist* 4 (1846–7): 42–3.

56. Although Budden Chunder Chowdaree (Badan Chandra Chowdhury), the Indian sub-assistant surgeon and '*élève* of the Medical College', also signed the statement, his testimony alone, evidently, would not have sufficed. It was *European* endorsement that counted. See Esdaile, *Mesmerism in India*, pp. 43, 45, 48.

57. Esdaile, *Mesmerism in India*, pp. 57–8.

58. See the report in *The Zoist* 4 (1846–7): 21–50, 25. This sentence was omitted from *Mesmerism in India* (see pp. 58–9).

59. A total of seventy-three operations were performed under mesmeric anaesthesia over the first eight months. See Esdaile, 'Mesmeric Facts', in *Mesmerism in India*, pp. xxi–xxiii. On the prevalence of scrotal elephantiasis in Bengal, see *Esdaile, Mesmerism in India*, pp. 227–32.

60. Esdaile, 'Mesmeric Facts', in *Mesmerism in India*, pp. 64–5, 173–88.

61. See *The Zoist* 4 (1846–7): 294–5.

62. Esdaile, *Mesmerism in India*, p. 12.

63. The transfer of mesmeric influence to water was considered to be possible by many mesmerists, but the question was controversial even at the time. For Esdaile's defence of the concept, his procedure, and case reports, see Esdaile, *Mesmerism in India*, pp. 156–65. For a contemporary report that was generally supportive but pointed out that the mesmerized water 'had no effect on a European officer, who ventured to take a large draught of it', see 'Dr Esdaile's Mesmeric Feats', *The Zoist* 3 (1845–6): 386–7.

64. Extracts from the report of this committee were published (with editorial comments from John Elliotson) in *The Zoist* 5 (1847–8): 50–62.

65. See *The Zoist* 5 (1847–8): 62.

66. See Ernst, '"Under the Influence" in British India', pp. 1114, 1116.

67. For a petition to Lord Dalhousie signed by more than 300 'native' gentlemen, see *The Zoist* 6 (1848–9): 119–20.

68. See Winter, *Mesmerized*, pp. 206–10.

69. Although British surgeons did not initially find chemical anaesthetics very easy to use or even particularly dependable, Alison Winter has suggested that they welcomed them because they seemed more 'scientific'

than mesmerism. See Winter, *Mesmerized*, p. 176. Whether one agrees entirely with that argument or not, it cannot be doubted that mesmeric anaesthesia as applied by Esdaile needed considerably more time and manpower than the colonial government was willing to support, especially when a cheaper and apparently more reliable chemical means was available. On this point, see Ernst, '"Under the Influence" in British India', pp. 1117–18.

70. See, for instance, William Kroger's 'Introduction and Supplemental Reports', in James Esdaile, *Hypnosis in Medicine and Surgery* [orig. *Mesmerism in India* (1850)] (New York: Julian Press, 1957), pp. i–xxxvii; and L. Pulos, 'Mesmerism Revisited: The Effectiveness of Esdaile's Techniques in the Production of Deep Hypnosis and Total Body Hypoanesthesia', *American Journal of Clinical Hypnosis* 22, no. 4 (1979–80): 206–11. On the association with magic, see Ernst, 'Colonial Psychiatry, Magic and Religion'.

71. Esdaile, *Mesmerism in India*, p. 27.

72. Esdaile, *Mesmerism in India*, p. 20. For an account of Esdaile's dealings with 'one of the most famous magicians in Bengal', see Esdaile, *Mesmerism in India*, pp. 21–3. Elsewhere, he said that *jar-phoonk* (shamanic treatment(s) to drive out evil spirits) conducted by Indian folk healers was mesmerism pure and simple. See Esdaile, 'Second Half-Yearly Report of the Calcutta Mesmeric Hospital from 1st March to 1st September 1849', *The Zoist* 7 (1848–9): 353–63, 362.

73. Esdaile, *Mesmerism in India*, p. 60.

74. See *The Zoist* 6 (1848–9): 151. Emphases added.

75. When Esdaile returned to Britain, he tried to use mesmerism in medical conditions. In a report sent to *The Zoist*, Esdaile argued that Europeans were most susceptible to mesmerism when ill: 'The depressing influence of disease will be found to reduce Europeans very often to the impressionable condition of the nervous system so common among the Eastern nations' ('Dr Esdaile and Mesmerism in Perth', *The Zoist* 10 [1852–3]: 419–25, 422).

76. Esdaile, *Mesmerism in India*, p. 73.

77. Esdaile, *Mesmerism in India*, pp. 27–8.

78. Esdaile, *Mesmerism in India*, pp. 40–1.

79. Esdaile, *Mesmerism in India*, pp. 59, 264–5.

80. The 'higher mental manifestations' of mesmerism, Esdaile remarked, were eminently deserving of investigation, but that task could only be attempted where there was 'mental sympathy' between the mesmerist and his patient. See Esdaile, *Mesmerism in India*, p. 28.

81. Esdaile, *Mesmerism in India*, p. 248. Emphasis added.

82. Esdaile, *Mesmerism in India*, pp. 14–15. Emphasis added.

83. Esdaile, *Mesmerism in India*, p. 34. Emphasis in the original.

84. For samples of such statements, see Zaheer Babar, *The Science of Empire: Scientific Knowledge, Civilization, and Colonial Rule in India* (Albany: State University of New York Press, 1996), p. 8; Thomas Metcalf, *Ideologies of the Raj* (Cambridge: Cambridge University Press, 1995), p. 29; Winter, *Mesmerized*, p. 173.

3

CONFESSIONS OF THE UNFRIENDLY SPLEEN
Medicine, Violence, and That Mysterious Organ of Colonial India

SUDIPTA SEN

Sometime during the course of the nineteenth century, the spleen emerged as a meeting point for a set of convictions about the relative frailty of the body of poor Indians. A punctuation to this long story is well-documented with the controversy breaking out over the Ilbert Bill during the late nineteenth century—which for a moment threatened Englishmen with the prospect of a few Indian magistrates passing sentences on white Europeans, a provision that was opposed vehemently and ultimately thwarted. It also highlighted some of the more egregious forms of violence visited upon native Indian servants by their colonial masters which either went largely unpunished or produced trials that seemed to make a travesty of the laws of assault, battery, and manslaughter. Lawyers defending British subjects routinely argued that bodies of Indian servants were diseased and weakened and their spleens abnormally engorged, whereby routine physical corrections resulted in unfortunate accidents.[1] Such a view of the bodies of Indian servants and Indians in general, I argue in this chapter, has a long genealogy dating back to legal trials of the eighteenth and early nineteenth centuries concerning the beating and murder of slaves and servants. This has been so ever since coroner's inquests and medical evidence have been used to establish a particular normative view of the native Indian body and organs as afflicted by climate, negligent habits, and narcotic abuse. The spleen in the later nineteenth century became one of the most visible symbols of this historical construction.

This chapter takes up the pathology of splenic dysfunctions that originated in England, but was developed much further as a peculiarly tropical affliction by the medical practitioners of British India. In many instances it reinforced certain deep-seated notions of physical, biological, and racial differences between Europeans and natives, which were also reflected in the use of forensic evidence in criminal trials. It must be made clear that this is not simply an exercise to demonstrate how misguided or unfair the 'spleen defence' might have been in cases where Britons were acquitted of the charges of assaulting or beating servants to death. It would be inadvisable and nearly impossible for the present-day historian to try and determine ex post facto whether or not the medical evidence offered in each case was in good faith or consistent with the accepted medical standards of the day. Nor can we establish with any certitude what kind of role abnormally enlarged spleens might have played in the death of native servants and menials independent of the physical punishment administered to them by their colonial masters.

Irruption of the 'Spleen Theory'

A seemingly innocuous Bengali cartoon in the periodical *Sulabh Samachar* became infamous in the 1870s for raising a spectre of native sedition against the British Raj. In an editorial dated 7 July 1877 under the caption 'Our Spleen', the inexpensive weekly which had a circulation of more than 3,000, condemned the state of justice in British courts of law. It accused Englishmen of getting away with murder in cases where they had beaten native employees to their death, by claiming spurious medical evidence of ruptured spleens of their victims. On 29 December 1877 it followed up this charge with a pointedly sharp cartoon that depicted a European factory owner, labelled Mr Rogue, who had given a blow on the nose of a coolie causing his death.[2] The coolie lay dead with his wife crying over his corpse. An English surgeon, Dr Bribe had been called for a cursory post mortem. The assailant stood indifferently nearby, smoking a nonchalant cigar. It also showed a European judge and a jury made up of white men. The caricature voiced a long-term grievance nursed by many Indians that Europeans had the unquestioned right to assault servants and subordinates, without as much as a reprimand.

Such cartoons caught the eye of the Viceroy Lord Lytton, who made an example of them in pushing through the Vernacular Press Act of 1878 in the space of a single day, intending to clamp down severely on anti-British political opinion. Europeans had long since noticed the calumnies indulged by the native press. A mouthpiece of the European population in Calcutta, the *Englishman*, had expressed with alarm that even the judges of the Calcutta High Court were not above native censure. The *Englishman* saw such attacks as not only indecorous and 'puerile' but very likely 'fraught with incalculable mischief'.[3]

Lytton seems to have agreed. With this one singular provision of the Vernacular Press Act, he sought to muzzle all native journalists writing in their respective vernaculars. In a fiery speech given to the Council on 14 March 1787, he vented:

> Not content with misrepresenting the Government and maligning the character of the ruling race in every possible way and on every possible occasion, these mischievous scribblers have of late been preaching open sedition; and, as shown by some of the passages which have to-day been quoted from their publications, they have begun to inculcate combination on the part of the native subjects of the Empress of India for the avowed purpose of putting an end to the British Raj.[4]

The Lucknow newspaper *Oudh Akhbar*, protested vehemently that the law favoured Europeans against natives, and 'any indulgence to the former in matters of criminal justice which affects both life and property is not a mere indulgence to them, but, on the contrary ... oppression to the natives'.[5] Europeans and natives alike could with ease try and punish a native offender, but the crimes committed by Europeans were difficult to prosecute, because British justice was based on a crude distinction of race. Were the law to recognize no such distinctions, the paper argued, 'no European would have dared to use violence towards natives in every street and thoroughfare'.[6]

At the head of this public controversy was the legal defence adopted by many European residents in India whose servants had been injured or had died from physical beating. This became commonly known as the 'Spleen Theory'. The natives of India suffering chronically from malaria,

Kala Azar (Leishmaniasis), Dum Dum fever and the like, developed
inordinately enlarged spleens that ruptured at the slightest provocation. Frequent cases of Britons acquitted after having been charged with
assault or manslaughter in the death of native servants exacerbated an
already heated controversy that came to a head in 1883. The Ilbert
Bill was originally designed to recognize certain administrative changes
that had taken place since the 1870s. It proposed that first-class magistrates, session judges, and justices of peace in parts of the Indian interior
provinces (generally known as the *mofussil*) should be given permission
to try the class of people known as the 'European British Subjects'.
Until this time, only the High Courts of Bombay, Madras, and Calcutta
had exercised such authority, and most magistrates, session judges, or
the justice of the peace were of European extraction. However, the
ruckus over the new bill made it evident that there was indeed a small
number of qualified Indian judges in the country, who might now be
in a position to try Europeans and inflict sentences ranging from a fine
to imprisonment. This very possibility created a tumultuous outrage,
stoking racial fears among many British residents.

Even as the bill was being presented by the liberal Viceroy Lord
Ripon, successor to Lytton, a huge controversy had erupted in the
print media.[7] Opinion was squarely divided among the men who ruled
India. The measure had been endorsed in principle by stalwarts such
as Barrow Herbert Ellis, Sir Richard Temple, and the Commander in
Chief, Lord Napier. On the opposite side of the debate was the conservative Fitzjames Stephen, who defended the right of Europeans, based
on English personal law, not to be tried by natives. Ripon was worried
about the growing incidence of lawlessness from an increased presence
of young European freebooters and vagrants in India, who often flouted
the law in their dealings with natives.[8] The bill infuriated the European
community, especially in Calcutta, who came together as a body to
denounce and reject the measure. Aptly labelled as the 'White Mutiny'
of 1883, the widespread disturbance was based on the contention that
Indians belonged to an inferior race and were, therefore, incapable
of discerning what constituted 'misbehaviour' among people of the
European race. As the act took effect, and there was news of an Indian
magistrate sending an Englishman to prison for assaulting a native, the
English in Calcutta, in the words of a contemporary observer, acted
as if the 'foundation of the world were broken up'.[9] During the years

1883–5, the public outrage vented in Calcutta over the indictment of R.A. Fuller for beating a servant made it plainly evident that the Europeans of British-India were never going to accept the affront of being tried by an Indian judge or magistrate in any court of law.

Racialized Law

R.A. Fuller, a lawyer no less, had beaten the groom of his stable, Katwaroo, to death. The facts of the case are as follows. Mr Fuller, an English pleader at Agra, was about to drive to Church with his family on a Sunday. When his carriage was brought to the door, the groom was not in attendance. Mr Fuller struck Katwaroo with his open hand on the head and pulled him by the hair to the ground. As Mr Fuller and his family drove to Church, Katwaroo got up and went into an adjoining compound where he died immediately.

Mr Fuller appeared before the joint magistrate of Agra, R.J. Leeds, charged with an indictment under section 323 of the Indian Penal Code for 'causing hurt' to Katwaroo. It appeared from the testimony of the medical officer who had conducted the post mortem that the groom had expired from a rupture of the spleen. The spleen of the victim had been so morbidly enlarged that even a slight blow or a fall would have been sufficient to cause fatal damage.[10] The evidence did not show any other assault. Mr Fuller was found guilty of 'voluntarily causing what distinctly amounts to hurt', and sentenced to pay a fine of Rs 30, or undergo fifteen days of confinement.

There was some doubt as to the degree by which the spleen had been distended so that even a 'moderate' amount of force would lead to death. Witnesses testified that Fuller had not slapped Katwaroo but had indeed kicked him in the stomach. But Joint Magistrate Leeds asserted: 'It is prima facie improbable that a European would kick his servant in the stomach.'[11] Britons were as a race, moderate and restrained, he reasoned. Delinquency and unpunctuality had provoked the action. At this point, Governor General Lord Lytton famously intervened with a special minute suggesting that the government should come to the aid of poor native servants abused by their European masters. Expressing his abhorrence of such beatings, Lytton wanted European masters not to treat 'their native servants in a manner in which they would not treat men of their own race'.[12] However, Lytton did acknowledge the peculiar physical condition of the native inhabitants of India. Britons should know better than to heap abuses on Asiatics, he argued, who were 'subject to internal disease which often renders fatal to life even a slight external shock'.[13] The Fuller case saw much attention devoted to medical evidence on the exact cause of death. Katwaroo had clearly died from a ruptured spleen. The magistrate did not believe the eyewitness reports of the deceased being kicked in the stomach. The defence had argued that no offence had been committed 'as the law authorized a master to inflict moderate chastisement on his servant'.[14]

The Fuller incident drew the ire of the vernacular press, most of all in Bengal. The Bengali middle-class intelligentsia defied the fear of sedition and began to vent their outrage at the blatant racial discrimination in the courts of law. A typical satirical piece penned incognito under the pseudonym 'Aprakash Gupta' ('unpublished and hidden') by the printer, journalist, and children's author Upendrakishore Raychaudhuri ran as a letter to the editor of a local Bengali periodical titled 'Spleen-Protector':

> In our country everybody has an enlarged spleen. The spleens of Indians burst at the first punch or a kick from white sahibs. Our deaths are of course no great loss, but it is indeed regrettable that sahibs have to go and stand witness at the courts, spend money on lawyers, sometimes even subject themselves to imprisonment and fines. Thus we have devised a broad steel belt called a 'spleen-protector' that can be easily worn by natives; it is also fitted with sharp spikes. With this on, the spleen can withstand kicks from the sturdiest English boot. It is cheap. As an experiment we let a coolie wear this 'spleen-protector'. You can see the results in the photograph above. From now on if sahibs just buy our spleen-protectors for each of their coolies, laborers and servants, they would be able to use their hands and feet on them freely and without worry. We are also developing a similar 'spleen-protector' for the head. This is because we are now hearing from European physiologists that natives do not really have brains inside their skulls, only spleen. This is why even when we are injured in the head, our spleens rupture.[15]

Such outrage, the likes of which led to widespread censorship of Indian public opinion in subsequent years, not only indicates the rise of seditious literati stung by the biological affront of racial inequality, but also, more pertinently for this paper, the bodies of the governing and the governed as overtly racialized caricature. Not just in the native editorials, mockeries and jibes were also flying in the Anglo-Indian press in northern India. The 1884 *Oudh Punch* gave a voice to the ultimate victim of this entire travesty of justice, the spleen itself:

> The spleen complains that it has a very deadly foe in the fist of rampant Anglo-Saxons, and no system of medicine, English or native, can prescribe anything which may make it strong enough to stand the blows of its adversary. ... Under these circumstances, spleen earnestly prays that it may not be placed in the bodies of natives, where its fate is sealed.[16]

The *Behar Herald*, a prominent weekly, advertised the Ilbert Bill as 'a new and installable remedy for chronic enlargement of the spleen'.[17] These and many other examples attest that the organ itself had indeed become a figure of speech for the infirmity of servile native bodies.

The English Malady

Knowledge of the human spleen had been associated since antiquity with Greek medicine, especially Galen, who described it as the *mysterii pleni organon*—an organ full of mysteries—which ultimately served to balance impurities of the liver.[18] The spleen was the refuge of emotions and passions, and the source of laughter, happiness, and delight. It was also responsible for attacks of anger, ill-temper and malice, and sudden impulses. It was the organ that controlled pride, courage, and impetus, and yet at the same instance, was the hidden seat of evil and disrespect. The function of the spleen was to remove melancholia, along with aiding purification of blood and digestion. The classical image of the spleen was tied to the humeral system of the Hippocratic Corpus, refined through the disquisition of Aristotle, who postulated that the live human body was a microcosm essentially governed through the four main elemental organs: heart, brain, liver, and spleen.[19] The spleen was associated with black bile and the earth, and was supposed to draw the watery part of the food from the stomach, just as the gall bladder drew bile from the liver. In *De Partibus Animaliam*, Aristotle argued that the spleen helps concoct nutrients by its heat, withdrawing superfluous humour from the stomach.[20] During the latter half of the seventeenth century, following the widespread reception of William Harvey's systemic study of the circulation of blood, followed by Marcello Malpighi's findings of the capillary structure of organs under prototypes of the microscope, the importance given to the study of blood as the vital and corruptible element in the human body raised the importance of the spleen as

an organ.[21] In the old Galenic scheme of the human body, it was held
that the useless bits of all that the body ingested was ultimately con-
verted into black bile,[22] essential to the metabolism that tied what the
Greeks had described as πνεῦμα or 'air in motion' to the movement
of human blood.[23] This view of the function of the spleen persisted
for many subsequent centuries. The spleen, it was believed, attracted
through its large vein the viscous and muddy juices generated by the
liver, which was excreted into the stomach without much change.[24]

Harvey's anatomical findings about the circulation of blood and the
pneumatic function of the heart did not entirely dispel the Galenic
theory of the ebb and flow of bodily humours, and the bilious attributes of splenetic blood remained a staple in medical discourse.[25]
Nathaniel Highmore, for instance, who made one of the first detailed
anatomical studies of the spleen, and wrote about splenic capsules, was
in fact convinced that the bilious excretions from the spleen disgorged
into the stomach were the true cause of melancholia. This became a
generally accepted view of the common disorders caused by the spleen
and its humours.

The spleen was considered to be one of the primary organs
responsible for particular bodily and mental states, including anxiety,
depression, exhaustion, digestive disorders, nervous spasm, and the
like. It was also seen as vulnerable to inclement vapours that caused
hysteria in women and hypochondria in men. Hypochondria could
drain men forever of their vital powers, leading to debilitating bouts of
enervation.[26] In the seventeenth-century moods, humours and organs
were the subject of both literary and medical texts. Thus, Burton in his
celebrated tract *The Anatomy of Melancholy* (1621) explained in detail
the third form of the disease, 'hypochondriacal or windy melancholy'
derived from the liver, spleen, or internal membranes.[27] In fact the word
'spleen' itself became another name for what was typically known as
the 'English malady', a bundle of ills caused by a host of factors, both
climatic and habitual: moist air, variability of weather, rankness and
fertility of soil, richness and heaviness of food, and even wealth and
abundance from trade and commerce. Such causes and symptoms were
popularized in the seventeenth century by George Cheyne, who also
suggested that melancholia was the classic affliction of the city dweller.
The inactivity and sedentary nature of the 'better sort', along with the
sordid humours of living in crowded and unhealthy towns, brought

upon these 'atrocious and frightful symptoms' of distemper, previously unknown to the English country gentlemen of yore.[28] Overcrowding and squalor were now viewed as significant factors in the causes of death in London. Ever since the publication of John Graunt's *Natural and Political Observations Made on the Bills of Mortality* in 1662, followed by William Petty's *Observations on the Dublin Bill Mortality* in 1682, the correlation between disease and mortality patterns along with the cyclical nature of epidemics had become a subject of the bold new science of political arithmetic. These numerical tables helped tabulate variations in mortality rates by season, year, and stage of life.[29] Graunt commented specifically on the growth of the city of London and its impact on mortality figures.[30] He also grouped splenetic disorders with liver-grown and rickets. During the eighteenth century, deaths occasioned simply by 'spleen' or 'spleen and vapours' appeared routinely in these bills of mortality.[31]

Epic poet and court physician Richard Blackmore in 1725 wrote an influential tract on the spleen, insisting that natives of the British Isles owing to their peculiar constitution and habit of indulging in copious amounts of flesh and malt liquors, and their susceptibility to coughs, catarrh, and consumption developed over time a set of hypochondriac and hysteric affections commonly called splenetic vapours, which were chronic distempers affecting the mind and body in unison.[32] Afflictions of the lungs and spleen were thus rampant, causing chronic fevers. Such causes and symptoms taken together constituted the state known as the 'English Spleen'. Blackmore held that diseases of the spleen were in fact even more fatal among inhabitants of warmer climates, where it not only caused disorders of the temper, but ultimately lunacy and death. In England the spleen was the Achilles heel of the otherwise robust English constitution nurtured by a colder and more temperate climate. However, Blackmore suggested that it was not the splenetic serums that caused these maladies, but glands and fibres affected by the obstruction of small vessels. Shivers and distempers were a result of nerves excited by pestilential damp and deadly exhalations.[33]

The true functions of the spleen and its relationship to moods and humours were debated ad infinitum throughout the course of the eighteenth century. Many doubted whether the organ was vital to the human body and actually drank up the dregs and lees in the blood.

Blackmore mused that if the spleen was 'continually receiving, and not discharging such a black and foul sediment' then it was bound to 'swell to an immense size, in bodies so ever it is found'.[34] Till now the spleen had been viewed as a scavenger of nature that drained the thick parts of blood, much like a cistern or a sink, and when dissection revealed an inflamed spleen, the cause was unfailingly attributed to 'blood as the author of all the evil'.[35] Blackmore challenged this idea and pioneered the contention that these were ultimately disorders of the nerves related to irregularities of the spirit and the 'nervous juices', not the fault of the spleen by itself.[36] Distempers of hypochondria in men were caused by nerves that connected the spleen and the brain, which rendered them 'meager, thin and un-muscular', bearing a pale, livid, and saturnine complexion, and also a 'dark, suspicious and severe aspect'.[37] Such a condition not only made it difficult for patients to breathe, it also affected the mind and disturbed the 'superior commanding powers'.[38] Susceptible to tumours and excrescence, the spleen was neither useful nor necessary, and could easily be removed without vital consequences.[39]

John Midriff, a contemporary of Cheyne and Blackmore, tried to connect such nervous disorders not just to distress, but external causes, which he termed as the 'melancholy circumstances of the times'.[40] They affected businessmen engaged in the financial market, for example, those who had suffered grievous losses during the fall of the South Sea Bubble and other stocks. Capitalism had been unkind on the English gentlemanly corpus already touched with the spleen, and if medicine offered little remedy for its suffering during booms and busts of the market, it could at least seek the comfort of liniments applied to the abdomen.[41] Other observers of medicine such as William Stukeley argued that the spleen had an adverse effect on the digestive systems of sensitive men, causing chronic melancholy distempers that especially afflicted scholars and poets.[42] Stukeley railed against the lifestyle and luxuries of the English upper classes who had abandoned healthy country living, prescribing exercise, open air, and conversation.[43]

The eighteenth-century English spleen was thus already a much maligned and disputed organ, a site of convergence for conflicting views of humeral and anatomical details of the human viscera. Towards the closing decades of the century, however, nerves, along with arteries and veins, were emerging in medical discourse as much more pertinent to dysfunctions of the spleen. Robert Whytt, for instance, argued that these were not just results of the obstructions of the liver, spleen or mesentery, but a condition of the nerves.[44] Despite such dissenting opinion, the customary notion that climate, habits, and society had a fundamental impact on the spleen and its relation to the condition of both the mind and body persisted.

During the eighteenth century most people in England and Britain still believed that fevers and chills were caused by morbific matter blocking the circulation of blood.[45] The conventional term for such visitations was 'ague', derived from the Medieval Latin *febris acuta* and applied to all quakes marked by paroxysm and sweating incurring at regular intervals. Agues were known to be brought upon by airs and seasons, caused by diseases that were not identified at the time, including typhus, malaria, and influenza.[46] Physics were of the opinion that intermittent and continual fevers were caused by different kinds of ague that required different treatments: cure of salt draughts, laxatives, or the administration of nitrates. Common remedies and practices dating back to the medieval period abounded in the countryside: from poultices of hops and bay salt, to the use of charms, amulets, and a host of chirurgical practices. It was commonly believed that one could rid agues by transferring them to both animate and inanimate objects.[47] Items including horseshoes placed under the bed of the sick were nailed to trees. Halters taken from the bodies of executed highwaymen were known to drive agues away. Many of these were clearly associated with the practice of witchcraft.

The ingenuity of such remedies notwithstanding, agues continued to be seen as closely related to melancholy humours and obstructions of the spleen. Repeated agues were seen to have resulted in enlarged spleens, known popularly as 'ague cakes'.[48] These would later be associated with chronic malaria resulting in a condition known as 'cachexia', indicating a state of complete and fatal enervation. Thomas Sydenham in his *Medical Observations* (1676) recorded the incidence of distended bellies of children affected by the autumnal agues around the spleen.[49] The distention of spleens as a symptom of agues and fevers was thus a well-established fact in the medical annals of England and Britain during the age of mercantilism and imperial exploration, and not merely a figment of tropical origin. It is likely that generations of sailors, soldiers, and fortune-hunters travelling across the Atlantic brought the English spleen to the tropics.

Tropical Spleen

It is necessary to clarify here that the enlargement of the human spleen (splenomegaly) is known as a medical condition in response to certain kinds of adaptive physiological functions such as phagocytosis of abnormal red cells or antibody production. Fibrous and chronically distended spleens are often found in cases of hemolytic diseases such as recurrent malaria. 'Tropical splenomegaly' is still current as a medical term, which indicates the enlargement of spleens from malaria, leichmaniasis, schistosomiasis, lymphoma, and many other disorders.[50] During the late nineteenth century, when the effect of fevers on the spleen became a subject of acute debate, malaria ravaged parts of Bengal with unprecedented severity. In the 1870s it was estimated that 75 per cent of certain villages in eastern Bengal were affected with malaria, and in certain places it wiped out a quarter of the population.[51] The causes for such eruptions are many and subject to debate.[52] However, it is possible that a large number of Bengalis may very well have developed distended spleens, lending further credence to the endemic, tropical location of the disease. However, during the eighteenth century, the pathogenic vectors such as plasmodia that we readily isolate today in the laboratory were not known, and thus not pertinent to observation or diagnosis. The dread of exotic fevers and its effect on the European spleen long preceded and thus compounded the fear of the malarial parasite.

There was a renewed effort to understand and prepare for fatal diseases known to seafarers and travellers during the second half of the eighteenth century. James Lind, who served as a naval surgeon on the coast of Guinea, and lived to write about his experiences, became a household name, and his *Diseases of Hot Climates* went through five editions between the years 1768 and 1808. Lind revived the notion that fevers in tropical climate were caused by noxious vapours released from marshes and moist soil. Lind recounted a number of symptoms for tropical afflictions incidental to Europeans: loss of complexion, indigestion and weakness of the stomach, enfeebled constitution, frequent fits of colic, or hardness of the spleen, liver, and the bowels.[53] He warned against the dangers of sudden exposure to the temperate climate of England to those returning from the tropics suffering from hardness of the liver, spleen, or abdomen. The coast of Bengal, Lind observed, was one of the places 'most fatal to Europeans' where the English had set up factories.[54] During the rainy season, large parts of the country were inundated with the waters of the Ganges, and the resulting slime and mud emitted noxious vapours heated by the sun. Europeans who had scarcely arrived succumbed most to the diseases that appeared after the rains, particularly distempers that were remittent and intermittent, accompanied by 'violent rigors' and flux of the bile.[55]

Alan Bewell has suggested that during these years there was rapid advance in the study of climate, natural history, and the distribution of plants and animals across the globe, and this shaped the idea of a new geography of medicine.[56] Differences in latitude and climate, in a fashion reminiscent of Montesquieu, became the determinant conditions for the incidence of disease and death. These factors created a heightened awareness of the fragility of European constitutions in proximity to foreign bodies and substances, to new plants and animals, and new natural environments such as marshes and jungles.[57] As John Leyden, an assistant surgeon in the East India Company's service, who later served as a judge in Madras observed: 'It is not every constitution that can resist the combined attack of liver, spleen, bloody flux and jungle fever, which is very much akin to the plague of Egypt, and yellow fever of America.'[58] Unfamiliarity, distance, heat, and humidity contrived to lay the basis of what became a paradigmatic medical topography of the tropics.[59] The entire East Indies as a geographical territory became associated with certain forms of disease and degeneration. Dutch medical accounts from Batavia circulated in India during the eighteenth century offered comparative notes on a wide set of symptoms for the effects of latitude and climate on unsuspecting bodies. One such text was the *Account of the Diseases, Natural History, and Medicines of the East Indies* (1769), translated from the original Latin of James Bontius, who served as a physician to the Dutch settlement at Batavia. Bontius led a detailed enquiry into epidemic and pestilential diseases that ravage the East Indies, arguing that fever and delirium tremens were caused principally by a 'thick, viscid, pituitous humor' that seized the nerves at night.[60] Native bodies manifested these humours differently. Not only their bodies, but their very habits were indicative of the joint afflictions of miasma and vapour inducing languor, listlessness, and a propensity towards alcohol, all of which affected their organs over time. Dissection of native bodies that had been consumed with the cholera morbus showed that their internal organs had been wasted by 'rioting morbific matter'.[61] Native intestines and mesentery in the Indonesian archipelago, Bontius argued, were even more diseased than their livers weakened by the consumption of the destructive indigenous arrack. As the Javanese drank water after the consumption of alcohol, they received into their bodies the noxious vapours arising from the earth. A diseased native liver was not just a sign of the excessive consumption of inferior alcohol, but humour and air that weakened its foundations and made it vulnerable to obstruction.[62]

Bontius's conviction that diseases of the tropical East were a result of the convergence of internal and external factors provided a new and succinct explanation of symptoms and causes, etiology, and pathology in places like British India. When Bontius argued that the 'fevers of India' were both symptomatic and continual and a result of putrefaction of vital humours, he casually replaced the word Indies with India. Native bodies of India, much like those in the Far East, were repositories of symptoms, visible reminders of the combined effects of heat, humidity, fevers, and weakened internal organs:

> It is common for people in this country to waste in their flesh, and grow lean without any manifest cause; no fever, or at most a very slow one attending. There is no considerable pain; only a little weight is felt about the navel and hypochondria. This disorder, besides an obstruction in the bowels, has often for its cause some latent fault in the meseraic veins, or the substance of the mesentery, where abscesses frequently are formed, as I have more than once observed upon dissection. ... Thus reduced to the last degree of extenuation, the native heat being entirely extinguished, the miserable mortals die.[63]

Eighteenth-century accounts available from coastal settlements, garrisons and forts in India reveal a similar conflation of humours and anatomy during this period. Curtis's *Digest* (1807) of diseases from India, for instance, that contained detailed evidence collected around Fort St George, Madras, by Dr Paisley, who studied the frequency and violence of spasmodic cholera, asserted that endemic causes and epidemic outbreaks were intimately related.[64]

Dissecting the Spleen

During the era of the territorial expansion of the East India Company's state in India, when garrisons and cantonments were proliferating in the countryside, military surgeons began to arrive in much greater numbers. During this period, post mortem dissection or 'morbid anatomy', as it was commonly called, became a widespread tool in the search for the causes of the deadly Indian diseases. Military surgeons were among the first medical men who had an extensive opportunity to study the anatomy and internal organs of natives and Europeans side by side. They had the unique and extensive opportunity to test clinical observations through a plethora of fresh corpses.[65] James Annesley, who rose through the ranks in the Madras European Regiment during the first decades of the eighteenth century and served in the field and city hospitals for more than two decades, observed in his much-cited *Researches* that army physicians and surgeons stationed in India acquired an unique opportunity to study both Europeans and natives suffering from the same diseases. They had the means of 'advancing our knowledge of diseases' because they had more or less complete control over their patients, especially natives, and they had the power to conduct post mortem examinations freely.[66] Morbid anatomy, one might argue, led to a vigorous focus on the most visible organs. Cadavers arriving from the ravages of pestilence and famine were plentiful, and native stomachs, livers, mesenteries, and spleens were subjected to this new, invasive scrutiny. This flurry of anatomical observations, displaced, superseded, or simply absorbed older theories of vapour and humour. In Bengal, in particular, where the fear of malaria was the greatest, dissection rejuvenated a lively discourse about climate, miasma, and their visible effects on the vascular structure of the spleen.

Annesley himself conducted extensive investigations into malaria, and his dissections revealed that both livers and spleens in India were affected by habitual exposure to the disease.[67] While he was convinced that climate, heat, effluvium, and constant exposure to noxious miasma produced different kinds of fevers, such factors had a combined effect on the human body and its internal organs including the stomach, liver, and the spleen.[68] These diseases not only enervated the body but also produced in many Europeans exposed to marshy, nocturnal, exhalations certain 'depressing passions of the mind'.[69] Annesley observed in his dissections that fevers, remittent, intermittent, and malignant, resulted in tenderness and tumefaction of the epigastric and hypochondriac regions of the liver.[70] Over time, these conditions also affected the spleens of Europeans till they became habitually diseased. Native spleens in these parts were typically enlarged and sensitive as a result of fevers occurring in 'low, marshy, or thickly wooded situations'.[71] Residents of Bengal in the lower delta, who had come from elsewhere, especially from more elevated altitudes and salubrious climates, developed characteristically vulnerable spleens.

Military and civil surgeons became increasingly obsessed with the spleens of natives. This interest burgeoned after the publication of William Twining's landmark treatise, *Observations on Diseases of the Spleen, Particularly on the Vascular Engorgement of That Organ Common in Bengal* (Calcutta, 1828). Twining, a surgeon attached to the Calcutta Hospital, drawing upon records produced by his predecessors William Russel and John Turner, chief medical officers, concluded that enlarged spleens were a highly visible result of the frequent outbreak of fevers in India, especially in the deltaic regions of Bengal. In a much quoted and discussed passage, he shared with his readers the gist of his copious record of the various states of engorgement of the native organ:

> The tumefaction of the spleen occasionally comes on very suddenly, in the course of remittent fevers, in Bengal; and in a few days the enlargement can be seen as well as felt, extending far below the cartilages of the left false ribs. The degree of enlargement which takes place is variable; it is very common to see the spleen extending downwards on a level with the umbilicus; and laterally, from its usual situation, as far as half way between the cartilages of the ribs and navel. In extreme cases the diseased spleen fills more than half the belly, extending to the right of the navel, while its lower extremity reaches the left iliac region. Several cases of this enormous tumefaction may be seen every year in Calcutta; and some of them recover.[72]

Ultimately, the enlargement of the spleen was related to the climatic and miasmal character of the lower Ganges delta. The humidity and heat contributed to these alarming tendencies:

> The progress of vascular engorgement of the spleen is more or less rapid, according to the injury which the constitution may have suffered from damp climate, and the nature and duration of the fevers which the patient may have recently suffered.[73]

Twining further observed that enlarged spleens had become endemic to the native constitution, most visible in children suffering from diseases and debility. I quote this passage at length to demonstrate the complex logic behind his observation:

> Enlargement of the spleen sometimes appears as an idiopathic disease in children, and in persons of delicate and feeble constitution; and is produced by the combined influence of a damp climate, variable temperature, want of exercise, unsuitable clothing, and insufficient nourishment. During the slow and silent influence of long-continued grief and distress of mind, the secretions generally appear to be perverted, the cutaneous circulation becomes languid, healthy transpiration obstructed, and then we often find enlargement of the spleen take place in Bengal. The disease when dependent on such causes is always difficult to cure. The most part of the cases of vascular engorgement of the spleen in this country follow intermittent and remittent fevers: and tumid spleen, may be stated as the most invariable consequence of acute and debilitating diseases among children of weak constitutions in Bengal. The same sort of enlargement takes place here in the spleen of adults, in consequence of various debilitating diseases.[74]

Twining went on to argue that the internal organs of the body were affected by frequent congestive fevers because of the 'low and damp situations' in tropical regions, in the delta of great rivers, and in the marshy foothills. Lack of drainage and imperfect ventilation were all contributing factors.[75] Certain peculiar symptoms present in native constitutions were actually long-term responses to such a pestilent environment. However, native bodies remained very susceptible to splenetic afflictions, which often developed without any palpable enlargement or sensitivity of the spleen.

Twining's findings became a standard for surgeons and physicians interested in tropical diseases. Their popularity underscores the fact that an etiological explanation for the weakness and malady of the native body had already taken hold of the medical and forensic discourse during the first part of the nineteenth century, empirically verified by the tumescent spleen that routinely appeared in anatomical dissection. An enlarged spleen was not a condition in itself, but a symptom of a much more pervasive Indian malady. In his lengthy compendium, *Clinical Illustrations of the More Important Diseases of Bengal* (1832) Twining argued that while dissection did provide a unique opportunity to observe the state of internal organs among natives, it was only a partial view. In the early visitation of the disease, which often proved fatal at a much later stage, the 'actual disorganization' bore 'no resemblance to the condition of the same organs at an earlier period of the disease'.[76] This is a striking observation, because it shows that he was looking for symptoms of malaria in natives who had died from other diseases. Twining thought that post mortem observations in some sense could be misleading:

> We must not forget that morbid anatomy only affords useful informa-
> tion, when the appearances observed, are compared with the symptoms
> which formerly existed; as the actual morbid condition during life,
> and even that condition which had been chiefly instrumental in the
> destruction of life; is often evanescent, so that we find but slight traces
> of it on dissection.[77]

By the middle of the nineteenth century, there were many eager ama-
teur enthusiasts of the Indian spleen waiting to get their hands on suitable native patients with the endemic trait. Alexander Carnegie, a tea planter's assistant in Assam, experimented in 1866 with hundreds of coolies in his charge, proving that they all had terrific spleens. Much of his prescriptions, however, proved to be more fatal than the disease itself.[78]

There is much more to be said about the genesis of the late nineteenth-
century spleen theory, especially the clinical verification of a racially qualified physical attribute, straddling the notional divide between ide-
ology and pathology. In the last instance, this idea of a weakened spleen and of weakened organs in general would become part of an established view, not only among Europeans but also among the educated natives of India. However, while the idea of the vulnerable spleen did emerge through the early anatomical pursuits of colonial medicine, the assertion that the bodies of poor natives in India were invariably feeble and ailing, also gained much currency through the use of forensic evi-
dence in trials conducted by the early colonial courts of law in British India. The remaining section of this chapter will explore the admission and use of medical evidence in the Supreme Court of Judicature, established in Calcutta in 1774 to underline a few important and related points. The idea that the bodies of natives, especially native servants, were repositories of weak components, vulnerable to miasmal

degeneration and tropical intrusion, was an old and established medical opinion by the second half of the nineteenth century. These ideas had been disseminated through the work of medical topographers of the East Indian Company, who began the task of classifying bodies, climates, and diseases of the tropical latitudes.[79] These ideas created an ideal context for a convergence of medical and legal discourses, leading to a forensic differentiation between the bodies of natives and Europeans, and especially between the bodies of masters and servants. Such distinctions further reinforced the characteristic pathology of the Indian spleen, which would be so forcefully brought to public attention in the context of heightened racial antipathies of the British Raj in later nineteenth century.

Correction of Servants

Douglas Haynes has argued in his fine study of the colonial advancement of medicine in the imperial tropical frontier that the drive toward the eradication of pathogens can be related to the fears of a damaged European constitution in exile. Haynes suggests that the persistence of disease often marked the limits of European civilization, and in constructing the tropics as a space afflicted with disease the discourse of medical advancement and hygiene fabricated its own perceptions of danger and triumph.[80] In a similar vein, Nancy Stepan has elucidated how tropical locales and native bodies during the latter half of the nineteenth century became the standard referents of an accepted pathogenic state.[81] In the context of India and the Caribbean, as Mark Harrison has demonstrated, tropical medicine bestowed the tools, practices, and the will for Europeans to overcome the fear of disease and the environment.[82] The rise of the discipline of tropical medicine and its quest for ascendancy over the organic and microbial world, I would argue, were also related intimately to the urge to discipline the bodies of native subjects in many parts of the British empire. There is a long and untold history here of the discrete points at which power and fear converged, illuminating how the views of climate, bodies, and organs were assimilated into an overarching and long-term set of colonial prejudices. There are surely dissonant histories at stake here: sequestration of bodies in ships, hospitals, barracks, and prisons, and changes in the pattern of microbial and viral exposure, but also the intimate histories of clinical observation at close quarters, bringing the English lancet and the microscope in close contact with the skin, organs, tissue, and cells of natives whose bodies came under the direct purview of the colonial medicinal state. The history of the rise of morbid anatomy in the long nineteenth century on this score demands much further scrutiny.

During the early years of the establishment of British rule in India, the class of natives who came most frequently into contact with Britons were native servants. Corporal punishment of servants during this time was an accepted practice in India as it was in England. It is not hard to imagine that the menial denizens of the Indian society, typically inferior in caste status and social hierarchy, were particularly vulnerable to what Britons in India referred to as 'moderate correction'. Soon after its founding in 1774, the judges and juries of the Calcutta Supreme Court had to deal with a number of cases concerning the excessive disciplining of slaves and servants.

William Jones, the doyen of Orientalist scholars and one of the first judges of British India, addressed this very issue during his second charge to the Calcutta Grand Jury delivered on 10 June 1785, highlighting the case of a slave girl in Calcutta beaten to death by her master.[83] Jones argued that a master had the right by law to 'correct' his servant with moderation. If during such correction the servant in question died by accident or 'misfortune unseen' the master in question was not guilty of any crime. However, if such correction was excessive, unreasonable, and cruel, then the servant did have a case for reparation. If the servant in question died during such punishment then the master was liable for charges of manslaughter or murder. It had to be seen, however, whether a fatal blow had indeed been struck in 'a sudden burst of passion', whether there was any 'violent provocation', or whether the weapon used that was likely to kill. The distinction between manslaughter and murder was of fundamental interest to Jones and the jury. A charge of murder could only be admitted if it was proven that there was clear, calculated intention or the 'coolness of blood', and that the assailant had administered an injury directly intended to destroy life and not simply exceeded the limits of moderate chastisement. Murder, Jones reminded the jury, was a charge based on the notion of mens rea, or malice aforethought, based on the 'malignity of heart' or a clear intention to do mischief. This could be ascertained by a careful comparison of the fault with the correction, the 'age and condition of the person stricken', the force of the striker, and the danger posed by the instrument used. In such cases Jones reasoned that servants and slaves stood precisely on the same grounds as would have a medieval serf, 'villain or a knave', vis-à-vis the lord during feudal times.

Jones's address reveals a certain intrinsic ambiguity in the laws relevant to the punishment of servants in an essentially alien context. In a certain respect these views were consistent with the reigning legal opinion of the day expressed succinctly in William Blackstone's legal commentaries, that rights and wrongs of individual legal subjects were both *absolute* and *relative*.[84] Relative rights of individuals were based on four archetypal relations in society: husband and wife, parent and child, guardian and ward, and master and servant. In each of these categories, the superior had the right to punish the inferior. In this particular context, however, not only was Jones wittingly comparing an Indian servant to a feudal slave or a serf, he was also refraining from providing any definition that could establish an accepted measure of 'moderate' physical chastisement of native servants. Moreover, it was not clear what kind of provocation *warranted* such correction. After all, standards of insolence and insubordination were specific to particular societies and periods of human history. Was Jones directly comparing colonial Bengal to feudal Britain? Or was it simply reason by analogy? And most pertinently, how was a jury supposed to determine the 'age and condition' of native servants, especially whether they could withstand the average blow of an Englishman or a prescribed number of strokes from a whip or a cane? This last question becomes even more insistent in the context of the main argument advanced by this chapter, that is, by contemporary medical standards native Indian bodies were established as weak, sickly, and vastly inferior.

Much as they were in England, servants, slaves, and dependents in India were subject to severe physical censure on occasion. There was widespread use of the bamboo rattan and the dreaded native bullwhip, the *korah*. Not only menials and servants, but members of large elite households were flogged and castigated for insubordination. When William Bentinck, the governor general of India passed the resolution (Regulation II, Act of 1834) to abolish the widespread use of flogging as routine punishment, especially in the East India Company's army, he was convinced that while it was an accepted and widespread practice in India, the whip was a barbaric instrument that had no place in a

civilized and enlightening government.[85] In the preamble to the Act of
1834, Bentinck stated that flogging was not efficacious for the actual
prevention of crime; it was degrading, and it affixed marks of infamy,
ultimately robbing a person of an honest livelihood.[86] He reasoned that
flogging, often injudiciously and unnecessarily inflicted, was in the end
a 'grievous and irredeemable wrong':

> It is becoming and expedient that the British Government, as the
> paramount power in India, should present in its own system the
> principles of the most enlightened legislation, and should endeavour, by
> its example, to encourage the Native States to exchange their barbarous
> and cruel punishments, of maiming, of torture, of loss of limb, for
> those of a more merciful and wise character, by which the individual
> may be reformed and the community saved from these brutalizing
> exhibitions.[87]

In contemporary England as well, much like fathers and husbands who
reserved the right to beat their wives and children, masters had the
right to beat servants for misbehaviour and negligence.[88] There seems
to have been a degree of relative impunity in this regard throughout
the Georgian period in England. It is reasonable to assume, therefore,
that during the period of British expansion in India, the beating of
servants was considered routine. However, intrusive forms of control
and discipline were being engrafted on older ones, and this reconfiguration of legitimate punishment was based on new medical rules
of thumb. As charges of immoderate correction against Englishmen
began to appear before the Calcutta Supreme Court, extant laws on
the limits of permissible correction began to be tested. In a number of
cases, European defendants charged with assault or murder were able
to plead that that they did not know the full effect or severity of their
actions on the bodies of native servants, which may have been debili-
tated by disease and insalubrious habits. Such pleas were often supported by the medical testimony of military surgeons who presented
post mortem reports on the morbid anatomy of natives. Legal and
medical evidence converged in such cases, articulating an overarching
forensic view of the weaker and vulnerable Indian body. These cases
help us reconstruct the long-term socio-pathological construction of
native anatomy that would ultimately produce the caricature of the
European boot and native spleen during the Ilbert Bill debates of the
late nineteenth century.

Morbid Anatomy in the Colony

The coroner's inquest became a routine feature of criminal prosecutions in late eighteenth-century British India, especially in cases involving natives against Europeans. During this period dissection had emerged as an advanced tool in the study of human anatomy in western Europe. As Andrew Cunningham has elucidated in great detail, the anatomist was at the forefront of both medical and biological research.[89] Autopsy, which included both vivisection and dissection, along with gross and microscopic anatomy, was an important tool of this new science. Anatomy was also a public spectacle. Anatomical theatres had sprung up in all major European cities, especially London, displaying its fine instruments and the manual dexterity of the surgeons in cutting through slippery remains of human viscera.[90] After 1761 the Padua anatomist Giovanni Battista Morgagni's comprehensive treatise on the *Seats and Causes of Diseases*, based on the observation of pathological changes in cadavers through systematic autopsy, became widely available. Although he believed in the primacy of bodily humours, Morgagni's emphasis on localized pathology, along with Albrecht von Haller's study of muscular and neural fibres detailed in his conspectus *Elementa Physiologiae Corporis Humani* (1755–67), further helped differentiate the function and purpose of vital organs, and encouraged new forms of nosology and etiology.[91] The publication of Thomas Baillie's *Morbid Anatomy* in 1793, with its brilliant copperplate illustrations (including a section on the diseased appearance of the spleen), marked a further step in the graphic illustration of the internal structure and the function of the human body.[92] By the turn of the century, the value of a meticulous pathology of tissues and membranes was reaffirmed in the studies of the Parisian army surgeon Marie Francoise Xavier Bichat, a pioneering scholar of morbid changes. Historians of medicine credit Bichat with having established the objective foundations for the systematic analysis of the effect of disease on the human anatomy. He certainly advanced the notion that diseases are caused by morbid changes taking place in tissues internal to each specific organ that constitute the basic machinery of the human body.[93] In his *Anatomie General* (1822) Bichat classified tissues according to nineteen discernible varieties, which became the subsequent standard: cellular, nervous, arterial, venous, exhalant, absorbent, osseous, medullar, cartilaginous, fibrous, muscular, mucous, and so on.

Following Bichat's findings, as more physicians opened up cadavers for clues, they increasingly began to find that such diseases were not the results of humour or climate, but causes lurking within the very organs and tissues. Bichat's studies of specialized body parts prepared the groundwork for what Foucault would later call the anatomical-clinical gaze, a gaze that transformed the individualistic, experiential, patient-centred medicine of the eighteenth century. Clinical anatomy was reordering the very relationship between death and illness, treating disease not just as residing in symptoms and morbid tissue, but as integral to the living body itself.[94]

Native bodies in early colonial India came under a similar and early regimen in the context of forensic medicine. Surgeons, especially military surgeons in India, had an extraordinary opportunity to explore the new frontiers of morbid anatomy. Such familiarity led to the rising frequency of forensic investigations in the context of criminal trials, where ideas of anatomy, epidemiology, racial characteristics, climate, and the colonial hierarchy of masters and servants converged and shaped certain fundamental dispositions of the law. Under the auspices of the Supreme Court of Judicature, the office of the coroner and the department of inquest became routine in criminal investigations in the 1790s, and both civil and military surgeons were brought in to offer testimonies based on their knowledge of morbid anatomy. In many cases where servants or dependants had been beaten, flogged, or kicked to death, inquiries into the internal injuries and haemorrhage were accompanied with a dissection of the stomach, spleen, and other organs where anatomists searched for traces of opium, marijuana, alcohol, cholera, or malaria in support of the forensic argument that physical castigation was only one cause of death among many.[95] Despite the fact that certain antipathies of race were clearly at work, bolstered by biological certitudes of the later nineteenth century, racial discrimination that we routinely associate with blood or skin does not seem quite enough in explaining this peculiar staging of the surgical expertise and medical knowledge in supporting the legal right of Britons to punish native Indian servants. During the controversy over the fragility of the Indian spleen in the 1880s, discussed at length in this chapter, *both* Britons *and* the educated Indian *literati* were debating the terms of physical subordination of Indian subjects *as servants*. Colonial courtrooms, therefore, in effect reproduced certain deep-seated forms of subordination, recapitulating not only a concise history of the forensic (that is, both medical *and* legal) but also an abiding Orientalist, meta-tropical, and colonial discourse targeting indentured and diseased Indian bodies. The spleen ultimately became its most derisive synecdoche. The archives of this peculiar story can be traced all the way back to the Calcutta Supreme Court of the last decades of the eighteenth century, to the office of the coroner, the department of inquest, the superintendents of police, the testimonials of civil and military surgeons, and to all-European grand and petty juries who sat in judgment of their roguish peers. It is the prehistory of this pervasive colonial fear of disease and insubordination, taken together, that must be exhumed and dissected once again if we are to understand the convoluted history of why the occasional deaths of servants beaten by their white masters were nothing more than unfortunate accidents waiting to happen.

Notes

1. On the history of European violence towards Indian servants, see Jordana Bailkin, 'The Boot and the Spleen: When Was Murder Possible in British India?' *Comparative Studies in Society and History* 48, no. 2 (2006): 462–93.
2. *Sulabh Samachar*, 29 December, 1877.
3. *The Englishman*, 25 July 1876.
4. Lady Betty Balfour, *The History of Lord Lytton's Indian Administration, 1876 to 1880* (Longmans, 1899), pp. 512–13.
5. *The Oudh Akhbar*, 16 May 1877.
6. *The Oudh Akhbar*, 16 May 1877.
7. See Uma Dasgupta, 'Crime, Law and the Police in India, 1870–80', *Indian Economic Social History Review* 10, no. 4 (1973): 333–70.
8. Elizabeth Kolsky, *Colonial Justice in British India: White Violence and the Rule of Law* (Cambridge: Cambridge University Press, 2009), pp. 10–11.
9. Arthur Hobhouse, 'Native Indian Judges', *Contemporary Review* (June 1883), reprinted (London: William Reeves, 1883), p. 18.
10. See Edwin Hirschmann, *The Ilbert Bill Controversy as a Crisis in Imperial Relationships* (PhD diss., University of Wisconsin, Madison, 1980), p. 41.
11. *Government v. R.A. Fuller*, Accounts and Papers of the House of Commons, pp. 8–9. See *Parliamentary Papers* 1877, vol. LXIII.
12. Charles Edward Buckland, *Bengal under the Lieutenant-Governors: Being a Narrative of the Principal Events and Public Measures during Their Periods of Office, from 1854–1898*, vol. 2 (S.K. Lahiri & Co., 1901), pp. 667–71.
13. Buckland, *Bengal under the Lieutenant*-Governors, p. 670.

14. *Government v. R.A. Fuller.*

15. See Upendrakishore Raychaudhri's letter to the editor of *Prabasi*, in *Upendrakishore Samagra* (Kolkata: Dey's Publishing, 2001), p. 901.

16. *The Oudh Punch*, 29 January 1884, quoted at length in Bailkin, 'The Boot and the Spleen': 481.

17. Hirschmann, *The Ilbert Bill Controversy*, p. 263.

18. See Andi Petroianu, 'Historical Aspects of Spleen and Splenic Surgeries', in *The Spleen*, edited by A. Petroianu (Hilversum, the Netherlands: Bentham Science Publishers, 2011), pp. 3–19.

19. E.H. Ackernecht, *A Short History of Medicine*, revised edition (Baltimore: Johns Hopkins University Press, 1982), p. 53.

20. See the notes in W. Ogle, trans., *Aristotle on the Parts of Animals* (Kegan Paul, Trench and Co., 1882), p. 208.

21. Ackernecht, *A Short History of Medicine*, p. 118. Malpighi's studies of human organs under the microscope and his descriptions of the structure of the major human organs were published in the early tracts of the *Philosophical Transactions* of the Royal Society. See Roy Porter, ed., *Cambridge History of Medicine* (Cambridge: Cambridge University Press), p. 140.

22. Lois N. Magner, ed., *A History of Medicine* (New York: Marcel Dekker, 1992), p. 91.

23. Porter, *Cambridge History of Medicine*, p. 139.

24. Henry Gray's introduction in H. Gray, *On the Structure and Use of the Spleen* (J.W. Parker and Son, 1854), p. 4.

25. In fact, Harvey's own study of the heart was to a degree indebted to Galen. See Thomas Wright, *William Harvey: A Life in Circulation* (Oxford and New York: Oxford University Press, 2013), pp. 109–111; Magner, *A History of Medicine*, p. 201.

26. See Lennard J. Davis, *Obsession: A History* (Chicago: University of Chicago Press, 2008), pp. 36–8.

27. Robert Burton, *The Anatomy of Melancholy*, edited by Thomas C. Faulkner, Nicolas K. Kiessling, and Rhonda L. Blair, vol. 1 (Oxford: Oxford University Press, 1989), p. 120.

28. Gorge Cheyne, *The English Malady: Or, A Treatise of Nervous Diseases of All Kinds* (London: Printed for G. Strahan & J. Leake, at Bath, 1734), p. ii.

29. Andres A. Rusnock, *Vital Accounts: Quantifying Health and Population in Eighteenth-Century England and France* (Cambridge: Cambridge University Press, 2009), p. 33.

30. See chapter 9, 'On the Growth of the City' in Graunt, 'Natural and Political Observations', in *Collection of Yearly Bills of Mortality, from 1657 to 1758 Inclusive* (London: A. Miller, 1759), pp. 27–9.

31. *Collection of Yearly Bills of Mortality*, pp. 119–33.

32. Richard Blackmore, *Treatise of the Spleen and Vapours: Or Hypocondriacal and Hysterical Affections, with Three Discourses on the Nature and Cure of the Cholick, Melancholy and Palsies* (London: J. Pemberton, 1726), pp. iii–iv.

33. Blackmore, *Treatise of the Spleen*, p. xii.

34. Blackmore, *Treatise of the* Spleen, p. 6.

35. Blackmore, *Treatise of the* Spleen, p. 183.

36. Blackmore, *Treatise of the* Spleen, pp. 307–9.

37. Blackmore, *Treatise of the* Spleen, p. 15.

38. Blackmore, *Treatise of the* Spleen, p. 24.

39. Blackmore, *Treatise of the Spleen*, p. 53.

40. John Midriff, *Observations on the Spleen and Vapours* (London: J. Roberts, 1721), p. v.

41. Midriff, *Observations on the Spleen and* Vapours, p. 23.

42. David Boyd Haycock and William Stukeley, *Science, Religion and Archaeology in Eighteenth-Century England* (Woolbridge: Boydell, 2002), pp. 68–9.

43. William Stukeley, *Of the Spleen, Its Description and History, Uses and Diseases, Particularly the Vapors, with their Remedy* (London: Printed for the author, 1723), p. 70.

44. Robert Whytt, *Observations on the Nature, Causes, and Cure of those Disorders Which Have Been Commonly Called Nervous, Hypochondriac, or Hysteric* (Edinburgh: Printed for T. Becket and P.A. de Hondt, London, and J. Balfour, Edinburgh, 1765), p. 108.

45. Mary J. Dobson, *Contours of Death and Disease in Early Modern England* (Cambridge: Cambridge University Press, 2002), p. 313.

46. Thomas Short, *A General Chronological History of the Air, Weather, Seasons, Meteors* (London: T. Longman & A. Millar, 1749), p. 250, and Dobson, *Contours of Death and Disease*, pp. 310, 329. See also Charles Creighton, *Epidemics in Britain*, vol. 2, *From the Extinction of Plague to the Present Times* (Cambridge: Cambridge University Press), p. 318. Of particular relevance here is Sir Robert Talbor's classic text, *Pyretologia, A Rational Account of the Cause and Cure of Agues* (London: R. Robinson, 1672).

47. Thomas Joseph Pettigrew, *On Superstitions Connected with the History and Practice of Medicine and Surgery* (London: Churchill, 1844), pp. 79–80, 92

48. Creighton, *Epidemics in Britain*, pp. 318–19.

49. See Thomas Sydenham, *Medical Observations Concerning the History and Cure of Acute Diseases*, in *The Works of Thomas Sydenham*, edited by William Alexander Greenhill (London: Sydenham Society, 1848), p. 91.

50. For reference, see G.V. Gill and N. Beeching, *Lecture Notes: Tropical Medicine* (Hoboken: John Wiley & Sons, 2011), p. 49.

51. Randall M. Packard, *The Making of a Tropical Disease: A Short History of Malaria* (Baltimore: Johns Hopkins University Press, 2010), p. 4.

52. See Ira Klein, 'Development and Death: Reinterpreting Malaria, Economics and Ecology in British India', *Indian Economic and Social History Review* 38, no. 2 (2001): 162.

53. James Lind, *An Essay on Diseases Incidental to Europeans in Hot Climates* (London: T. Becket and P.A. de Hondt, 1768), p. 290.

54. Lind, *An Essay on Diseases Incidental to* Europeans, p. 87.

55. Lind, *An Essay on Diseases Incidental to* Europeans, pp. 88–9.

56. Alan Bewell, *Romanticism and Colonial Disease* (Baltimore: Johns Hopkins University Press, 1999), p. 36.

57. Bewell, *Romanticism and Colonial Disease*, pp. 23–4.

58. See *The Poetical Works of Dr. John Leyden* (London and Edinburgh: W. P. Nimmo, 1875), p. lxxxi.

59. David Arnold, 'Introduction: Tropical Medicine Before Mansion', in *Warm Climates and Western Medicine*, edited by David Arnold (Amsterdam: Rodopi, 2003), p. 9.

60. James Bontius, *An Account of the Diseases, Natural History, and Medicines of the East Indies, Translated from the Latin of James Bontius, Physician to the Dutch Settlement at Batavia* (London: T. Noteman, 1769), p. 1.

61. Bontius, *An Account of the* Diseases, p. 28.

62. Bontius, *An Account of the* Diseases, p. 30.

63. Bontius, *An Account of the* Diseases, p. 48.

64. Charles Curtis, *An Account of the Diseases in India: As They Appeared in the English Fleet, and in the Naval Hospitals at Madras, in 1782 and 1783* (Edinburgh: W. Laing, 1807), pp. 56–7.

65. See Mark Harrison, 'Racial Pathology: Morbid Anatomy in British India', in *The Social History of Health and Medicine in Colonial India*, edited by Biswamoy Pati and Mark Harrison (London: Routledge, 2009), pp. 176–7.

66. James Annesley, *Researches into the Causes, Nature and Treatment of the More Prevalent Diseases of India: And of Warm Climates Generally*, 3rd ed. (London: Longman, Brown, Green and Longmans, 1855), p. 3.

67. Annesley, *Researches into the Causes*, p. 42.

68. Annesley, *Researches into the Causes*, pp. 39–40.

69. Annesley, *Researches into the Causes*, p. 47.

70. Annesley, *Researches into the Causes*, p. 540.

71. Annesley, *Researches into the Causes*, p. 541.

72. William Thomson and William Twining, eds, *A Practical Treatise on the Diseases of the Liver and Biliary Passages* (London: Ed. Barrington & Geo. D. Haswell, 1842), pp. 296–7.

73. William Twining, *Clinical Illustrations of the More Important Diseases of Bengal* (Calcutta: Baptist Mission Press, 1832), pp. 277–8.

74. Twining, *Clinical* Illustrations, p. 297.

75. Twining, *Clinical Illustrations*, p. 297.

76. Twining, *Clinical Illustrations*, p. v.

77. Twining, *Clinical Illustrations*, p. v.

78. Bailkin, 'Boot and the Spleen': 478.

79. Sudipta Sen, *Distant Sovereignty: National Imperialism and the Origins of British India* (London and New York: Routledge, 2002).

80. Douglas Melvin Haynes, *Imperial Medicine: Patrick Manson and the Conquest of Tropical Disease* (Philadelphia: University of Pennsylvania Press, 2001), p. 8.

81. Nancy Leys Stepan, *Picturing Tropical Nature* (Ithaca, New York: Cornell University Press, 2001), pp. 88–94.

82. Mark Harrison, *Disease and the Modern World: 1500 to the Present Day* (Hoboken: Wiley, 2013), p. 87.

83. *The Works of William Jones*, vol. 5 (London: J. Stockdale and J. Walker, 1807), pp. 9–10.

84. William Blackstone, *Commentaries on the Laws of England*, vol. 3, 16th ed. (London: A. Strahan, 1825), p. 138.

85. John Rosselli, *Lord William Bentinck: The Making of a Liberal Imperialist, 1774–1839* (Berkeley: University of California Press, 1974), pp. 320–1.

86. Imperial Legislative Council, India, *Abstract of the Proceedings of the Council of the Governor-General of India, Assembled for the Purpose of Making Laws and Regulations* (Calcutta: Office of the Superintendent of Government Printing, India, 1863–1907), p. 21.

87. Imperial Legislative Council, *Abstract of the Proceedings of the Council of the Governor-General*. See the discussion of the 'Whipping Bill', 17 February 1864.

88. Men in England had the right to subject women, children, and servants to moderate correction in direct proportion to the aggravation caused, as long as beatings did not draw blood and the instrument by which it was administered was not thicker than a man's thumb (hence the expression 'rule of the thumb'). See Anthony Fletcher, *Gender, Sex and Subordination in England, 1500–1800* (New Haven: Yale University Press, 1995), pp. 192–3.

89. Andrew Cunningham, *The Anatomist Anatomis'd: An Experimental Discipline in Enlightenment Europe* (Farnham, Surrey, England; Burlington, VT: Ashgate, 2010), p. 19.

90. Cunningham, *Anatomist Anatomis'd*, p. 41.

91. Magner, *A History of Medicine*, p. 227.

92. Mathew Baillie, *The Morbid Anatomy of Some of the Most Important Parts of the Human Body* (Walpole, N.H., printed by G.W. Nichols, for W. Fessenden, Bookseller, Brattleborough, Vermont, 1808), pp. 155–6.

93. See Mary Ann G. Cutter, *Reframing Disease Contextually* (Boston: Kluwer Academic Publishers, 2004), p. 42.

94. Foucault develops this argument much more systematically in *The Birth of the Clinic* (New York: Routledge, 2003), pp. 177–9. See also Harrison, *Disease and the Modern World*, p. 57.

95. See, for example, the testimony of surgeon John Fleming in *King v. Humphrey Stuart Gordon* for the flogging death of Mansa in Rani Talau, Bihar, 16 June 1785. See also the testimony of Thomas Casement, assistant surgeon of the 31st Battalion, Bengal Army in *King v. James MacLean* for the assault and battery of Karim Khan in Ramnagar, Benares, on 18 December 1788, and the account of a civil surgeon, Dr Thomas Marten in *King v. William Townsend Jones* for the murder of Shariat Ullah in Calcutta on 10 December 1789 (Hyde Papers, National Library, Kolkata, Rare Books Division: Reports, vols 23, 27). The criminal cases referred to here are from the voluminous diaries of Justice John Hyde (1775–95). These cases are beyond the purview of the present chapter. They deserve a much more detailed and extensive study.

II

ENACTMENTS OF THE MEDICAL

4

STATE MEDICINE OR MEDICAL STATE?
A Prison Epidemic in Colonial Burma, 1881

JONATHAN SAHA

The historiography on medicine in colonial contexts has become increasingly sophisticated and nuanced over the last thirty years. Imperial hagiographies consisting of Whiggish narratives chronicling Western medical improvements and their intrinsically beneficial effects for colonized populations have, of course, long been discredited. But since these stale histories have been dispensed with, the rigours of postcolonial critical thinking have continued to drive the field forward, unsettling some of the certainties and assumptions about colonial medicine. In the process, the role of the colonial state in the history of Western biomedical practice has been substantially, although perhaps inadvertently, diminished. It is not my intention to contend in this chapter that the state should simply be 'brought back in',[1] but instead to demonstrate that recent advances in state theory provide historians with the tools to conceptualize the relationship between the state and Western medicine in colonial contexts in innovative ways. In the light of these novel approaches, it is necessary for historians to more carefully locate the medical vis-à-vis the colonial state.

In the late 1980s and 1990s historians of colonialism most often approached Western medical practices as strategies for establishing the authority of the colonizer over the colonized.[2] This authority was conceived of broadly, encompassing not only material authority over the subject population, but also moral authority.[3] It is impossible to do justice to the diversity and detail of this literature, which was always informed by in-depth empirical research and has been sensitive to the contingent historical contexts of both developments in medicine and the nature of colonialism at any given point in time. Nevertheless, it is instructive to note the ambiguous place of the writings of Michel Foucault in framing much of this work conceptually. For both Megan Vaughan in *Curing Their Ills* and David Arnold in *Colonizing the Body*, Foucault's theorization of power/knowledge provided a starting point for their own theoretical frameworks. Vaughan borrowed Foucault's terminology of biopower to understand Western medical conceptions of 'African' illness, and Arnold applied Foucault's focus on the body to examine colonial contests over medical practice in India. However, both authors distanced themselves from Foucault's nebulous conception of power as capillary and ubiquitous, favouring instead to focus on the colonial state.[4] In these histories, Western medicine was usually synonymous with state medicine in a colonial context.

Recent historical research has complicated this image and revealed some of the profound ambiguities of Western medical practices in colonial contexts. Although neither Arnold nor Vaughan ignores indigenous medical practices—indeed local medicine plays an intrinsic role in both of their books—historians have since sought to explore the interactions between Western and local medicines in greater detail. The concern of historians began to shift away from the use of Western medicine by the colonial state increasingly to the social and cultural histories of a plurality of medical practices and knowledge under colonialism.[5] This newer focus has taken historians down a number of different avenues. Both sides of the exchange of ideas between Western medicine and indigenous medicine that went on during colonialism have been researched. The appropriation of indigenous medical practices by colonial doctors has been revealed in fields as diverse as the use of mesmerism as an anaesthetic, to the collection of materia medica.[6] But a more developed strand of research has been the study of the diverse engagements of indigenous populations with Western medicine.[7] These studies have moved quickly beyond the exploration of resistance to its implementation, although this remains a rich vein for historical research.[8] Instead a greater range of interactions has been explored, revealing how aspects of Western medicine were appropriated into local understandings and refigured by local actors.[9] It is now increasingly apparent that the colonial state had no monopoly over the uses of Western medicine. Nor is it any longer self-evident that Western medicine was distinct from indigenous medicine, even within the medical institutions of the colonial state. Western medicine is increasingly understood to have been a 'contested site' rather than as straightforwardly synonymous with state medicine.[10]

The focus of histories of colonial medicine has begun to shift still further from the state with justified concerns emerging about the limitations of the implicit territorial frames that historians have usually worked within. Warwick Anderson raised this as a problem as early as 1998. He noted that despite the undoubted influence of postcolonial thought on historical writing in the field, the vast majority of published research remained firmly within the confines of national boundaries.[11] His own research on the history of colonial medicine in the Philippines attempts, successfully in my view, to collapse the binary between metropole and periphery by exploring them as part of the same history, with the Philippines being used as a 'colonial laboratory'.[12] Of course, historians of tropical medicine have long moved between Britain and India in their writings, and not all have done so because of a desire to retain the critical edge of postcolonial approaches. But the spatial framework has shifted further and increasingly global perspectives are being preferred.[13] Not that this shift has been universally welcomed. Sarah Hodges is correct in her concerns that the move to explore global medicine has been, for some, a retreat from postcolonial theory; a retreat that has introduced (or reproduced) universalizing conceptions of health that overlook the importance of asymmetrical configurations of power based upon discourses of difference.[14] In addition to Hodges' concerns, I would note that the role of states, and colonial states especially, has been further diminished, having been usurped by international and supranational entities as the focus of medical histories.

These trends in the history of colonial medicine have tended to lead historians away from examining the state. Returning to earlier works which did focus primarily on the state, such as Lenore Manderson's study of sickness in colonial Malaya, this shift may seem to be justified. Nearly all these earlier authors pointed out the inconsistency, incapacity, and often the lack of will within colonial states' attempts to implement their policies. For instance, Manderson argues that there was a structural contradiction to colonial medicine in Malaya. State policies often exacerbated the very illnesses they were attempting to combat.[15] Likewise, Warwick Anderson has argued that for the Filipinos, colonial medicine was contested, negotiated, and marked by apathy in its implementation.[16] Even in the work of those who have focused on the state directly, it was a limited and dysfunctional agent. So, given these trends in the historiography, how should we conceptualize the relationship between the state and Western medicine? Was the colonial state simply one ambivalent actor in the 'contested site' of Western medicine? Was the colonial state merely an ineffectual conduit for global medical developments? Instinctively I am drawn to disagree with both positions and argue that the state had a more important historical role, but the historiography offers little in the way of useful models for evaluating the relationship between the colonial state and Western medicine. This may in part be because theorizations on the state have had little direct influence on the writings of historians of colonial medicine.

A great deal of excellent work has been completed over the last thirty years reconceptualizing the modern state in ways that provide an opportunity to explore the relationship between the colonial state and Western medicine from a different perspective. Philip Abrams's essay on the state, in which he argues that scholars must take seriously the state's ideological and mythical qualities, is justifiably seen as a milestone for new approaches to the state. Following on from this crucial insight, Timothy Mitchell has argued that the state, as a mythical and imagined entity, was made through myriad everyday practices. These conceptualizations have led to a raft of anthropological studies of the postcolonial state in South Asia, exploring how the state was experienced and manifested as an imagined, quotidian entity.[17] Placed in this framework, the colonial state should not be treated as an a priori historical agent in the spread of Western medicine. Instead we can reverse the usual historical enquiry. Rather than examining the state's deployment of medicine—a line of investigation that seems bound to turn up instances of ambivalence and failure—it might prove fruitful to examine how Western medicine shaped the making of the colonial state.

In this chapter I attempt to apply this approach to a particularly disastrous episode in the history of colonial medicine in British Burma; a devastating prison epidemic that broke out in Thayetmyo jail in the summer of 1881, resulting in the deaths of over one-hundred inmates.

This event may be justifiably described as a failure of colonial bio-politics and the state's use of Western medicine to preserve the lives of those under their care. Certainly all the medical interventions made to arrest the spread of the deadly disease (the disputed nature of which is discussed later) were ineffective. However, this episode also reveals the centrality of medical knowledge and practice to how colonial officials performed and enacted the state. The official enquiry into the epidemic demonstrates that Western medicine informed the disciplining of state practices, regardless of officials' unavoidable awareness of the failure of Western medicine in the case at hand. The epidemic provides us with a window into how the colonial state was shaped by medicine. In the context of this volume, this chapter will remind readers that the history of medicine, as a disputed, shifting, and contingent category of knowledge and praxis was entangled with the constitution of numerous social artefacts, of which the colonial state was but one important example.

The Prison

The jail at Thayetmyo was opened to little fanfare in December 1867. In contrast to many of the prisons of colonial Burma at the time, the jail had been especially constructed for its purpose and was not a pre-existing building that had been adapted. The principal importance of the jail was its location, Thayetmyo being situated on the border with the still independent Upper Burma ruled by the Konbaung Dynasty from their court at Ava. The jail was thus a visible symbol of the presence of the colonial state in a district remote from the colonial centre at Rangoon and on the fringes of British territorial control. The area was also one which during the nineteenth century and early twentieth century became associated with banditry and unrest for the British.[18] For these reasons, ensuring that the 250 prisoners did not escape was at the top of prison officials' concerns about the new jail, and it was noted at its opening that 'strict discipline' would be essential. But the health of the prospective prison population was also made a marker of how the jail's success would be judged.[19]

At its opening British colonial officials questioned whether metropolitan penal institutions could be transplanted to different climatic conditions without having negative consequences on the inmates' health.

The superintendent commented upon its opening that, 'The whole gaol has been extremely well built and will last for many years, but whether its manner of construction will be prejudicial or not to the health of the Burmese prisoners confined in it is a question which will require time for its solution.'[20] For the first thirteen years of the new prison's existence, during which the capacity and population of the jail increased to over 400, the answer seemed to be that the prison had no detrimental effects on the health of its prisoners. Mortality in the prison was reported to be low in comparison to the other carceral institutions of Lower Burma, excepting the years 1873 and 1877, when there were cholera outbreaks in the province, and the year 1879, when the jail's ice machine exploded killing the prisoners who were working with it.[21] However, in June 1881 a seemingly unstoppable, apparently unknown, and usually fatal disease, that at its zenith afflicted roughly a third of the prison population, spread suddenly. The epidemic led to the very architecture and daily routines of the prison being subjected to medical investigation by a specially appointed committee. By November 1881 the prison had been evacuated, temporarily closed, and many of the convicts suffering from the disease were released.

In the history of this prison outbreak we have the historiographic problem of state medicine in microcosm: colonial state institutions were crucial sites in which Western medicine was practised on colonized populations, but the results were ambiguous, occasionally disastrous, and often negligent. Colonial prisons have been seen by historians as exemplary state spaces in British India, and as such they have been conceptualized as an 'enclave' of Western medicine. As David Arnold has argued, the prison was a site in which the state could get access to the bodies of the colonized in order to perform medical practices, such as vaccinations. State institutions were also a site of medical knowledge generation as colonial medical officials experimented in these spaces, developing new medical practices and theories.[22] Indeed, Ian Brown has argued that ensuring the health of prisoners was an underpinning imperative for prison officials in colonial Burma. As a result they produced a large body of statistical evidence on convict health.[23] However, as historians have shown in a host of different contexts, colonial prisons were often chaotic and dysfunctional institutions. Peter Zinoman has aptly described the prison in colonial Vietnam as 'ill-disciplined'.[24] Arnold's own work also detailed the corruption, resistance, and daily negotiations between staff and inmates endemic to prison life in nineteenth-century colonial India.[25] This complexity also applied to medicine. As Satadru Sen has shown, for the penal colony in the Andaman Islands, medicine was not simply imposed on 'docile' convict bodies, but was instead a site of contestation and resistance to penal discipline.[26] Taking these arguments even further, the failures of colonial medicine in the French imperial penal system led the anthropologist Peter Redfield to argue that the state established its authority by having power over death, rather than through biopower.[27] Medicine has been viewed by historians as intensively practised in state institutions and important to colonial ideologies, but at the same time being compromised and neglected.

Reconciling these two features of the history of colonial prisons is not easy. One might be tempted to argue that it was simply the difference between theory and practice: official desires for order compromised in the messy realities of implementation, the story of good intentions gone badly wrong. Such explanations circle around the capacity of the state to act, suggesting that even in its 'enclaves' Western medicine was applied in a piecemeal fashion. But medicine's role in state institutions is not best understood in terms of success, failure, and state incapacity, in even the case of the devastating Thayetmyo prison epidemic. Rather than primarily examining state institutions as sites in which attempts were made to impose medicine on the bodies of the colonized, I think it is more helpful to explore the ways medicine structured state institutions. This formulation moves us away from simply considering how successfully medicine was applied by the state, to considering the place medicine had in enacting the state. Indeed, medicine was more important for disciplining state actors and how they performed their state duties, than it was for maintaining the health of convicts. Of course the two were different sides of the same process. Medically informed state practices were expected to have beneficial effects for the inmates. Nevertheless, as we shall see, the emphasis of the investigation into the Thayetmyo prison epidemic was to examine whether the institution and its routine were medically sound and reform any aspects found wanting. In other words, the outbreak exposes the role of medicine in establishing norms for penal institutions in Burma, and disciplining the otherwise 'ill-disciplined' prison. In this way, medicine structured how the state was enacted and envisioned,[28] even when it was clearly having little positive impact on the health of those under its care.

The Epidemic and the Investigation

On 22 June 1881 Dr Dalzell, the newly appointed Superintendent of Thayetmyo Jail, treated a patient suffering from an unusual disease that he called 'acute oedema'. This rather obtuse and crudely descriptive medical definition was used because he could not find a pathological cause for the illness and its symptoms, which consisted of a large degree of swelling on the body and face. Four days later, a second prisoner was admitted with what appeared to be the same illness. Dalzell treated both cases with iron, nourishing foods, and purgatives, apparently with some success. Things began to take a dramatic turn for the worse on 24 July, when during the Sunday parade, Dalzell noticed a third prisoner who had extensive swelling all over his torso and legs. The prisoner was immediately sent to the prison hospital but died suddenly that night. His post mortem examination failed to reveal the nature of the disease and the numbers of prisoners suffering from the illness began to sharply spiral upwards. From a prison population of 472 in July, within just three months 62 inmates had died from the disease, 52 had been admitted to the prison hospital, and a further 92 were suffering from the condition but could not be admitted to the now overflowing hospital.[29] Under the pressure of the rising numbers of ill inmates, prison routines broke down. In a perversion of the panoptic design of the prison, the central tower was transformed into a makeshift hospital and on the platform around it, intended originally for surveillance, latrines were housed.[30]

During the epidemic between June and October, five colonial medical officers visited Thayetmyo jail and attempted to diagnose the illness. They did not reach a consensus as to its nature and, although each doctor had his own opinions about its causes and spread, no one made a confident claim to know what the disease was. Attempts to treat the disease were equally unsuccessful. The symptoms were varied, but the outcome was almost invariably death. The most common symptoms were swellings, these occurred at various parts of the body but primarily the face, legs, and arms. The sufferer usually became 'despondent', lost their appetite, became 'anaemic in appearance', and often developed vomiting and diarrhoea. Eventually fluids began to fill the chest causing the heart to struggle and stop.[31] Given the very visible symptoms of the disease, the proximity in which prisoners were kept to each other, and the rapidity with which deaths occurred, the prison must have made an unimaginably appalling and desperate scene. In the face of what officials referred to as the 'mysterious disease',[32] the prison authorities and colonial doctors were singularly impotent.

At one level of analysis the colonial doctors' attempts at identifying the cause of this epidemic constituted a particularly indeterminate episode in the social construction of medical knowledge. Although various terms were used to refer to the disease, such as 'acute oedema' and 'epidemic dropsy', most medical officers called the illness beriberi: a nutritional disease that we now understand to be caused by a thiamine (vitamin B1) deficiency, one particularly common among people whose diets consist predominantly of polished white rice. Whilst many of the symptoms described by the medical officers are consistent with those of beriberi, I have no interest in engaging in a retrospective diagnosis of the epidemic here, particularly since understandings of beriberi were highly contested at the time of the outbreak. Indeed, the terms 'acute oedema' and beriberi were used interchangeably by some contemporary doctors in India.[33] Moreover the aetiology of beriberi was disputed in Britain, with a debate running into the early twentieth century over whether it was a disease of location or a disease of diet.[34] Medical understandings of beriberi were more complex still in British India during the late nineteenth century, as it was often put together with epidemic dropsy (caused by argemone oil poisoning), which has similar symptoms. In India at this time the term 'beriberi', encompassing both diseases, was understood to be a disease of location, caused by climatic and environmental factors.[35] As Joanna Barnard's recent study has shown, within British Burma beriberi was an elusive disease that appears only sporadically within colonial archives. It emerged as a discrete diagnosis through changing understandings of nutrition in the early twentieth century and by being identified in particular spaces, including prisons.[36] Beriberi was a highly contested diagnosis. The medical officers investigating the epidemic in Thayetmyo jail recognized the symptoms of the disease, but they, like most medical people, were unsure of its cause and treatment. The debates over whether the illness was brought on by the immediate conditions, climate, contagion, or diet, were played out in their correspondence.

Despite their inability to arrest the rising mortality in the jail, the primary task of the various medical officials sent to Thayetmyo was to assess whether the prison and its routines were at fault, and if they were, how they might be rectified in the future. The earlier explanations made by prison officials tended to downplay the role of the jail itself in spreading the disease. Dalzell, for instance, did not view the prison as being either a primary cause for the disease or even a notable factor in its spread. This was unsurprising given that he was the newly appointed superintendent of the prison, and that the outbreak had occurred within months of him taking the post. Rather than lay the blame on the management of the prison, which would implicate himself as having been negligent, he argued that the disease was a contagious one that resulted from the unhealthy state of the prisoners *before* they entered the prison. Under later questioning he was asked to justify his belief in the unhealthy prior state of the prisoners. He answered, 'I first ascribe it to the poverty of the district, and consequent bad condition of health in which the men were admitted into the jail, as indicated by their appearance, and by my knowledge of the condition of the district generally.'[37] By stressing the contagious nature of the disease and the frailty of the population of Thayetmyo, Dalzell was attempting to eliminate the prison as a factor in the epidemic. The illness in his opinion was not caused by the prison conditions rather it was caused and spread by a contagious illness originating outside the jail.

Dalzell's stance was challenged first by Dr Kelly, the inspector general of prisons for British Burma, who visited the jail a month into the epidemic, just as it was reaching unmanageable proportions. On viewing the sickness amongst the prison population, he came to believe that the illness was caused by malnutrition. He immediately ordered that milk be introduced for the sick and that the diet of the prisoners be investigated. He argued that the food being supplied to the prison was of an inferior quality and laid the blame on the contractor and Dalzell for failing to procure better supplies. Kelly claimed that on his visits to the prison, he twice found the meat to be principally bone and the vegetables to be partly inedible. On the first occasion Dalzell had told him that the food was generally good and that this had been an exception, and on the second occasion Dalzell had fined the food contractor, although Kelly contended that he had not been fined enough. However, like Dalzell, Kelly eliminated all other aspects of prison life from being causes of the outbreak.[38] This may have been because in many respects, Thayetmyo prison was being managed in the usual fashion. As Kelly was the inspector general of prisons, locating the cause of the disease in the prison regime more broadly would have raised questions about his own role. Blaming the outside contractor for a poor supply of food emphasized local origins for the disease whilst deflecting attention from the general penal system.

Both Dalzell and Kelly were colonial doctors directly involved in prison management, and it is revealing that their own aetiologies of the disease reflected their proximity to potential blame. Whether or not this was a deliberate attempt to absolve themselves from responsibility, their immediate experiences of the disease and their bureaucratic positions will have informed their perspective when examining the nature and causes of the disease. It is worth identifying these influences as a reminder that medical investigations in history are often conducted within personal and micro-political contexts. In Burma, careers and reputations were on the line. It is further revealing that it was a colonial official without medical training and not directly employed in the penal system, the commissioner of the Irrawaddy division, who first suggested that the prison regime itself might have been a crucial factor in the epidemic. After visiting in early October, the commissioner called for a committee to be formed to investigate the outbreak. Faced with an exponential rise in the number of suffering inmates and a mortality rate at 36.6 per cent, Dalzell was forced to support the recommendation for the formation of a committee.[39]

The committee that was set up was headed by Dr Griffith, the civil surgeon of Rangoon, with considerable experience in Burma, and he was joined by the civil surgeon of Prome, Dr Chatterjee, and a surgeon, Dr Frenchman. The report that they produced on the prison epidemic provides us with the greatest detail on the nature of the disease and the daily routines in the jail before and during the outbreak. It is interesting that most of the published research on the history of colonial prisons in Burma has been written based on evidence found in investigative reports into failures and disruptions in the penal system, although none have looked at reports into epidemic outbreaks specifically.[40] Such reports were moments of official reflection on the running of prisons, outside of the normal bureaucratic routine of gathering information for annual reports, an activity which had become increasingly systematized and banal by the end of the nineteenth century. But these one-off reports are more than repositories of primary sources. They were moments in which the normative standards for state institutions were discussed and performed,[41] and medicine was vital to this process. The committee of medical officials sent to investigate the outbreak of beriberi in Thayetmyo jail were not only sent to recommend how the disease might best be combated, they were sent to pass a judgment on the conduct of prison officials, the standard of prison buildings, and, where necessary, to apportion blame. The investigation and its report had more than an air of legal proceedings about them. It is the formation of this committee, and how it conducted the investigation, that is demonstrative of the role medicine played in structuring the routine enactment of the state. Rather than conceptualizing this as a moment in which state medicine was deployed, it is better to understand it as an episode in which a state institution was disciplined according to emergent medical norms.

In the process of investigation, many different objects were brought under the medical gaze, not only the bodies of the colonized: the convicts' food; the prison's air flow and water supply; the architecture of the prison buildings; the quality of the soil; the convicts' bedding; and the rigours of prison discipline. Each was assessed according to implicit normative standards determined by what was deemed medically acceptable. In attempting this, the first problem the committee faced was the dearth of administrative paperwork. Griffith complained that the poor recording of the prison's day-to-day running had seriously hampered their investigations, pressing for improved archiving.[42] In the face of a lack of primary sources, the committee turned to scientific measurements and then to interviews to ascertain (or generate) the facts.

Given the colonial state's general governmental predilection for quantifiable evidence in the late nineteenth century, it is unsurprising that measurement was the first stage in investigating the prison.[43] The architecture of the prison was assessed for the space it allowed for inmates, the amount of air they had, and how rapidly this air supply was replenished, and it was found wanting: 'The prisoners get 36 square feet of superficial area per head, or ... 432 cubic feet of air per head.

In order to keep the air in the ward to its natural standard of purity, it should be changed at least six times an hour. ... This ... cannot possibly take place.'[44] In this same fashion the nutritional value of the food was calculated, with the committee commenting on the relatively high amount of nitrogenous substances to non-nitrogenous substances.[45] The quality of the drinking water was also criticized as it had not been filtered (although there was a dispute between the members of the committee over the merits of hard water over soft water). This performance of scientific objectivity in the medical officers' investigation was tempered by inquiries into the 'customary practices' of the Burmese. When commenting on the lack of air flow, the committee asked 'whether a masonry jail with a corrugated iron roof is suited for Burmans, who are accustomed to live in well-ventilated bamboo huts'.[46] When discussing the variety of the food, it was queried whether Burmans would eat a balanced diet without *ngapee*, a fish condiment, which had been banned in the jail following the 1877 cholera epidemic. And during the analysis of the prison's water quality, it was suggested that rather than from wells, water should be sourced from rivers in accordance with 'Burmese habit'.[47] In this way the medical gaze, which the prison was subjected to during the investigation, sought out both scientific and social data upon which to judge the institution, employing the now familiar methods of colonial governance: enumeration and ethnography.[48]

Following this preliminary investigation, the committee then interviewed the prison staff, some prisoners, and local notables in order to ascertain more information on the prison routine as well as further evidence of the customary habits of the local Burmese population. However the principal witnesses were Dalzell and Kelly, who were grilled on their responses to the crisis and their medical explanations for the epidemic. Dalzell's claim that the prison had played no part in the epidemic came under rigorous scrutiny, particularly over whether the architecture was suitable for the hot temperatures experienced in the Thayetmyo area. Griffith led the questioning:

> Griffith [G]: When going round the jail and inquiring of the prisoners we ascertained that they were in the habit of selecting, if possible, the position next to the doors as being cooler; did you know this?
> Dalzell [D]: No, I never noticed it ...
> G: When you first came to Thayetmyo where did you reside?
> D: By the river, in a pucca [masonry] building.

> G: Did you find it hot there?
> D: Yes, I found it very hot at night.
> G: Did you leave that house? What was the reason?
> D: On account of its bad surroundings and also on account of its heat.
> G: Did you suffer in health there?
> D: Yes.
> G: In what way?
> D: I lost weight and eventually suffered from fever.
> G: Taking into account the habits of Burmans, living as they do inside bamboo huts, do you think the present accommodation in a masonry building is likely to prove prejudicial to the health of men already in bad health on admission?
> D: Yes, I do.[49]

Through this rather personal and seemingly aggressive cross-examination—although it is hard to tell for sure from the transcript—Dalzell was forced to partly concede his assertion that the jail had no impact on the disease. The universalizing elements in medical knowledge were deployed by Griffith to make Dalzell openly acknowledge the likelihood that Burman bodies experienced the heat in the same way as his had. But to win his point fully, Griffith also had to guard against the potential defence of the Burmese alterity, which he did by referring to Burman 'habits'.[50] Similar lines of questioning were pursued not only with Dalzell but also with other colonial officials involved in the prison, concerning the water supply, the quality of the food, the prohibition on ngapee, and the accusations of parasites infesting the convicts' bedding. The point of these inquiries was not only to ascertain the cause of the disease (indeed, some lines of enquiry had nothing to do with the epidemic), but to judge whether the actions of officials had been correct according to established medical knowledge and practice.

Although the committee had highlighted in the body of its report a number of problems with the prison, they were unable to come to a firm conclusion on the causes of the epidemic. Despite the prison's air supply and food quality being deemed questionable, they were ultimately not thought to either be at blame for the disease or to be evidence of official neglect. As a result, the recommendations made in the report were rather banal and practical: the ill were to be released; water was to be sourced from the river; the diet was to be improved with a greater variety of foods and more nutritious foods; and all prisoners were to be removed temporarily to a camp outside the prison whilst it was cleaned. The chief commissioner of Burma's response to the report was equally pragmatic, arguing that since the disease did not appear to be contagious, the prisoners could be sent to other prisons in Burma rather than camped by Thayetmyo prison where escape to Upper Burma would be easy. However, he took issue with the report's suggestion that the jail's poor air supply had any effect on the disease, and particularly the claim that Burman homes were better ventilated: 'The Committee have apparently not penetrated any of these huts or they would have found Burmans sleeping within inner walls and inside thick cotton mosquito curtains where the air would hardly be less close than in jail wards.'[51] This final, authoritative piece of ethnographic insight (coming as it did from the highest-ranking official in the colony) further exonerated the jail for responsibility for the epidemic.

The medical investigation had done its job. It had not found the cause of the outbreak, but it had ascertained whether the prison was medically unfit for habitation, and whether the routine had been neglectful of the prisoners' health. The chief commissioner reflected on the events, 'We cannot acquiesce in the prisoners continuing to die as they have during the last 18 months at Thayetmyo, even though the wards and ventilation are in complete accordance with hygienic rules.'[52] It is the latter part of the chief commissioner's reflections that has often been overlooked by historians of colonial medicine. Colonial medicine was not only about maintaining the health of those under the state's care, a task in which on occasions it failed. Medicine also provided a normative standard for disciplining state practices and institutions. In this case it was found that despite the high death toll, medical standards had been met.

* * *

It has become a commonplace understanding within the historiography on colonial Burma that the colony was treated as a neglected appendage to British India; a 'skinny state' from which more was extracted by imperial power than was invested into it.[53] The usual chronology has it that it was not until the annexation of Upper Burma in 1885–6 that the colonial state was developed in any meaningful way, and even then it has been noted that the British remained reluctant and slow to develop the colony's infrastructure, preferring to rely on already established institutions in the older Presidencies of British India wherever possible. The devastating epidemic in Thayetmyo jail, as well as the gradual, pragmatic, and economically minded official response to it, could be seen to attest to this overarching neglect. State medicine was, in this construal of events, ineffectual. But even in this case it is clear that medicine was of greater importance to officials than such an interpretation allows for. Whilst the report into the epidemic showed that the colonial regime clearly had concerns over the health of the prison's inmates, and implicitly suggested worry over how the prison might be perceived by the populations, the primary imperative was to discipline the prison regime (and any errant officials) according to normative medical discourses. The role of medicine in shaping state practices and institutions, ineffective and underinvested as they may have been, has been overlooked by historians.

The report into the Thayetmyo prison epidemic was only a symptom of a broader and deeper development in how the colonial state was performed in Burma from the 1870s through to the 1890s. In this period a range of medical institutions were opened, including numerous hospitals, dispensaries, a lunatic asylum, medical classes, leper asylums, vaccination depots, lock hospitals.[54] These were often underfunded and small-scale state institutions which had, perhaps, a minimal impact on the Burmese population at large, but their existence was indicative of the greater government of India and metropolitan oversight that the colony was subjected to.[55] It was necessary for the government of Burma to be able to demonstrate that British Burma had at least basic medical institutions. However, more interesting than state institutions with explicitly medical purposes were the non-medical state officials and institutions that had progressively more medical roles. Courts increasingly had to handle medical evidence.[56] Correspondingly, policemen had to be taught how to collect such evidence.[57] Village headmen were instructed to ensure that their villages were sanitary, and trained to do so.[58] Census workers attempted to enumerate the numbers of lepers, lunatics, and others suffering from a number of medical afflictions.[59] If and when state officials failed at these tasks, they could become the target of bureaucratic discipline.

Put simply, to perform and enact the state bureaucracy, state actors often had to behave according to medical rules. Of course, as the other chapters in this volume amply demonstrate, medical knowledge and praxis were not stable and unchanging. The reader should not interpret this chapter to be suggesting that medicine was a prior, preordained category shaping state practice. Instead, I would urge that when locating the medical in relation to the colonial state, the history of the two should be conceptualized as co-constitutive.[60]

Although I do not want to overstate the comparatively piecemeal development of the colonial state in Burma in the nineteenth century, it is nevertheless important to note that at the same time as the state bureaucracy expanded and became more specialized, medical practices became more ubiquitous across its various branches. Western medicine may not have been furthered or successfully imposed on subject populations by the colonial state, but, in nineteenth-century Burma at least, the colonial state was increasingly structured according to medical ideas.

Notes

1. Peter B. Evans, Dietrich Rueschemeyer, and Theda Skocpol, eds, *Bringing the State Back In* (Cambridge: Cambridge University Press, 1985).
2. This approach undoubtedly has earlier antecedents, not least Frantz Fanon's essay 'Medicine and Colonialism', in *A Dying Colonialism*, translated by Haakon Chevalier (Harmondsworth: Penguin, 1970), which has had a mixed but profound impact on the historiography (Richard C. Keller, 'Clinician and Revolutionary: Frantz Fanon, Biography and the History of Colonial Medicine', *Bulletin of the History of Medicine* 81, no. 4 [2007], 823–41).
3. For some influential examples, see Daniel R. Headrick, *Tools of Empire: Technology and European Imperialism in the Nineteenth Century* (Oxford: Oxford University Press), which although not dedicated to medical history, does bring in the role of medicine in sustaining colonial rule; Lenore Manderson, *Sickness and the State: Health and Illness in Colonial Malaya, 1870–1940* (Cambridge: Cambridge University Press, 1996); David Arnold, ed., *Imperial Medicine and Indigenous Societies* (Manchester: Manchester University Press, 1988); Roy Macleod and Milton Lewis, eds, *Disease, Medicine and Empire: Perspectives on Western Medicine and the Experience of European Expansion* (London: Routledge, 1988); Megan Vaughan,

Curing Their Ills: Colonial Power and African Illness (Stanford: Stanford University Press, 1991); David Arnold, *Colonizing the Body: State Medicine and Epidemic Disease in Nineteenth-Century India* (Berkeley: University of California Press, 1994).

4. Arnold, *Colonizing the Body*; Vaughan, *Curing Their Ills*.

5. This shift has been noted recently in South Asian historiography by Waltraud Ernst, 'Beyond East and West: From the History of Colonial Medicine to a Social History of Medicine(s) in South Asia', *Social History of Medicine* 20, no. 3 (2007): 505–24, and was pre-empted in African history earlier by Megan Vaughan, 'Healing and Curing: Issues in the Social History and Anthropology of Medicine in Africa', *Social History of Medicine* 7, no. 2 (1994): 283–95.

6. See Waltraud Ernst, 'Colonial Psychiatry, Magic and Religion: The Case of Mesmerism in British India', *History of Psychiatry* 15, no. 1 (2004): 57–71, and Hans Pols, 'European Physicians and Botanists, Indigenous Herbal Medicine in the Dutch East Indies, and Colonial Networks of Mediation', *East Asian Science, Technology and Society: An International Journal* 3, nos 2/3 (2009): 173–208.

7. For a recent historiographic overview of work on indigenous medicine in South Asia, see Projit B. Mukharji, 'Symptoms of Dis-ease: New Trends in the Histories of "Indigenous" South Asian Medicines', *History Compass* 9, no. 12 (2011): 887–99.

8. For some examples drawn from different parts of the British empire in South Asia, see Ira Klein, 'Plague, Policy and Popular Unrest in British India', *Modern Asian Studies* 22, no. 4 (1988): 723–55. Niels Brimnes, 'Variolation, Vaccination and Popular Resistance in Early Colonial South India', *Medical History* 48, no. 2 (2004): 199–228; Maitrii Aung-Thwin, 'Healing, Rebellion, and the Law: Ethnologies of Medicine in Colonial Burma, 1928–1932', *Journal of Burma Studies* 14 (2010): 151–85.

9. Again, as a sample of the range of literature drawn from around colonial South Asia, with differing concerns, see Biswamoy Pati, 'Siting the Body: Perspectives on Health and Medicine in Colonial Orissa', *Social Scientist* 26, nos 11/12 (1998): 3–26; Chie Ikeya, 'The Scientific and Hygienic Housewife-and-Mother: Education, Consumption and the Discourse of Domesticity', *Journal of Burma Studies* 14 (2010): 59–89; Guy N.A. Attewell, *Refiguring Unani Tibb: Plural Healing in Late Colonial India* (Hyderabad: Oriental Longman, 2007).

10. Poonam Bala and Amy Kaler, 'Introduction: Contested "Ventures": Explaining Biomedicine in Colonial Contexts', in *Biomedicine as a Contested Site: Some Revelations in Imperial Contexts*, edited by Poonam Bala (Lanham: Lexington Books, 2009), pp. 1–9.

11. Warwick Anderson, 'Review Essay: Where Is the Postcolonial History of Medicine?' *Bulletin of the History of Medicine* 72, no. 3 (1998): 522–30.

12. Warwick Anderson, *Colonial Pathologies: American Tropical Medicine, Race, and Hygiene in the Philippines* (Durham: Duke University Press, 2006).

13. See, for instance, the shift in geographical scale between Mark Harrison, 'Tropical Medicine in Nineteenth-Century India', *The British Journal for the History of Science* 25, no. 3 (1992): 299–318 and Mark Harrison, 'Disease, Diplomacy and International Commerce: The Origins of International Sanitary Regulation in the Nineteenth Century', *Journal of Global History* 1, no. 1 (2006): 197–217.

14. Sarah Hodges, 'The Global Menace', *Social History of Medicine* 24, no. 3 (2011): 1–10.

15. Manderson, *Sickness and the State*, p. 230.

16. Anderson, *Colonial Pathologies*, p. 6.

17. Philip Abrams, 'Notes on the Difficulty of Studying the State', *Journal of Historical Sociology* 1, no. 1 (1988): 58–89; Timothy Mitchell, 'The Limits of the State: Beyond Statist Approaches and Their Critics', *The American Political Science Review* 85 (1991): 77–96; Stuart Corbridge, Glyn Williams, Manoj Srivastava, and René Véron, eds, *Seeing the State: Governance and Governmentality in India* (Cambridge: Cambridge University Press, 2005); C.J. Fuller and Véronique Bénéï, eds, *The Everyday State and Society in Modern India* (London: Hurst and Company, 2001); Thomas Blom Hansen and Finn Stepputat, eds, *States of Imagination: Ethnographic Explorations of the Postcolonial State* (Durham: Duke University Press, 2001); Lloyd I. Rudolph and John Kurt Jacobsen, eds, *Experiencing the State* (New Delhi: Oxford University Press, 2006).

18. Thayetmyo is situated close to the north-west of the Pegu Yoma mountain range, often used as a launch pad and space of retreat during anti-colonial revolts. Whilst not holding quite the same resonance as the 'infamous' Tharrawaddy District to the south of the Pegu Yomas, it was seen as a troublesome place. See James C. Scott, *The Art of Not Being Governed: An Anarchist History of Upland Southeast Asia* (New Haven: Yale University Press, 2009), pp. 167–72; Matrii Aung-Thwin, *The Return of the Galon King: History, Law, and Rebellion in Colonial Burma* (Athens: Ohio University Press, 2011); Parimal Ghosh, *Brave Men of the Hills: Resistance and Rebellion in Burma, 1825–1932* (London: Hurst and Company, 2000). The area was known during the 'pacification' because of the bandit Bo Shwe who operated there. See Charles Crosthwaite, *The Pacification of Burma* (London: Edward Arnold, 1912).

19. *Annual Gaol Report for 1867*, India Office Records, British Library, London [hereafter IOR], V/24/2409, pp. 180–1.

20. *Annual Gaol Report for 1867*, pp. 180–1. For a discussion of the broader conceptual problems that are raised by the practical difficulties colonizers experienced transplanting 'modern' disciplinary institutions, see Martha Kaplan, 'The Panopticon in Poona: An Essay on Foucault and Colonialism', *Cultural Anthropology* 10, no. 1 (1995): 85–98.

21. 'Report on the Cause of Excessive Mortality from Dropsy in the Thayetmyo Jail', 4 November 1881, *Burma Home Proceedings*, IOR, P/1596, p. 3.

22. Arnold, *Colonizing the Body* and 'The Colonial Prison: Power, Knowledge and Penology in Nineteenth-Century India', in *Subaltern Studies VIII: Essays in Honour of Ranajit Guha*, edited by David Arnold and David Hardiman (Dehli: Oxford University Press, 1994), pp. 148–87. Also see, for an interesting example of this process in lunatic asylums in British India, James H. Mills, *Madness, Cannabis and Colonialism: The 'Native-Only' Lunatic Asylums of British India, 1857–1900* (Basingstoke: Macmillan, 2000), pp. 43–65.

23. Ian Brown, 'Death and Disease in the Prisons of Colonial Burma', *Journal of Burma Studies* 14, no. 1 (2010): 1–20.

24. Peter Zinoman, *The Colonial Bastille: A History of Imprisonment in Vietnam, 1862–1940* (Berkeley: University of California Press, 2001), pp. 13–37.

25. Arnold, 'Colonial Prison'.

26. Satadru Sen, *Disciplining Punishment: Colonialism and Convict Society in the Andaman Islands* (Delhi: Oxford University Press, 2000).

27. Peter Redfield, 'Foucault in the Tropics: Displacing the Panopticon', in *Anthropologies of Modernity: Foucault, Governmentality and Life Politics*, edited by Jonathan Xavier Inda and Peter Redfield (Oxford: Blackwell, 2005), pp. 50–82. This conceptualization has parallels with some theoretical approaches which also modify Foucault's work. See, Giorgio Agamben, *Homo Sacer: Sovereign Power and Bare Life* (Stanford: Stanford University Press, 1998); Achille Mbembe, 'Necropolitics', *Public Culture* 15, no. 1 (2003): 11–40.

28. Prisons in British-India were intended as highly visible state institutions projecting the colonial state's moral and material authority; see Clare Anderson and David Arnold, 'Envisioning the Colonial Prison', in *Cultures of Confinement: A History of the Prison in Africa, Asia and Latin America*, edited by Frank Dikötter and Ian Brown (Ithaca: Cornell University Press, 2007), pp. 304–31.

29. 'Report on the Excessive Mortality in the Thayetmyo Jail', IOR, P/1596, pp. 8–12.

30. 'Report on the Excessive Mortality in the Thayetmyo Jail', IOR, P/1596, 3.

31. 'Report on the Excessive Mortality in the Thayetmyo Jail', IOR, P/1596, pp. 11–12.

32. 'Proceedings of the Chief Commissioner in the Judicial Department', 21 April 1882, Burma Home Proceedings, IOR, P/1802.
33. See, for example, F.D.S. Fayrer, 'Acute Œdema: Beri-beri' (1880), Pamphlet 7402, Foreign and Commonwealth Office Collection, University of Manchester.
34. See, for instance, the following debate: Neil Macleod, 'Can Beri-Beri Be Caused by Food Supplies from Countries Where Beri-Beri Is Endemic?' *British Medical Journal* 2, no. 1911 (1897): 390–2; D.C. Rees, 'Beri-Beri a "Place" Disease, Not a Food Disease', *British Medical Journal* 2, no. 1916 (1897): 747–8.
35. David Arnold, 'British India and the "Beri-Beri Problem", 1798–1942', *Medical History* 54 (2010): 300–2.
36. Joanna Barnard, 'Placing Beriberi on the Map: Rice, Vitamins, and Colonial Health in Burma, 1867–1940' (PhD diss., University of Nottingham, 2014).
37. 'Report on the Excessive Mortality in the Thayetmyo Jail', IOR, P/1596, Appendix.
38. 'Report on the Excessive Mortality in the Thayetmyo Jail', pp. 9–10.
39. 'Report on the Excessive Mortality in the Thayetmyo Jail', p. 12.
40. Ian Brown, 'A Commissioner Calls: Alexander Paterson and Colonial Burma's Prisons', *Journal of Southeast Asian Studies* 38, no. 2 (2007): 293–308; Ian Brown, 'A Shooting Incident at Insein Prison, Burma, in 1947', *Journal of Imperial and Commonwealth History* 37, no. 4 (2009): 517–35; James Warren, 'The Rangoon Jail Riot of 1930 and the Prison Administration of British Burma', *South East Asia Research* 10, no. 1 (2002): 5–29.
41. Ann Laura Stoler, 'Colonial Archives and the Arts of Governance', *Archival Science* 2, no. 1 (2002): 87–109.
42. 'Report on the Excessive Mortality in the Thayetmyo Jail', pp. 1–2.
43. Arjun Appadurai, 'Number in the Colonial Imagination', in *Orientalism and the Postcolonial Predicament: Perspectives from South Asia*, edited by Carol Appadurai Breckenridge and Peter van Der Veer (Philadelphia: University of Pennsylvania Press, 1993), pp. 114–135.
44. 'Report on the Excessive Mortality in the Thayetmyo Jail', p. 2.
45. 'Report on the Excessive Mortality in the Thayetmyo Jail', p. 8.
46. 'Report on the Excessive Mortality in the Thayetmyo Jail', pp. 2–3.
47. 'Report on the Excessive Mortality in the Thayetmyo Jail', p. 9.
48. Bernard Cohn, *Colonialism and Its Forms of Knowledge: The British in India* (Princeton: Princeton University Press, 1996); Nicholas Dirks, *Castes of Mind: Colonialism and the Making of Modern India* (Princeton: Princeton University Press, 2001).
49. 'Report on the Excessive Mortality in the Thayetmyo Jail'.

50. For more on the changing relationship between bodily difference, climate, and disease, see Mark Harrison, '"The Tender Frame of Man": Disease, Climate and Racial Difference in India and the West Indies, 1760–1860', *Bulletin of the History of Medicine* 70, no. 1 (1996): 68–93; David Arnold, 'Race, Place and Bodily Difference in Early Nineteenth-Century India', *Historical Research* 77, no. 196 (2004): 254–73.

51. 'Proceedings of the Chief Commissioner in the Judicial Department', 21 April 1882, Burma Home Proceedings, IOR, P/1802.

52. 'Note by Mr. C. Bernard, Chief Commissioner, British Burma, on the Thayetmyo Jail', 28 September 1882, *Burma Home Proceedings*, IOR, P/1803.

53. Mary P. Callahan, *Making Enemies: War and State Buildings in Burma* (Ithaca: Cornell University Press, 2003); D.G.E. Hall, *Burma* (London: Hutchinson's University Library, 1956); Robert H. Taylor, *The State in Burma* (London: C. Hurst and Co., 1987); John F. Cady, *A History of Modern Burma* (Ithaca: Cornell University Press, 1958).

54. Atsuko Naono, *State of Vaccination: The Fight Against Smallpox in Colonial Burma* (Hyderabad: Orient BlackSwan 2009); Jonathan Saha, 'Madness and the Making of a Colonial Order in Burma', *Modern Asian Studies* 47, no. 3 (2013): 406–35; Jonathan Saha, '"Uncivilized Practitioners": Medical Subordinates, Medico-Legal Evidence, and Misconduct in Colonial Burma, 1875–1907', *South East Asia Research* 20, no. 3 (2012): 423–43; Penny Edwards, 'Bitter Pills: Colonialism, Medicine, and Nationalism in Burma, 1870–1940', *Journal of Burma Studies* 14 (2010): 21–58.

55. For an example of this creeping metropolitan oversight, see Sally Swartz, 'The Regulation of British Colonial Lunatic Asylums and the Origins of Colonial Psychiatry, 1860–1864', *History of Psychology* 13, no. 2 (2010): 160–77.

56. For instance, see the debates surrounding criminal lunatics in Saha, 'Madness in Colonial Burma', and the use of medical evidence in cases of gendered violence in Jonathan Saha, 'The Male State: Colonialism, Corruption and Rape Investigations in the Irrawaddy Delta, c. 1900', *Indian Economic and Social History Review* 47, no. 3 (2010): 362–72. For a broader, British-India-wide discussion of the use of medico-legal evidence in courts, see Elizabeth Kolsky, '"The Body Evidencing the Crime": Rape on Trial in Colonial India', *Gender and History* 22, no. 1 (2010): 109–30 and Joanne Bailkin, 'The Boot and the Spleen: When Was Murder Possible in British India?' *Comparative Studies in Society and History* 48, no. 2 (2006): 462–93.

57. See the issues arising from the use of the Rangoon hospital by the police gathering medical evidence discussed in Saha, '"Uncivilized Practitioners'". Also see 'Guidance for Criminal Investigations (Medical)', May 1891, Burma Home Proceedings, IOR/P/3808.

58. 'Sanitary Condition of Villages', November 1878, Burma Home Proceedings, IOR/P/1132.

59. 'Report on the Census Operation in Burma', December 1891, Burma Home Proceedings, IOR/P/3810.

60. I have elsewhere made a similar argument regarding the law and the state. See Jonathan Saha, 'A Mockery of Justice? Colonial Law, the Everyday State and Village Politics in the Burma Delta, c.1890–1910', *Past and Present* 217, no. 1 (2012): 187–212.

5

'DR. KAR I PRESUME!'

'Medical' Narratives from the Jarawa Tribal Reserve

VISHVAJIT PANDYA AND MADHUMITA MAZUMDAR

Any attempt to write a narrative of the contemporary history of biomedicine among the Andaman Islanders has more often than not proved to be a tortuous exercise.[1] Part of the reason for this is that biomedicine as it has been historically introduced among the indigenous communities of the Andaman Islands—the Ongees, Jarawas, and the Great Andamanese—has stubbornly eluded the archive.[2] The scattered traces and labyrinthine trails one follows to address standard conventions of historical or anthropological research have often led to dead ends or more positively to new questions that have muddled the verities of foundational categories and assumptions about the 'medical'.

The state archives of the Tribal Health Department remain difficult to access, while the search for 'reliable informants' is rarely rewarding. Tribal health and welfare functionaries face the hazard of violating service rules if found to be purveying information to the press or to any outsider without official sanction.[3] Published records from the health department are often a statistical compilation of the numbers, sex, and age group figures of tribal patients receiving hospital care either at the local primary health centre or the G.B. Pant Hospital in Port Blair. There are no epidemiological studies or reports of specific pathologies. A point made compellingly by Elizabeth Matthews, superintendent of the G.B. Pant Hospital, Port Blair, in her brief study of the health care for the Jarawas in what she described as a period of transition.[4]

What one does get, however, are conventional 'demographic and health profile reports enumerating anthropometric data under heads such as body structure, total content of body fat, body surface area or other measurable statistics related to basal metabolic rates, blood groups, and blood pressure'.[5] These discrete pieces of information have rarely been put together as the kind of holistic health care reports or specific epidemiological studies Matthews talked about. Many of the parameters of contemporary research studies continue to be mere replications of older colonial reports.[6]

More complex issues of tribal health or tribal medicine enter public discourse only in the context of crises, such as the successive outbreaks of pneumonia, measles, malaria, and a hepatitis E epidemic among the Jarawas.[7] Such discussion, it must be noted, has been possible only after 1997, when the Jarawas came out into regular contact with the outsiders. The implications of regular contact, which had already become the subject of widespread debate, acquired a sense of urgency with the sudden and rapid outbreak of successive epidemics and apocalyptic visions of the 'dying savage'. In these times too all that got reported through information provided by the state or discussed in the local, national, and international media were mortality figures. State medical bulletins churned out figures to reassure anxious rights groups around the world that timely and effective medical intervention had ensured the long-term survival of groups, such as the Jarawas, who were perpetually deemed to be on the brink.[8]

Yet, there has seldom been any information or discussion of what this 'medical intervention' might have been. What kind of treatment or what kinds of medicines were deployed to control successive epidemic outbreaks? What kinds of checks were undertaken before the introduction of these medicines? Was there any resistance to the introduction of these medicines among the Jarawas? Who were the specialists involved and what kind of policies did they formulate in case of future occurrences? Is there any clearly formulated tribal health/medical policy that is reviewed and revised in the context of the increasing event of contact between the indigenous Andamanese such as the Jarawas and outsiders?[9] All these questions proved to be rhetorical in the face of restricted archival access and limited public discourse.

It is in this context that our relentless search for 'traces' of the time of the Jarawa epidemics' yielded an unexpected surprise. We happened to chance upon a recently published popular ethnography of the Jarawas in Bengali, written by a state medical practitioner Dr Ratan Chandra Kar. It needs to be pointed out that the book titled *Andamaner Adim Janajati Jarawa* or the 'Primitive Tribes of the Andaman Islands, the Jarawas' is not the first of its kind to be written by a state functionary.[10] In fact, as we were to find, Dr Kar's book followed closely on the publication of two other popular ethnographies of the Jarawas written by a field anthropologist of the state tribal welfare organization, the AAJVS. Dr Kar's locus standi as the more respected ethnographer derived in large measure from his status as a medical functionary responsible for successfully implementing a regime of biomedicine among the Jarawas. His unparalleled service towards these 'primitive people' of the Islands and his unceasing compassion for their plight we were told, earned him a special commendation from the lieutenant governor of the Islands on Republic Day (26 January), 2000. The people of the Islands were meant to appreciate Dr Kar's ability to bridge the civilized world and that of the primitive, borne out by the fact that the once endangered Jarawas were now on a new demographic curve.[11]

Dr Kar, however, was not a local islander or settler. He was born and raised in the Ghatal subdivision of Medinipore district in West Bengal. His professional career in medicine took shape in Kolkata, where he graduated from the Nilratan Sircar Medical College in 1981. His first posting as a medical practitioner of the government of India was in Nagaland. Here he was involved in delivering medical services to the Konyak Nagas. In September 1988 he was transferred to Port Blair as a medical officer to the Island administration. It was in this capacity that Dr Kar began to participate in the first-ever medical services provided to the Jarawa. From 1989 to 1993 Dr Kar was involved in work among the Great Andamanese. In 1998 the Island administration constituted a special Jarawa Welfare Group in which Dr Kar was appointed a member. It was during his stint with this medical team that Dr Kar was able to enter each and every Jarawa hut in the forests of the South and Middle Andamans. He was able to establish his reputation not only as an able medical practitioner but a trusted friend of the Jarawa.[12]

The title of Dr Kar's book made it clear that he didn't want to position it as a medical memoir. Simply called 'The Primitive Tribe of Andamans, the Jarawas', the book claimed to be an authentic account of a people the author had the privilege of knowing with a degree of intimacy and erudition. The blurb and the preface complemented each other in claiming for Dr Kar a certain kind of ethnographic authority unmatched by other observers in the field. For ten long years Dr Kar was able to observe the everyday lives of the primitive Jarawa, understand their customs, practices, social norms, dietary habits, and their indigenous medical practices. The experiential depth of his knowledge made his observations of the community a first of its kind and hence a significant ethnographic event. The writer of the foreword to his book, the late Priten Roy, a veteran journalist of the Islands, reinforced this claim with the argument that the 'stone-age Jarawas' were the subject of deep and ever-widening curiosity all over the world. By sharing his invaluable ethnographic insights with his readers, Dr Kar was fulfilling a commendable social and cultural obligation. Mr Roy hoped that Bengalis not only in the subcontinent but globally would embrace and appreciate Dr Kar's unique endeavour.[13]

This chapter is woven around a close reading of Dr Kar's book as an ethnographic text that doubles up as a medical memoir. It seeks to develop the argument that Dr Kar's 'medical memoir' cum ethnography could be read as much as a realist account of a lesser-known culture as a narrative of the state's self-representation as sole and undisputed custodian of its 'primitive' population. It also serves as an unwitting trail into the complex and contingent presence of the 'medical' in the tribal reserve forests of the Andaman Islands. This chapter seeks to address one of the key concerns of the volume by exploring the 'enactments of the medical' in sites and conditions that disavow any easy or stable understandings of what the editors in their introduction describe as the 'out-there-ness' of the medical. In the absence of formal archival records and difficulty of access into the Tribal Reserves, the elusive trails of 'medical enactments' in the Andaman Islands are at best followed through the larger trajectories of the Indian state's relationship with its subjects belonging to the Particularly Vulnerable Tribal Groups (PVTGs) as it has sought to pacify, confine, control, and protect them over the last six decades. The terms and timing of Dr Kar's medical intervention among the Jarawas must be seen in that context.

As an ethnographic text, Dr Kar's account follows the conventions of realist ethnography but without any disciplinary restraints.[14] There are the usual chapters on ethnogenesis, composition, social welfare concerns, quotidian life, and material and spiritual culture of the

community he studies. But all of this is framed within a more intimate narrative of his larger 'medical' accomplishments. Although put
together as a seamless whole, the textual organization of the book with
its twelve chapters could be broadly classified around three heads—
history, medical journal, and ethnography. The first two chapters
constitute the historical, the next set of three chapters are evidently
extracts from Dr Kar's medical diaries, while the final four chapters are
Dr Kar's ethnographic descriptions of the early identity of the Jarawas,
their indigenous medical practices, their camps and dwelling practices
in the forest, their demographic statistics, and lastly a detailed account
of their daily lives.

Broadly speaking, chapters invoking Dr Kar's intersubjective
engagement with his individual Jarawa patients are followed by more
ethnographically informed descriptions of them as a bounded 'primitive'
culture—as abstract historical others defined by dichotomies and
essences. The first chapter titled 'Amar Katha' (My Story) sets the
larger tone of the narrative by invoking two key events in the contemporary history of the Jarawas: their coming into friendly contact with
the Outsider and the steady increase in their population following their
eager acceptance of biomedical intervention. The momentous event of
the Jarawas coming out of the forest and accepting the friendship of
the Outsider is closely woven around the story of the young Jarawa boy
Enmei, whose fortuitous accident on the fringes of the Jarawa reserve
forest in Middle Andamans occasioned the first systematic attempt by
the state to treat the Jarawa within the confines of a modern medical
facility in Port Blair.[15] Enmei's stay at the G.B. Pant hospital in Port
Blair became a cause célèbre not only for the medical establishment
in Port Blair but for the Island administration at large. The state had
at last accomplished the task of establishing friendly contact with the
Jarawas, putting an end to centuries of endemic conflict. Enmei was
hailed as a messenger of peace and sent back to the forest with the task
of persuading the rest of his community to trust the Outsider and avail
of the new medical services provided to them.[16]

It was in this context, writes Dr Kar, that the Island administration gave him charge of introducing a mobile dispensary in the Jarawa
Tribal Reserve and later of managing the newly established ward for
the Jarawa at the Kadamtala hospital in the Middle Andamans.[17]
Dr Kar describes this phase of his life as marking the golden period of his

medical career. His three major accomplishments during this period were first, his medical team's ability to enter each and every Jarawa hut in the forest interiors and deliver medical aid, ensure the quick removal of two phases of threatened epidemics among the Jarawas, and finally ensure a 30 per cent increase in their numbers, a feat unparalleled when compared to the steady demographic decline of the two other groups the Great Andamanese and the Ongee.[18]

Notwithstanding the fact that the veracity of these claims demand scrutiny, what is interesting is Dr Kar's skilful interweaving of these facts with his introductory autobiographical note. Dr Kar appears as both individual hero and the committed state functionary. His autobiography is merged with that of the state narrative, whose voice he both internalizes and celebrates.

As part of the exercise of reading Dr Kar's account as a kind of popular ethnographic text, this chapter tries to draw attention to its rhetorical and narrative dimensions, its marks of enunciation and its strategies of communicating effective ethnographic authority. It does not attempt a straight translation of the text, but tries to draw out three interweaving narratives that tease out the dilemma involved in writing about biomedical practice in a context where its presence is inherently contingent and ambivalent.

The first section focuses on the rhetorical strategies invoked in presenting the narrative of the first encounter. Section two draws out the 'medical' component of his ethnography with an account of his time spent with the Jarawas as part of the first medical team introduced into the reserve. Section three delves into Dr Kar's real 'fieldwork' experience in a Jarawa campsite in order to draw out the underlying tensions of the larger structure of the book that struggles to combine the heroic story of a Dr Livingstone in the forest with that of the dispassionate ethnographer and the compliant state functionary.[19]

This chapter tries to develop the argument that Dr Kar's ethnography of Jarawas opens up a possibility of locating the 'medical' in the realm of a contingent yet pervasive presence of the state in the forest. It draws upon insights from recent writings that have sought to reconceptualize states as 'culturally embedded and discursively constructed ensembles'.[20] Aradhana Sharma and Akhil Gupta argue that instead of looking at states as 'pre-constituted entities that perform given functions, it is more fruitful to show how these are

produced through everyday practices'.[21] Focusing on everyday practices opens up a vast terrain of sites and contexts through which states
might be anthropologically examined. Thinking about how states are
culturally constituted, how they are substantiated in people's lives,
and about the sociopolitical everyday consequences of these constructions involved moving beyond macro-level institutional analysis of
the state and looking into, among others, bureaucratic practices and
encounters and public cultural texts.[22] These studies also encourage
us to look at modern states as 'embodied forms'.[23] Such a perspective acquires a special relevance in the context of the Andaman Islands
where the imperative of tribal welfare drives the state to create spaces
of interaction and power (the Jarawa Reserve for instance) that are
inherently 'corporal formations' created and sustained through the
deployment and regulation of bodily practices. Tribal Reserves in the
Andaman Islands continue to be places where the state through its
agents of welfare reaches deep into the communities' interior spaces,
into the recesses of daily life and acquires what has been described
as a distinct corporal habitus.[24] It tries to explore the ways in which
Dr Kar's ethnography offers a fleeting glimpse into the corporal habitus
of the state in the forest wherein biomedicine and the 'primitive body'
co-constitute themselves through a contingent assemblage of discourses
and practices which defy the certitudes of foundational categories and
the disciplinary imperatives of the archive.

Narratives of Encounter

It was the 11th of December 1998, the day of the Jarawas' first
encounter with a state medical practitioner. I still remember the day
very vividly. We set out on a little a dinghy towards the Jarawa camp
of Lakralungta ... we had to reach medical services to this part of the
Jarawa camps in the Middle Andamans. ... After sailing westwards for
about half an hour, Lakralungta suddenly appeared before our eyes ...
what a beautiful location it was on the west coast of the Middle
Andamans! As we sailed a little further up, we spotted a large group of
jet-black naked people staring at us in bewilderment![25]

Immediately after this dramatic description of the first encounter, Kar
turns to a different line of questions. From where did these Negritos
come to these isolated Islands? For how many thousands of years have

they lived here? Kar tells his readers that these were the questions whirling in his head as the dinghy was slowly anchored on the beach. Dr Kar felt he had suddenly become a curious anthropologist![26] At that moment a small group of Jarawa children scrambled onto the dinghy and started grabbing the coconuts and bananas that the medical team had brought for them. A few minutes later, after having collected their 'gifts' from the shore, they ran back to their huts. Following them Dr Kar and his team walked up the beach towards those huts. They could not see much from the distance as huge swirls of smoke rose up in the air and clouded their vision for a few minutes. As the smoke cleared the team stood face to face with the huge group of Jarawas staring at them in awe and suspicion. They kept asking the tribal welfare officer who accompanied Dr Kar and his team and who was familiar to them whether Dr Kar could be trusted as a friend. On repeated reassurances they allowed him to enter their huts. Armed with a small box of bandages and antibiotic ointment, Dr Kar treated his first Jarawa patient. He wondered if he had made a sudden and unsolicited entry into their world of medicine! In his words, 'from that day on my medical career took a new turn'.[27] Interestingly enough, Dr Kar's narrative seemed to suggest that all went well from this initial moment of mutual discomfiture. The relative ease of the encounter, we are told, was ensured by the presence of the tribal welfare officer, who was known to this group of Jarawas. Once the Jarawas were convinced that Dr Kar was a friend, they willingly allowed him into their huts. The dramatic build-up to the moment of the first encounter with its ominous signs of suspicion and fear is pleasantly resolved in the course of the next few paragraphs.[28]

Notwithstanding the occasional moments of self-doubt, Dr Kar's memoir goes on to record subsequent trips into the Jarawa huts; each one of seemingly greater significance than the other. Dr Kar provides extensive details of these 'fables of rapport' that serve to provide a counterpoint to possible questions relating to the legitimacy of his presence in the forest.[29] Such questions of legitimacy are addressed through two interesting strategies: one, through descriptions of those moments in these encounters where his Jarawa patients displayed positive signs of affection towards him and, second, through a careful recording of Jarawa curiosity about the new experience of medical care accorded to them.[30]

In the month of March 1999, Dr Kar tells his readers, he had the
most memorable experience during his third visit to the camp of
Lakralungta. During this visit his team set up a little mobile clinic
on the edge of the forest. While some willingly came out of the forest to get themselves examined or receive specific treatments, Dr Kar
was compelled to trudge into the interiors to treat those whose health
conditions were more fragile.[31] In the course of one of these visits,
Dr Kar seemed to have lost his way. He had tried to reach the beach
clinic by himself but was unable to retrace the route through which
he had walked in. As he struggled to find his way, he encountered a
group of Jarawa men who on seeing his predicament took him along
the route they used to come to the beach. This sharing of their own
route with a stranger, was according to Dr Kar, unprecedented. They
would never have done it for anyone else. But this was not all. There
was more help coming his way as he fell on the way and hurt his
right leg. The fall was so sharp that it immobilized him completely
and he couldn't stand on his feet for the next one hour. To his utmost
surprise all the group members sat around him and waited anxiously
until the pain subsided and he was able to walk again. Dr Kar tells us
that the incident was to leave an indelible impression on his mind and
strengthen his growing conviction that the Jarawas were able to 'feel'
like us![32]

With the growing acceptance of the medical team in the forest,
the tribal welfare officers were able to bring many Jarawa men and
women for further treatment into the hospital at the settlement of
Kadamtala. Here Dr Kar writes, the Jarawa were exposed to a more
complex medical regime with regular periods of stay in the hospital
and a fuller exposure to a whole new range of medical instruments and
practices. Dr Kar introduces a new element into his narrative from this
point on. This is not about descriptions of Jarawa unease or resistance
to the new medical environment, but a clear and emphatic statement
of the Jarawas' sense of wonder and curiosity about a world of things
unknown to them and a happy acceptance of much of it.[33]

Dr Kar tells us that the Jarawas' medical experience at the
Kadamtala hospital says much about the nature of the impact of
their contacts with the Outsider. The Jarawas, he says, are given to
mimicry. Although housed in a separate ward away from the main
hospital building meant for the non-tribal settlers, Jarawa children in

particular were seen to be keen to move out of their isolated rooms and play with other children in the hospital courtyard. As far as the adult patients were concerned, many of them were seen to seek the company of medical staff and offer help in doing little errands. They displayed a remarkable spontaneity in establishing relationships with doctors, nurses, and all the other staff deputed to help them. They were ceaselessly curious about all that was going on around them in the various wards. The telephone and the stethoscope were two objects that aroused their greatest curiosity. Medical staff were keen to indulge their curiosity by allowing them to pick up phones or play with the stethoscopes when doctors were away! Some of the more adventurous among them would sneak into the laboratory and urge Dr Kar to let them peer into the microscope or look at all the little bottles around it. Others were drawn into the hospital kitchen where smells of alien spices filled the air and burnt their noses! Many would scramble out rubbing their eyes and vow to never return again. When Dr Kar took them to the department of radiology to get X-rays done, many would ask him to show them the plates and demand explanations about what all of it said about their illness.[34]

Dr Kar's anecdotal rendition of these little vignettes of the Jarawa experience of biomedicine at Kadamtala adds up to his overall narrative of personal accomplishment. He is able to win the affection of his patients, arouse their sense of curiosity, command respect, and ensure the continuance and legitimacy of the state medical project for the Andamanese PVTGs. Dr Kar juxtaposes this 'affective' encounter with the Jarawas at the Kadamtala hospital with background narrative of continuous conflict between the Jarawas and settlers residing on the fringes on the reserve forests in Middle and South Andaman.[35] Most of these conflicts centred on complaints about Jarawa youth entering the villages and looting and vandalizing whatever came their way. From wristwatches to utensils to bananas and coconuts, villagers complained that nothing could be kept safe from bands of marauding Jarawa men and women who entered their homes anytime, any day. The situation went out of hand when it was observed that a group of Jarawas from the reserve of Middle Andamans had set up their camp right on the edge of the Andaman Trunk Road (ATR). Tribal welfare staff feared that this was indicative that vehicles and commuters on the road were likely to be their next targets. Two cases of looting were soon reported. One was on the 14 October 2000 and the other was on the very next day. It was at this point that Dr Kar and his team decided to intervene. The objective was to persuade the Jarawas to remove their campsite from Dhani Nullah on the fringes of the ATR to interiors of Lakralungta where it was originally set up. The task, he argues, was a difficult one and they had to resort to deception and false promises to convince the Jarawas.[36]

Although the removal of the Jarawa camp back into the interiors of the forest was regarded to be a significant success, incidents of conflict and what was deemed as 'unpredictable' behaviour on the part of the Jarawas continued unabated. Thus while there were reports of the Jarawas dancing and doing their best to please the visiting Tribal Welfare Minister, there were simultaneous reports of them entering nearby villages and picking up whatever they could. More surprisingly there were attacks on the tribal welfare staff themselves when some of them refused to accommodate a large group of Jarawas on the small dinghy in which they were travelling.

Dr Kar reports these incidents as part of his dilemma in confronting what seemed to be a wholly unexpected situation. The very same tribal elders who met him at the Kadamtala hospital and seemed to be completely at ease with the villagers around them were found to be resorting to acts of looting and violence in another context. The narrative of Jarawa conflict with the villagers, however, fails to record the numerous cases of poaching in the forest. Tribal welfare officials remain fully aware of the fact that the seemingly random incidents of violence are part of the Jarawas' own strategies of defence against the constant intrusion of settlers into the tribal reserves.[37]

The Jarawas in Dr Kar's narrative are 'like us' in one context and 'alien and unknown' in another. They are individual men and women with names and distinctive personalities in the hospital but a primitive tribe outside its confines, given to inexplicable hostility and violence against the very same people who they befriended in the course of their medical treatment. The juxtaposition of stories about a grief-stricken Jarawa mother mourning the death of her only child in a hospital in Chennai and that of a group of Jarawa men and women attacking commuters on the ATR apparently without provocation bring out a complexity in Dr Kar's narrative which he himself sets out to unravel in the concluding chapters of his book. It is here that we find Dr Kar struggling to present the Jarawas within the framework of an 'alterity' that is both radical and amenable.[38]

Narratives of Triumph

Kar and his team were able to face up to the challenges of a series of medical crises that affected the Jarawas during this period. Many of the afflictions suffered by the Jarawas were deemed to be post-contact conditions. Between 1998 and 2003, the community underwent a series of illnesses including severe cases of tuber poisoning (1998), measles (1999), mumps (2000), malaria (2001), and Hepatitis E (2002–3).[39] Apart from these severities, there were chronic cases of respiratory tract infections, skin diseases, and bone injuries. Clearly each of these particular conditions demanded different kinds of medical treatment, hospital stays, and health regimens. Dr Kar studiously avoids any discussions of these. All that we are told is that notwithstanding widespread anxieties about the mortality of the Jarawas during the outbreak of diseases such as measles, the team led by Dr Kar was able to limit the number of deaths to just a few. We are also told that despite some rare occasions of resistance to medical intervention, Jarawa patients were on most occasions receptive to most forms of treatment, many of them smilingly accepting the pain of intramuscular and intravenous injections![40]

Readers expecting to get a sense of the debates within the tribal health establishment relating to the application of specific forms of drugs on a people completely unaccustomed to any forms of biomedicine are sorely disappointed. There is absolutely no discussion on what could be described as some of the most critical issues in the health care of indigenous communities. Medical department records are out of bounds for outsiders, and all that one gets to know of the state's thinking on these issues are periodic statements about the feasibility or not of putting these communities through a full-scale regime of biomedicine or combining biomedicine with other more natural or alternative medical practices.[41]

Dr Kar's narrative on the health crises affecting the Jarawas between 1998 and 2003 seems to be curiously de-contextualized. He appears to be operating on a purely personal capacity with a small and dedicated team of tribal welfare staff. There are no recorded moments of self-doubt, of things going wrong or of concern about the larger implications of these crises in shaping the structure of medical care. The description of the diseases and their relation to the experience of contact, however, is underscored repeatedly. The first case of tuber poisoning that happened in 1998, for instance, was related to the fact that the Jarawas belonging to the Middle Andamans had ventured out from their familiar gathering spots in the forest and entered areas around the village of Kadamtala, where they picked up tubers from grounds that were polluted with toxic waste. Similarly the hepatitis-E epidemic that struck the community in 2002 was related to the fact that the community had come out of their forests and drank from a polluted source. The scourge of malaria too was related to their coming into frequent contact with road workers along the (ATR). Dr Kar argues that the propensity of Jarawa youth to venture out of their familiar foraging spaces in the forest and come out into the settler villages was particularly evident ever since the Enmei incident of 1998. Some sections of the community residing around the villages of the Middle Andamans were often seen to build their huts in locations where contact with all kinds of outsiders, tourists included, was inevitable. In most such cases, the Jarawas were compelled by tribal welfare staff to relocate their huts deeper into the forests and to return to more familiar foraging practices.[42]

The overall sense that one gets from this rendition is that notwithstanding the series of severe medical crises that faced Dr Kar and his team, morbidity rates within the community were remarkably small. In the course of his ten-year stint among the Jarawas, Dr Kar says that only ten members of the community lost their lives, five of whom were not directly under his care. Although there was widespread anxiety among international tribal rights groups such as Cultural Survival about the Jarawas' imminent death in the face of the measles epidemic of 1999 and after, Dr Kar proudly proclaims that most of these fears proved to be unfounded. A third of the community of 260 may have been afflicted, but the medical team's relentless work ensured their full recovery and survival.[43]

Unlike the chapter that recorded the first encounters between the Jarawas and Dr Kar's medical team, the chapter on the specific health crises facing the community between 1998 and 2003 reads more like a public medical report addressed not merely to the Island administration in Port Blair but to various civil society groups critical of the Indian state's policies of tribal welfare in general and medical care in particular. It is a sanitized chronology of medical crises, a dispassionate account of possible causes, general statistics of recovery and mortality, and finally a general statement of satisfaction that all problems were successfully addressed. Dr Kar's final reflections are on the need of preventive and promotive health care for the indigenous communities. There appear clear points of tension in these recommendations. On the one hand there is a stated need to address issues of nutrition, hygiene, and lifestyle while on the other there is a caveat that any change of lifestyle must not interfere with existing cultural practices. Yet the case for a more systematic application of biomedicine was compelling—the project of 'preventive and promotive' health care hinged on it. Dr Kar observes that although a regime of vaccination has not been introduced among the Jarawas so far, the time had come to think of introducing it at some level. The Jarawas had in the course of the last few decades become a high-density population with an experience of contact with the outsider. In these circumstances it was advisable to consult experts on the issue of an aggressive or selective regime of vaccination. There were fears that that Jarawas in the coming years could be vulnerable to more deadly viruses and diseases such as small pox, typhoid, and viral hepatitis. All these concerns, he argues, had to be debated within the frames of biomedical practices introduced among indigenous communities in other parts of the world.[44]

Modern biomedicine demands the adoption of specific nutritional and hygienic standards. Yet Dr Kar argues that such standards cannot override the practices and procedures involved in a lifestyle sustained by indigenous medical regimes. He makes the point that although the Jarawas had demonstrated their acceptance of modern biomedical practices, there was always the fear that any rapid imposition of conditions could prove to be counterproductive.[45]

The case for biomedicine is made but with a certain 'ethnographic sensitivity'. Dr Kar grounds his observations on what he describes as his first-hand experience of the community with whom he had interacted as a participant-observer. In arguing his case for a certain kind of a medical regime for the Jarawa, Dr Kar combines in himself the authoritative voice of the modern medical practitioner and an engaged ethnographer. The sections that follow are indicative of the conscious ethnographic turn he undertakes in his work. The titles of these sections include 'The Traditional Medical System of the Jarawas', 'The Ancient Identity of the Jarawas', 'Jarawa Habitats and Camps in Present Times', 'The Population of the Jarawas', and finally, 'The Daily Life of the Jarawa'. These sections are further subdivided into short chapters each giving us a short ethnographic record of customs, habits, diet, festivals, ritual practices, funerary rites, and so on. All these are meant to draw his readers into a world they would have never been able to enter.[46] Dr Kar's singular achievement as a medical practitioner is his ability to chronicle the life of the Jarawa in the forest, as participant-observer and classical ethnographer. In his very meagre bibliography at the end, among the three books he refers to are the colonial ethnographer Maurice Vidal Portman's two volume classic, *A History of Our Relations with the Andamanese*.[47] Dr Kar is evidently aware of the significance of keeping Portman as a final reference point in the context of the historical legacy and iconic status Portman continues to enjoy in the Islands.

Narratives of Legitimacy

Dr Kar's month-long stay among the Jarawas in a camp adjacent to theirs from 11 December 2001 was, according to him, the most significant phase of his career as a medical practitioner. This was particularly because the period marked the beginning of a phase of uneasy truce between the Jarawas and settlers after a year-long spate of violent encounters. According to Dr Kar, the pretext for this violent phase was a sudden rise in the frequency of Jarawa visits into the neighbouring villages. The initial demands were for tobacco and betel nut, to which many young Jarawa men were addicted, but soon these became occasions for random loot and plunder. Dr Kar cites settler accounts of these attacks to make the point that the Jarawas were emboldened by the constant reassurances they got from the welfare staff that in spite of their 'misdemeanors' they would not be subject to any form of retaliatory attack by the villagers. The tribal welfare staff would be there to 'protect' them. Towards the end of 2001, however, the acrimony of the past year seemed to have subsided and the tribal welfare team found it opportune to enter the Tribal Reserve and initiate a systematic study of quotidian life in the forest, of indigenous culture, and medical practice.[48]

Dr Kar prefaced this section of his narrative with the following observation:

> In my opinion, in the context of the Jarawa contact, conflict and cultural exchange with the Outsider, this was a significant development. It was a rare opportunity to live close to the primitive community and learn about their grievances and aspirations or even research them as anthropological subjects. This was to be an adventure![49]

Dr Kar's team included a Tribal Welfare Officer, a member of staff each from the Anthropological Society of India, the Botanical Survey, and the Zoological Survey, members from the Andaman and Nicobar police, and a couple of male attendants to help with cooking and cleaning routines at the campsite. The chosen camp was Hu-Lele in the Jarawa Tribal Reserve of the Middle Andamans. Part of the reason for choosing this campsite was Dr Kar's familiarity with its members, many of whom were treated by him. Some of the team members, however, continued to remain sceptical about the kind of reception they would receive in spite of repeated assurances from Dr Kar. As the dinghy anchored on the shore near the campsite, Dr Kar was persuaded to walk out first and inform the camp members about the reason, purpose, and duration of stay of the team there.

In Dr Kar's own words, the exercise proved to be a particularly easy one.

> On reaching Hu-Lele *chadda* (a campsite or a cluster of huts), I beckoned a group of young Jarawa men who stood close by. ... I told them I would stay there for a few days with my friends—I would look after those who were ill and give them medicines. I asked them if they had any objections to this arrangement? At this the Jarawa men looked at me and smiled warmly. Some of them expressed their delight by dancing a little jig, while others called on their families to help us put up our tents.[50]

In the days that followed, Dr Kar and his team formed themselves into small groups with specific research interests. Dr Kar's own interests led him into researching what he took to be the Jarawa's indigenous medical practices. In an interesting shift of tone, Dr Kar's narrative on Jarawa medicine moved from the counter-modern romantic strain of the earlier chapter where he celebrated the simple, childlike innocence of these people to a predictably modern voice of censure of the 'primitive' predicament. To be fair to him, however, the Jarawa medical practice gets a mixed report card. The Jarawas are praised for their remarkably effective management of reproductive processes while heavily censured for their 'weird' approaches to treat bodily 'pains'. For Dr Kar, Jarawa practices of treating coughs, colds, and fevers with strips of bark and leaves around the waist had no 'scientific explanation'. These were nothing but expressions of blind faith. He lamented the fact that they had nothing approximating the modern antibiotic in their traditional medicine. This made them more susceptible to infections.[51]

Yet, when it came to managing childbirth, the Jarawas, according to Dr Kar, seemed to be following perfectly rational methods. None of the young children he examined during his stay suffered from umbilical sepsis, nor where there any observed cases of post-partum haemorrhage among new mothers. The juices of *oro* leaves that women applied to stop post-childbirth bleeding had proven coagulant properties. Dr Kar's general assessment of the Jarawas' medical condition was that they were in general endowed with sturdy constitutions, had no congenital disabilities, no surgical problems, no instances of hypertension, diabetes, or unusual levels of cholesterol. In sum, the Jarawas were able to sustain the enduring attributes of a 'primitive body' relatively untouched by the scourge of modern constitutional dysfunctionalities.[52]

Yet, he concludes that the Jarawas remain deeply vulnerable to the consequences of sustained contact with the Outsider. Their emerging health problems were the first indications of the hazards of exposure to a world outside the forest as to the regime of modern welfare. The change in their dietary habits and their increased dependence on items of food provided by the welfare office proved to have a debilitating impact on their constitutions. Notwithstanding this mild critique of state welfare policy, Dr Kar argues emphatically that the state medical department deserved commendation for its ability to keep the Jarawas alive in their 'primitive innocence'! It had taken modern medicine to the 'primitive', but only to sustain its 'primitive' entity. Dr Kar is deeply sceptical of all opinions to 'mainstream' the Jarawa. Nor is he quite sure about the benefits of keeping them in 'isolation'. He charts out a possible midway, which he says is based on views expressed by the Jarawas themselves. The Jarawas, he argues, are willing to accept the inevitability of contact with the Outsider but only on their own terms.[53]

Notwithstanding the precariousness of his own position as an Outsider in the forest, Dr Kar interprets his access and acceptance in its interior spaces as testimony to the legitimacy of the state's custodianship of the Andamanese. It is a custodianship that is beyond scrutiny, debate, and public accountability. There is little need to archive its constitutive moments or its long-term consequences. Dr Kar's book is recognized and celebrated by the state not merely as a medical memoir or accessible popular ethnography but as reinforcement of its triumphant narrative of nurturing a 'primitive people' under the benevolent aegis of a modern state.[54]

* * *

Yet the positioning of Dr Kar's book as part medical journal and part ethnography, with the ethnographic element in some ways valued over the medical, sets up the points of tension that would eventually reveal the more fundamental tensions underlying the structures of state welfare policy in the Andaman Islands and the politics of knowledge informing it.[55] This chapter has attempted to explore these points of tension as part of a larger attempt to understand the constitutive discourses that continue to shape the state's relationship with its 'primitive' population. It has tried to argue how the state's representation of its medical policy towards the indigenous communities forecloses the possibility of scrutiny or debate. For such representations tend to overwhelm the medical content of policy with loud self-congratulatory platitudes. The 'primitive' Jarawa are positioned as embodying an amenable alterity—an alterity that only the state can access, know, and manage.[56]

Dr Kar's account reinforces the argument that medical discourses such as the state's anthropological discourse is about defining the boundaries of admissible debate. One of the enabling conditions for tribal welfare policy in the Andamans, he implicitly affirms, is about the importance of ensuring the legitimacy of the state's custodianship of its 'primitive' population. In this context, the realities of the complex, messy, and contentious terrain of medical practice among the indigenous communities is best left unstated. Successful medical practice needs to be measured in terms of population statistics on the one hand and projections of affective ties between medical practitioners and their patients on the other. Once that correlation is established all debate is deemed redundant.

Yet, any close reading of state medical discourse in the Andamans unwittingly reveals as much as it conceals. Dr Kar's narrative, for instance, offers a peek into the constitution of the medical in the complex arena of state practice in the forest interiors of the Andaman Islands where states, bodies, and divergent or incommensurable rationalities become entwined in contingent formations of power. It is in these intimate spaces that the heroic narrative of biomedicine shapes the 'primitive body' as both pristine and amenable. In doing so it also narrates its own complex self-fashioning in the forest as a practice that legitimizes its authority by eluding the bounds of defined categories, meanings, practices, and archives.

An exploration of the narrative structure and consequences of Dr Kar's ethnographic/medical memoir has thus allowed us to address some of the key concerns of this volume, particularly the question of the constitution of the 'medical'. Dr Kar's heroic narrative on the making of his 'medical authority' in the forest offers important insights into the contingent formations of the 'medical' in the interstices of tribal welfare practices in the Andaman Islands. The contingent, ambivalent and largely elusive configurations of the 'medical' among the Andamanese are reflective of the larger ambiguities informing the Indian state's relations with its 'primitive' populations. The 'medical' in such contexts often becomes an euphemism for the intrusive enactments of the state in the quotidian lives of these communities. Dr Kar's narrative affirms this 'corporal' presence of the state in the forest and celebrates the ways in which the everyday state, the anthropologized 'primitive', and the biomedical are shaped in relation to one another.

Notes

1. This chapter builds on the earlier work of Pandya on Onge and Jarawa experience of biomedicine. See, for instance, Pandya's '"Do Not Resist, Show Me Your Body!" Encounters between the Jarawas of the Andamans and Medicine (1858–2004)', *Anthropology and Medicine* 12, no. 3 (December 2005): 211–23 and 'Pain in All the Wrong Places: The Experience of Biomedicine among the Onge of Little Andaman', in *Medical Marginality in South Asia: Situating Subaltern Therapeutics*, edited by David Hardiman and

Projit Bihari Mukharji (Routledge, 2012), pp. 59–84. It also brings together insights developed from field and archival work undertaken by Pandya and Mazumdar in connection with an Economic and Social Research Council (ESRC)-funded collaborative research project with Clare Anderson, titled 'Integrated Histories of the Andaman Islands' (2009–12).

2. Although referred to as 'Primitive Tribes' until late, the five indigenous communities of the Andaman and Nicobar Islands are now designated as Particularly Vulnerable Tribal Groups or PVTGs. Official population figures for the five communities are: the Great Andamanese, 61, the Onge, 115, Jarawas, 452, Sentinelese, estimated 50, and the Shompen of the Nicobar Islands, 220 (*A and N* [A Quarterly from Andaman Nicobar Islands Administration], May–July 2016, p. 3).

3. There have been exceptions to this rule as a recent field research undertaken by Pandya brought out valuable information from field pharmacists associated with the Andaman Adim Janjati Vikas Samiti (AAJVS), the tribal welfare organization of the Islands.

4. Elizabeth Matthews, 'Health Problems and Healthcare in the Transition Phase', in *Jarawa Contact: Ours with Them, Theirs with Ours*, edited by R.K. Bhattacharya, K.K. Mukhopadhyay, and B.N. Sarkar (Calcutta: Anthropological Survey of India, 2002), pp. 155–60.

5. *A and N*, p. 3.

6. See, for instance, the ethnographic surveys of Colonel E.H. Man, *On the Aboriginal Inhabitants of the Andaman Islands* (first printed 1883), reprint (Delhi, 1975), pp. 16–20. Man's researches on the Andamanese physiognomy and medicine followed the *Notes and Queries* format laid out by the British Association for the Advancement of Science (BAAS).

7. All of these were seen as classic 'post-contact' diseases commonly afflicting people living in complete or relative isolation.

8. The most anxious and earnest critic of the Indian government in this regard as been Survival International, a human rights organization established in 1969. The Survival campaign drew attention to the fact that diseases such as measles were responsible for wiping out many tribes worldwide following contact with outsiders.

9. It may be noted here that on 23 July 2003 the Tribal Welfare Department did organize a day-long workshop to formulate a standard medical practice regime. Two of the recommendations made were to inoculate all newborns and maintain regular records. But the recommendations made therein were never really implemented and eventually 'dismissed' by the 2004 Jarawa Expert Committee report.

10. Ratan Chandra Kar, *Andamaner Adim Janajati Jarawa* (Port Blair: Amrapali Publications, 2009).

11. A recent newspaper report celebrates the fact by quoting that the Jarawa population had recorded a 62 per cent growth since 2001. See http://timesofindia.indiatimes.com/city/kolkata/Jarawa-numbers-up-62-in-15-yrs/articleshow/52814739.cms, last accessed 21 July 2017.

12. Kar, *Andamaner Adim Janajati*, 'Introduction'.

13. Kar, *Andamaner Adim Janajati*, 'Abataranika' (Preface).

14. For a discussion of the nine conventions of realist ethnography, see G.E. Marcus and D. Cushing, 'Reading Ethnography as Text', *Annual Review of Anthropology* 11 (1982): 25–69.

15. See, among others, Vishvajit Pandya, *In the Forest: Visual and Material Worlds of Andamanese History (1858–2006)* (Lanham, Maryland: University Press of America, 2009), pp. 291–7.

16. Pandya, *In the Forest*, pp. 291–7.

17. Kar, *Andamaner Adim Janajati*, pp. 15–16.

18. According to a recent press release by the Ministry of Tribal Affairs, New Delhi, the numbers of the Jarawa population had gone up from 240 in 2001 to 375 in 2010 (*The Daily Telegram*, Island Administration, Port Blair, 8 December 2010).

19. Dr Livingstone (1813–1873) was a medical missionary associated with the London Missionary Society and was an explorer in Africa.

20. Aradhana Sharma and Akhil Gupta, eds, *The Anthropology of the State—A Reader* (Blackwell, 2006), pp. 26–7.

21. Sharma and Gupta, *Anthropology of the State*, pp. 26–7.

22. Sharma and Gupta, *Anthropology of the State*, pp. 26–7.

23. See, for instance, U. Linke, 'Contact Zones: Re-thinking the Sensual Life of the State', *Anthropological Theory* 6, no. 2 (2006): 205–25.

24. Marcel Mauss, 'Techniques of the Body', *Economy and Society* 2, no. 1 (1973): 70–88.

25. Kar, *Andamaner Adim Janajati*, p. 39.

26. Kar, *Andamaner Adim Janajati*, pp. 39–40.

27. Kar, *Andamaner Adim Janajati*, p. 40.

28. What Dr Kar wilfully ignored in his rendition of the first encounter was the fact that the relative ease of the Jarawa acceptance of his bandage and ointment treatment was because contact teams entering the Jarawa reserve from as early as 1984 always had a doctor who was deployed to treat arrow wounds with basic antiseptics. This was a practice welcomed and accepted by most.

29. Part of realist ethnographic strategy as discussed by Marcus and Cushing, 'Reading Ethnography as Text', pp. 33–4.

30. Kar, *Andamaner Adim Janajati*, pp. 42–5.

31. We, of course, have no idea how he was informed about this situation. As his vocabulary of the Jarawa language at that point must have been limited

to the occasional contacts at Lakralungta. (See M. Sreenathan, *The Jarawa Language and Culture* [Calcutta: Anthropological Survey of India, 2000].)

32. Kar, *Andamaner Adim Janajati*. For details of incidents such as these, see, chapters 4 and 5, pp. 39–56.

33. Jarawas were also keen to come to the medical facilities in large numbers, not only for the patient care they received but for the unusual levels of hospitality they enjoyed and the large number of gifts they acquired in the form of food items, clothes, and beads and trinkets of various kinds. See, Pandya, *In the Forest*.

34. Kar, *Andamaner Adim Janajati*, pp. 42–3.

35. Kar, *Andamaner Adim Janajati*, pp. 47–9.

36. Kar, *Andamaner Adim Janajati*, pp. 47–9.

37. See Pandya, 'Events, Incidents, Accidents: Rethinking Indigenous Resistance in the Andaman Islands', in *Savage Attacks: Tribal Insurgency in South Asia*, edited by C. Bates and A. Shah (New Delhi: Social Science Press, forthcoming).

38. The term 'alterity' as used in philosophy and social theory refers to the 'quality of state of being other'. It connotes the ways in which difference or otherness is socially and historically produced. More nuanced connotations of 'alterity' have been elaborated by, among others, Johannes Fabian, *Time and Other: How Anthropology Makes Its Subject* (Columbia University Press, 1993).

39. Medical details related to these epidemics were presented at a closed-door seminar in 2003, to which Pandya was invited as a speaker. In the document that was presented to participants, there was the following data: there were 49 reported cases of pneumonia, 95 cases of measles, 93 cases of malaria, and 12 cases of viral hepatitis. Antibiotic drugs such as ampicillin were used to treat pneumonia and measles, chlorquine, and primaquine for malaria, and symptomatic treatment was deployed for viral hepatitis E patients. The number of recorded deaths was one.

40. Kar, *Andamaner Adim Janajati*, p. 62.

41. For details, see, S.A. Awaradi, *The Jarawa Master Plan 1991–2021* (Port Blair: Andaman and Nicobar Administration, 1990). In this master plan, it was stated that health management for the Jarawas would need to have two aspects: one of fighting out the invasion of foreign diseases by employing modern medical treatment, and second encouragement of ethno-medicine. How these were to be put together was not discussed at this stage. All that was categorically stated was that a primary ship would be sent out to the tribal reserve once a week with a medical officer in charge. An extension officer from the tribal welfare agency, the AAJVS, would prepare a health report of the Jarawa population in that reserve

and present it to the medical officer, who would then decide on specific forms of treatment. Jarawa patients would get treatment on board and also retained there, if necessary. At this point it was still uncertain whether and how and what forms of modern medical treatment would be deemed appropriate (Awaradi, *Jarawa Master Plan*, pp. 176–7).

42. Kar, *Andamaner Adim Janajati*, pp. 62–3.

43. Kar, *Andamaner Adim Janajati*, pp. 64. Kar makes reference also to an article published in the *The Daily Telegraph*, London, titled, 'Modern World May Spell Death for Ancient Tribe', 19 September, 1999.

44. Kar, *Andamaner Adim Janajati*, pp. 67–8.

45. Kar, *Andamaner Adim Janajati*, pp. 67–8.

46. See chapters 7–11, Kar, *Andamaner Adim Janajati*, pp. 70–93

47. Maurice Vidal Portman (1861–1935) was a British naval officer who landed himself an appointment as officer in charge of the Andamanese in 1879. Portman researched and wrote extensively on the Andamanese. His best known work, *A History of Our Relations with the Andamanese*, being published in two volumes in 1899.

48. Kar, *Andamaner Adim Janajati*, pp. 53–4.

49. Kar, *Andamaner Adim Janajati*, pp. 53–4.

50. Kar, *Andamaner Adim Janajati*, p. 54.

51. Kar, *Andamaner Adim Janajati*, pp. 70–3.

52. Kar, *Andamaner Adim Janajati*, pp. 70–3.

53. Kar, *Andamaner Adim Janajati*, pp. 70–3.

54. He expressed satisfaction at the fact that at the height of the international debates generated in the context of the epidemics, the *New Indian Express* despite its earlier criticism of the government finally came out with an editorial titled 'Government Holds Keys to Jarawa Survival' (20th October 1999), which for Kar was an acknowledgement of the efforts that were being put in by the tribal welfare department and the medical authorities in particular.

55. See, among others, Pandya, *In the Forest*.

56. Kar, *Andamaner Adim Janajati*, p. 140. See chapter titled *Paribartaner Pathe* or the 'Road to Change'.

III

RETHINKING DISCONNECTIONS AND CONTINUITIES

6

THE MAKING OF AN ECLECTIC ARCHIVE

Epistemologies of Global Knowledge in the Papers of J.P. Walker (1823–1906)

CLARE ANDERSON[1]

Lining the shelves in the basement of the Lloyd Library and Museum in Cincinnati, Ohio, Unites States of America, are 461 handwritten, leather-bound volumes, compiled by retired surgeon-general of the Indian Medical Service, Dr James Pattison Walker (1823–1906). Walker bequeathed the volumes, which he envisaged as the basis of a vast medical encyclopaedia, to the Lloyd Library, along with his extensive personal library and the considerable sum of £6,000.[2] The *Cincinnati-Times Star* wrote at the time: 'General Walker's collection of books and manuscripts is known to scientific men as one of the most valuable private collections. Its worth cannot be measured by money, for money could not purchase it or duplicate what was gathered in a long life of studious research.' The newspaper continued that the money was to be used for 'original investigations and literary compilations in the direction of the practice of medicine and pharmacy', most particularly the study of the specifications of medicine.[3] The Lloyd Library declined Walker's collection of books, because the conditions of his will prevented its rearrangement and classification as well as the exclusion of books not within the library's scope. Further, after a legal challenge to the will in Britain, the money did not make it to Ohio either.[4]

The Lloyd Library still exists in downtown Cincinnati. Curtis Lloyd and his brother John, two of the great American proponents of eclectic medicine, founded it in the mid-nineteenth century. It is devoted to botany (it has an internationally renowned herbarium collection of fungi) and to materia medica (pharmacology).[5] As Curtis explained shortly after Walker's death, Walker was 'personally a stranger' to him, but had known that the library was the largest and most complete collection of books on specific medicine in the world.[6] Specific medicine, which promoted the efficacy of employing a concentrated botanical remedy for each disease expression, was intertwined with eclectic medicine, which as its name suggests borrowed treatments and cures from a nineteenth-century medical culture 'marked by competing sects'.[7] Eclectic medicine was founded in the USA in the 1840s, part of an anti-elitist movement that claimed to democratize medicine, and it reached the heights of its popularity in the 1880s and 1890s. It favoured American botanical medicines, and drew in part on Indigenous American and other non-mineral botanical traditions.[8] Eclectic practitioners opposed purging, bleeding, and the use of mercury that was common in the nineteenth century, favouring a 'vital' approach, the correction of bodily imbalances. Across two oceans in colonial India, Walker was sympathetic to the eclectic approach, and was later described by one of the Lloyd librarians as 'truly Europe's greatest exponent of Eclecticism in every respect'.[9]

Before he began his great work of medical synthesis, J.P. Walker had a long Indian career. He served for over thirty years as a medical officer in jails in the Northwest Provinces (NWP) and Bengal, and for a brief two-year period as superintendent of the penal colony in the Andaman Islands. As well as his scripting of the Cincinnati volumes, his letters and reports appear frequently in the records of the Oriental and India Office Collections of the British Library and in the National Archives of India in New Delhi. He left his official papers (dated 1844–77) to St Thomas' Hospital, London.[10] And yet, there is a remarkable disconnect between these sets of records, for Walker's British Indian research experience barely appears in the voluminous American papers. If we are to understand Walker's work in India as an element of his interest in eclectic medicine, we are compelled to work across the national and imperial borders that usually underpin the institutional bases of archives, and often define and contain the parameters of research in the history of medicine.

This chapter argues that Walker's papers are significant for our understanding of the history of medicine in and of South Asia, as well as the development of eclectic medicine in the USA. It also explores what Walker's work means for a consideration of the larger relationship between the colonial and the global, in particular the multiple points of contact and layers of interaction (or apparent lack of them) between the history of medicine in India and the Atlantic world. Using evidence from Walker's work in India alongside his medical manuscripts, the chapter will suggest that during the nineteenth century, South Asian and American medical practices informed each other in important ways, with both produced in part out of European colonial encounters—with Indians, Africans, and indigenous Americans. Thus the chapter urges us to appreciate the significance of research across the intellectual and geo-political borders of history writing—medical, colonial, and global. In this way, we can take a fresh approach to the history of medicine by bringing together the historical anthropology of archive making—recognizing the importance of absence and elision as well as textual presence in imperial record-keeping—with 'new' imperial histories that have stressed the importance of transnational relationships, networks, and connections in the making of metropolitan and colonial societies.[11] Walker's papers enable us to gain insights into medicine as an historically contingent organizing principle of social worlds; as part of the materiality of the historical ontology described by the editors in the Introduction to this volume. In thinking through the place of this chapter in the larger theoretical frame of this collection, and, in particular, in thinking through the coloniality of colonial medicine, first, let us turn to Walker's illustrious Indian medical career.

J.P. Walker's Indian Career

Like many of his contemporaries serving in India, J.P. Walker was born in Scotland. He graduated in medicine from King's College in his home city of Aberdeen in 1842, became a member of the Royal College of Surgeons in 1844, and was appointed assistant surgeon in the Bengal Medical Department a year later, aged just 23. Initially, he was placed in medical charge of Indian regiments across Bengal, the NWP, and the Punjab. In 1848, he was appointed civil surgeon of Humeerpoore (NWP), an appointment that was interrupted by his service in the Anglo-Sikh Wars (for which he received the Punjab

Medal and Goojerat Clasp).[12] In 1850 he went back to the NWP and was transferred to Mynpoori.

During this period, civil surgeons worked in jails as well as with troops, with little distinction between medicine and social discipline. Changes to the penal and military regime had potentially significant health effects, for instance with respect to jail or barrack accommodation (wards, cells, ventilation), indoor/outdoor labour, prison or station transfers, transportation or service overseas, rations, the issue of tobacco and opium, and secondary punishment such as fettering, flogging, or the tread wheel. Resistance did too, as prisoners went on hunger strike or self-harmed, refused food, injured themselves, or deliberately caused and opened up sores to avoid work. And of course, prisons and barracks were spaces of medical enquiry where Indians could be scrutinized at close quarters, anthropometrically measured and vaccinated, and tropical diseases studied and treated. It is this blurring of the lines of distinction between colonial punishment, the military, and medicine in South Asia that led David Arnold to define colonial expansion as the colonization of the body.[13] Walker himself actively pursued district vaccination programmes against smallpox, mindful of the positive effects of prisoner inoculation in Bihar as well as amongst sepoys in the NWP.[14]

At the time of Walker's appointment to Humeerpoore in 1848, radical experiments in jail discipline were well underway. A major report into prison discipline in 1838 had generated little subsequent discussion or action. But, in 1845, the government directed the inspector of prisons, W.H. Woodcock, to draw up new rules, classify prisoners, reduce costs, and make prison labour profitable. Perhaps the most controversial subsequent innovation was the replacement of prisoners' per diem allowances with the common messing system, which prescribed that inmates of different castes, classes, and status should eat together. Prisoners across the Bengal Presidency had rioted each time government had attempted to introduce communal eating, with such resistance dating back to the late eighteenth century. Later on, in the 1850s, prisoners in Chuprah (in the Saran district of Bihar) had been joined by 3,000 townspeople in protest against it; in Gaya eighteen prisoners were killed during riots; and in Shahabad sympathetic townspeople set fire to the courthouse, destroying prison records. Against this background, the government of the NWP was understandably cautious in the withdrawal of money allowances. By 1846 it had only been successful in about half of prisons, against a background of riots and discontent.[15]

There were other experiments in jail discipline too. One of Walker's first innovations as civil surgeon in Mynpoori was to teach prisoners to read and write. Lessons took place on Sundays and every other evening. Woodcock reported with evident satisfaction that this was 'the only effort which as far as I am aware has ever been made towards the reformation of criminals by the improvement of their moral condition'. He described a visit to the prison in 1852:

> [W]e were surrounded by 150 prisoners, each with one or more books or slates in their hands, one more anxious than the other, to show his progress in education. About one-third of the prisons have been during the past eighteen months under instruction in reading and writing Nagree, some few in Persian and Hindee; and within the last twelve months forty prisoners have been released with a good knowledge of Nagree, none of whom could previously either read or write.

He added that there were six females in the jail at the time, and that they were the only literate women in the entire district.[16]

Innovations in jail discipline in the NWP included also the establishment of a central prison at Agra for long-term prisoners. From 1846 the jail was under the charge of inspector Woodcock, but his continued absence from Agra on jail business elsewhere held back the pace of change. In 1851, therefore, he recommended that J.P. Walker should replace him, writing that he was 'qualified through talent, temper and judgement, energy and zeal and the knowledge and interest in and of prison discipline'. The government of India agreed, and appointed Walker on a Rs 700 per annum salary with a house.[17] Woodcock's enthusiasm for the appointment was surely informed also by recent events unmentioned in his application. In March 1850 there had been a catastrophic incident after 250 Punjabi prisoners were placed in jail in the aftermath of the Anglo-Sikh Wars. They complained about their rations, and when a fight broke out with the guards, the guards killed and wounded seventy-five men. At the time, the government claimed that the NWP authorities tried to cover the incident up.[18] Meantime, the remaining Punjabi prisoners almost broke out of the jail,[19] and it was in this context that Woodcock requested a new superintendent.

At the time of Walker's appointment to Agra, with just under 3,500 inmates, and partially modelled on a radiating panoptican design, the jail was one of the largest and most innovative prisons in the world. Following his experiments in Mynpoori, Walker introduced lessons in literacy, and perhaps mindful of its success in Alipur near Calcutta, he also set up a lithographic press for the production of books and maps. The new inspector general of prisons, C.B. Thornhill, raved about his colleague: 'Although ... the worst characters in the country are assembled in one spot, the necessity for corporal punishment has almost ceased to exist, and breaches of discipline by violence are unknown.'[20] Walker busied himself with the task of moral reformation, publishing a Hindi copybook and a basic guide to reading and arithmetic. Both were printed at the jail press. He also oversaw the production of 10,000 copies of the vernacular storybook *Gouthun Seetha*, which explained the purpose of vaccination. He later wrote of its immense influence: 'I never did better service to the government of India, in the cause of prophylactic medicine, than in popularising vaccination.'[21]

Walker undertook medical experiments also, most importantly in the treatment of hospital gangrene. Previously, gangrene accounted for a quarter of all deaths in Agra jail, but using an application of burnt alum (antiseptic), Walker almost completely eradicated it. He also invented an ointment made out of powdered alum, catechu (an astringent extracted from acacia and used in ayuvedic medicine, *katha* in Hindi), ballot (extract of *berberis lycium*, or Indian barberry), opium, soap, and water. He claimed that it was effective in treating boils, bruises, sprains, swelling, and even ophthalmia (inflammation of the eye).[22] Walker's remedies were used in later attempts to improve the health of European troops in India.[23] His use of locally sourced remedies was far from unusual at the time, and European interest in existing pharmacopoeia was a significant aspect of Britain's colonization of India.[24] Less usual, however, was his great interest in eclectic medicine. It was said that Walker bought every book and periodical on American materia medica that he could find, that he used 'specific' remedies whenever he could get them, and that he ordered his medical apparatus from American manufacturers.[25] Walker had a private medical practice in Agra in the 1850s, and though the archives reveal nothing at all about his patients, we might speculate that his experience of prisoners and troops, and his knowledge of global medical trends informed the nature of his treatments there.

Walker went back to Europe on leave during 1855–6, and under the patronage of the East India Company, undertook a six-month tour of jails in England, Scotland, Ireland, and the French capital, Paris. His objective was to write a lengthy report on the improvement of prison discipline in India.[26] 'For the last 7 years,' he noted at the start of his trip, 'I have unceasingly and almost exclusively devoted my time and attention to the practical study and improvement of prison discipline in the North West Provinces of India.'[27] Walker subsequently recorded in great detail impressions of sixty prisons, houses of correction, reformatory and industrial schools, debtors' gaols, hulks, and military jails—for men, women, and juveniles. He was especially critical of the separate (cellular) and silent systems, which he saw as unworkable and at odds with prisoner reform; at this time, Agra kept prisoners in jail wards (the associated system).[28] He surmised: 'The general result of my enquiry is that if English penal institutions were transferred to India they would prove failures, more especially as regards construction, ventilation and conservancy arrangements.' Nevertheless, he intended to submit plans for reform to the government on his return to India.[29]

A severe attack of cholera, which left Walker 'prostrated', swiftly followed by the outbreak of the 1857 rebellion, and the breaking open of Agra jail, brought an abrupt end to his plans.[30] Inspector general of prisons, Thornhill, noted the 'admirable constancy and unflinching devotion' of Walker and his assistant, *daroga* (jailer) Lalla Muthoora [Muttra] Doss, as the guards and turnkeys turned against them, the jail was attacked, the prisoners released, and the iron bars and stores were plundered. The government lost 81,590 rupees worth of goods from that one jail during the revolt or, to put it another way, 117 times Walker's annual salary.[31]

No doubt Walker's medical and penal knowledge, his fluency in Hindustani, and his experience of managing Punjabi prisoners of the Anglo-Sikh Wars underpinned the government's subsequent decision to appoint him as the first superintendent of the Andaman Islands, which it occupied as a penal colony in March 1858.[32] Walker arrived in the Islands with the first batch of 200 convicts, accompanied by his trusted Agra daroga, Lalla Doss, and aided by Assistant Surgeon Alexander Gamach, Assistant Apothecary J. Ringrow, two Indian doctors, Nawab Khan and Kurreem Buksh, two hospital assistants, one hospital sweeper, fifty sailors of the Indian naval brigade and their lieutenant.

The settlement received over 3,500 convicts during the period to October 1859, when Walker resigned his position. Mortality rates were appalling, and almost half of all the convicts transported to the Andamans died during the first eighteen months of settlement. A small number of convicts fell foul of accidents, were killed by the Islands' indigenous peoples, or committed suicide. But many convicts were ill from the war and long periods of mainland incarceration before their transportation. The monsoon set in just after the first batch arrived; their tents were inadequate, they often had no choice but to work and sleep in wet clothes and bedding, and they suffered from diarrhoea, dysentery, and fevers. Most significant perhaps were the effects of malaria and ulcers, both caused by the demands of hard labour—the physical effort of clearing dense jungle, injuries from scratches and bruises, and the constant rubbing of fetters against skin that opened up sores, which then became infected.[33] Walker himself blamed the high rates of sickness on the mental state of convicts. He claimed that in the aftermath of their defeat in 1857, the rebels and mutineers were 'reckless and desponding' and cared little for their fate.[34] In 1859 visiting surgeon G.G. Browne agreed, noting parallels with the first Indian transportations to Arakan upon accession at the end of the First Burmese War of 1828. Many of the convicts had been unused to work, had been horrified at the ritual pollutions associated with crossing the sea, and had no hope of seeing their families again. This must, he reported, 'materially affect the sanitary condition of such a settlement as Port Blair'.[35]

It is notable that the first permanent structure in the Andamans was a hospital. It was elevated five feet above ground, and modelled on the Alipur jail hospital, in the hope of protecting convicts from what Walker described as 'damp malarious exhalations'.[36] Health and sickness were closely observed, and the convict hospital became an important space of medical enquiry. Walker and his assistants interviewed convict patients in the settlement hospital and produced detailed studies on their pre-conviction use of opium, marijuana, tobacco, and liquor. They concluded that the sudden withdrawal of narcotics and stimulants upon transportation had had a negative impact on health, and believed that the results of the hospital investigations could be generalized to the entire convict population.[37] In his treatments, Walker was sympathetic to the issue of 'native medicines', including purgatives and tonics. However, other doctors were not so enthusiastic.

Surgeon Browne described how 'a convict, who has a turn for quacking himself or his neighbours, may fool himself and them to the top of his bent'. He added: 'the demand is I believe considerable'.[38]

During the early weeks of settlement, more than a third of all the convicts in the Andamans tried to escape. Some believed that they could find a road to Burma and enlist with the 'Burma rajah' to bring down the penal colony. Walker's response in May 1858 was to execute eighty-one recaptured men in a mass hanging. Though Walker reported with satisfaction that this put an immediate check on escapes, the government of India was horrified. The president in council, J.P. Grant, wrote that the convicts should not have been punished so severely, and ordered him in future to flog and fetter absconders. So doubtful were Walker's actions that the government destroyed his records. For his part, Walker seemed baffled at the lack of mainland understanding of the reality of convict management in the Andamans. Things got even worse. First, a convict plot to assassinate Walker was only narrowly averted, and only after his assistant Lalla Doss was stabbed. Second, the government accused Walker of 'unprovoked aggression' against the indigenous Andamanese, which he was explicitly warned against.[39] Criticized from all quarters, dissatisfied with the long hours and low pay, and missing the financial benefits of his private medical practice in Agra, Walker resigned. 'I require a rest,' he wrote, 'after the physical and mental exertions of establishing and organizing this penal settlement.'[40] Captain J.C. Haughton, then magistrate of Moulmein, which at the time was also the destination for Indian transportation convicts, was appointed as his successor.

Walker went back to the mainland in 1859. He worked briefly as the medical storekeeper of Allahabad, and as the superintendent of the government press and the curator of government books in the NWP. In 1864 he served on the Indian jail commission, and was responsible for the complete revision of the Bengal jail rules, and the preparation of the first-ever complete set of Indian prison forms. At the time it was noted that the latter were more perfect than those existing in Europe and America, and that the innovation would allow India to take a central place in the production of global prison statistics.[41] In 1865 Walker was promoted to surgeon-major and took medical charge of the Bengal Sappers and Miners (engineer corps). He also served as secretary to the sanitary commissioners; who helped to frame the Contagious Diseases

Act of 1868. This formalized the compulsory detention and treatment of prostitutes for venereal disease during a period in which British and colonial practices were inextricably intertwined.[42] Walker became deputy inspector general of hospitals in the NWP in 1872, and retired in 1877 with the honorary rank of surgeon-general.[43] He returned to Britain, not to Scotland but to the Essex seaside resort of Clacton-on-Sea, where he lived for the rest of his life with his wife Frances Ann, until his death in 1906.

Walker's Eclectic Bequest

We do not know for sure when Walker began the process of compiling the medical papers now in the Lloyd Library, but from the dates of some of the news and journal clippings included in them, he likely began work in the 1860s and continued with his labours right up to the year that he died. The collection is huge; and is divided into volumes, notebooks, and newspaper-bound packets of press clippings. The volumes contain 21,795 numbered pages and 175,399 numbered entries, each written by hand. Walker divided them into five series, and he arranged and indexed them with care. The first set is *A Register of Specific and Best Treatment* (5 volumes), the second *Supplementary Notes on Jonathan Pereira's Materia Medica and Therapeutics* (57 volumes), the third *Notes on James Copland's Dictionary of Practical Medicine* (279 volumes), the fourth *Medical Notes* (144 volumes), and the fifth *A Thesaurus of Medical Words and Phrases* (31 volumes).[44] None of the volumes present any original research; they are wholly compiled from other sources. These include written notes, bibliographic references, clippings, proverbs, and even a few sketches and drawings. Topics are mentioned under different headings and are frequently cross-referenced. They offer observations, case histories and remedies on a range of topics: for instance cures for colds, the advantages of vaccination, and comments on valvular heart disease. There is a wide range of headings: 'stormy weather', 'scanty and timid applications in severe diseases', 'want of vital power', and 'drug-treatment', for example. Biblical quotes are scattered throughout the pages, and unsurprising in the context of nineteenth-century evangelical reformism, 'Satan', 'salvation', and 'superstition' each appears. The volumes are transnational in scope; they include material in ancient languages, as well as case studies from all over the world, including Europe, the Americas, and Asia. Accompanying the volumes is a small, alphabetized set of much smaller notebooks that seem to be Walker's first draft of the condensed, publishable version of his extensive labours. Finally, there are forty-six unsorted newspaper-wrapped bundles, which consist mainly of clippings from newspapers and journals, and which Walker evidently wished to consider for inclusion. Indeed, he left a number of pages in the volumes blank for this very purpose.

Compiled by an eclectic practitioner sympathetic to various schools of medicine, and with extensive professional experience in and knowledge of India, Britain, and America, overall the notebooks might be described as an astonishing snapshot into accumulated medical knowledge in the late nineteenth century. As a work in progress they also reveal something of the epistemology of medical knowledge, the way in which Walker synthesized notes, research, evidence, experience, and sources into a work of reference and planned for its publication. An archivist writing in the 1950s noted: 'The minute subdivisions and specified subject headings under each category are a veritable encyclopaedic index of therapy.' She added: 'Had he been living today his theories and comments would be of unusual modern interest.'[45] It is obvious that Walker knew that he would never complete his medical volumes, for his will specified that they be made accessible to physicians who would work towards a series of 'prizes' for their editing and publication. Walker divided his financial legacy (the £6,000 mentioned at the start of this chapter) into twenty-four prizes, arranged into three series of eight prizes each. He named a number of American physicians who might lead the work. Here, we find another part of the explanation for how the volumes ended up in Ohio. Walker's first choice was Dr Harvey Wickes Felter of Cincinnati. Felter was a distinguished proponent of eclectic medicine, a former chair of the city's Eclectic Medicine Society and a contributor to the *Eclectic Medical Journal* and *Eclectic Medical Gleaner*. He worked together with the Lloyd brothers, founders of the Lloyd Library and Museum, and especially John Uri, who was one of the most important pharmacists of the time.[46]

Walker hoped that Felter would oversee the first three prizes offered for the continuation of the compilation of notes and abstracts, according to the extraordinarily detailed plans in his will. The next three prizes were for the editorship of three books based on the manuscript—again

Walker specified in detail the exact contents and arrangement of each. Prizes 7 and 8 were offered for the composition and publication of a book of sermons (104 in number, each an hour long) and a book of daily litanies for the medical profession, questions and answers for surgeons, midwives, nurses, and chemists. Curtis Lloyd thought that only British doctors could undertake the latter, explaining that their American colleagues 'in general do not combine Professional matters with Religeous [sic] ideas.'[47] He added that, in his opinion, Walker's wishes and intentions for medicine 'bear an analogy to what was accomplished by Charles Darwin in the botanical world'. (Famously, Darwin had left money to Kew Gardens to produce the *Index Kewensis*, the formal register of all plant names, now known as *The International Plant Names Index*.[48]) Despite leaving thiry-five pages of detailed instructions, however, in the absence of his planned financial inducements, Walker's great work remains unfinished to this day.

Given Walker's long career in South Asia, it is curious that 'India' per se appears relatively infrequently in the dozens and dozens of newspaper-bound packets of clippings, cardboard boxes and notebooks—and the tens of thousands of hand written entries—that constitute the Lloyd Library's collection. There are a few references, including on the use of Indian hemp in the cure of melancholia in women and a brief reference to the practice of sati (the self-immolation of Hindu widows) in a discussion of whether suicide victims were necessarily insane. Most extensive, relatively speaking, is the heading 'leprosy', under which (unusually) Walker made Hindustani notes of Indian treatments. But in their inclusion of Walker's own knowledge and experience, these entries are highly anomalous to the rest of the collection. Despite his extensive experience of Indian jails (and the tour of English, Scottish, Irish, and Parisian prisons mentioned earlier), the heading 'prisoners' contains only the note: 'Tis not enough to help the feeble up, But to support him after', Sermon of Athens I, 1. While this certainly gives a religious context for his earlier efforts at prisoner education, a second category, 'prison surgeons', appears at the top of blank pages with the reference 'insert notes'. Perhaps Walker intended this page to take the form of that for 'ships surgeons', which contained five 1880s clippings from the *British Medical Journal*, together with two sets of instructions, the first to surgeon superintendents of government emigration ships (1866) and the second to passengers themselves (1882).[49]

However, given what we know of his three decades in India, it is likely that Walker's interest in eclectic medicine emerged out of and was inflected by his knowledge and use of 'native' palliatives and cures. It is clear from his writings on the treatment of hospital gangrene, his description of treatments for leprosy, and his supply of particular types of medicines to prisoners and convicts that he was sympathetic to their use. Little wonder, then, that Walker was a proponent of eclecticism, a supporter of its incorporative approach to and reliance on native plants and remedies. His approach was entirely in keeping with the larger medical appropriations that underpinned colonial encounters— between Europeans, South Asians, and indigenous Americans—and it would appear in this respect that knowledge circulated transnationally around the Atlantic and Indian Oceans as well as between metropoles and colonies. In this sense, Walker's Cincinnati archive might be read beyond its place in the history of eclectic medicine, and beyond the long Indian career of its author. Rather, the volumes are best inter-preted as part of a global history of medicine that drew together indig-enous American, South Asian, and other practices, each pragmatically adopted rather than theorized in or drawn from a singular intellectual frame of understanding.

* * *

Walker died in February 1906, aged 83. A few weeks later, a lengthy obituary appeared in the *British Medical Journal*. We read that Walker was 'able and distinguished', 'a man of talent and energy', who 'lived and served in stirring and critical times and circumstances'. He was intrepid, 'capable,' 'energetic,' and possessed with 'personal enthusiasm, honest earnestness, and marvellous influence'; 'a man of uncommon power, industry, courage, and decision of character. Whatever he did was done conscientiously, laboriously, elaborately, and efficiently'. His disastrous appointment in the Andamans was unmentioned in this tribute, though is easily read into a note that although some of his actions had been seen as rash or indiscreet, 'his censors have not always placed them-selves in his position, or fully realized the gravity of the emergency which occasioned the measures which he adopted'.[50] Walker is buried with his wife in Clacton. His grave is elaborate, stylistically more in keeping with London's Highgate or Calcutta's Park Street than a small cemetery in East Anglia. There is a tall column at the centre of the plot, enclosed with metal bars, and mounted with a towering statue of an angel holding a cross.

Walker's elaborate memorial belies his near-absence from the history of medicine. This is almost certainly in large part because his life's great work—a voluminous medical encyclopaedia of specific and eclectic medicine—was neither completed nor published. However, an appreciation of both his Indian career and his expansive notes for publication, or what we might describe as his archive-in-the-making, together offer a remarkable insight into the production of medical knowledge within a global frame. For once we look outwards from India, from North America and from Britain, and travel beyond and work across national archival borders to explore Walker's global interests and connections, we glimpse in his Indian innovations, in his European prison tours, and in his enthusiasm for American eclecticism a geographically expansive framework within which we might position medical histories of South Asia. This epistemological approach suggests that Walker's interests in 'native' remedies in India might be linked to his interest in specific and eclectic medicine and its incorporative approach to the palliatives and cures of indigenous Americans and African-Americans. This opens up to view a glimpse of the common ground between seemingly separate and disconnected parts of his life. To be sure, this helps us to understand medicine in and of India. However, it also assures Walker a central place in the construction of globalized forms of medical knowledge, enabling insights into the inter-sections between the local, the colonial, and the global.

Notes

1. This research was funded by the Economic and Social Research Council (ESRC), United Kingdom, as part of the collaborative international project 'Integrated Histories of the Andamans' (award no. RES-000-22-3484). I am grateful to the ESRC, to staff in the Wellcome Library and the Asian and African Studies Reading Room of the British Library, and to Anna Heran, curator of the Lloyd Library and Museum, for her assistance during my stay in Cincinnati (http://www.lloydlibrary.org/index.html).

2. At the time, noted as £6,000 with accrued interest—according to The National Archives' currency converter, this is equivalent to approximately £345,000 in 2010.

3. Lloyd Library, *Eclectic Medical Journal* 66, 10 (October 1906): 480–1 (reprinted from *Cincinnati Times-Star*, 20 August 1906).

4. Paice and Cross, 5 St Clements Inn, London, 25 April 1907, High Court of Justice, in the matter of the estate of James Pattison Walker deceased, Lloyd Library, Coll. 11, box 4, folder 40. See also, Corinne Miller Simons, 'Walker's Eclectic Collection in Lloyd Library', *The National Eclectic Medical Quarterly* (June 1950): 8.

5. See the Lloyd Library's website, at http://www.lloydlibrary.org/, accessed 27 April 2012.

6. Testimony of Curtis Lloyd, 30 January 1907, High Court of Justice, in the matter of the estate of James Pattison Walker, deceased, Lloyd Library, Coll. 11, box 4, folder 40.

7. I borrow this phrase from Roberta Bivins, *Alternative Medicine? A History* (Oxford: Oxford University Press, 2007), p. 35.

8. John S. Haller, *A Profile in Alternative Medicine: The Eclectic Medical College of Cincinnati, 1845–1943* (London: Kent State University Press, 1999); John S. Haller, *Medical Protestants: The Eclectics in American Medicine, 1825–1939* (Carbondale: Southern Illinois University Press, 1994); James C. Whorton, *Nature Cures: The History of Alternative Medicine in America* (Oxford: Oxford University Press, 2002), p. 47.

9. Simons, 'Walker's Eclectic Collection', p. 8.

10. Papers of Dr Pattison Walker, 1845–77, London Metropolitan Archives, St Thomas' Hospital Group [henceforth LMA], H01/ST/NC/017.

11. Clare Anderson, *Subaltern Lives: Biographies of Colonialism in the Indian Ocean World, 1790–1920* (Cambridge: Cambridge University Press, 2012); Durba Ghosh, 'Another Set of Imperial Turns?' *American Historical Review* 117, no. 3 (2012): 772–93; Alan Lester, 'Imperial Circuits and Networks: Geographies of the British Empire', *History Compass* 4, no. 1 (2006): 124–41; Ann Laura Stoler, *Along the Archival Grain: Epistemic Anxieties and Colonial Common Sense* (Princeton: Princeton University Press, 2009).

12. J. Pattison Walker, MD, civil assistant surgeon of Humeerpoor, 'A Contribution towards an Improved System of Prison Organisation in India' (manuscript), May 1849, LMA H01/ST/NC/17/005.

13. David Arnold, *Colonizing the Body: Sate Medicine and Epidemic Disease in Nineteenth-Century India* (Berkeley: University of California Press, 1993).

14. 'Extract Report of J.P. Walker, civil surgeon Mynpooree, 1851', *Indian Annals of Medical Science, or Half-Yearly Journal of Practical Medicine and Surgery* 2, no. 3 (Calcutta, Lepage and Co., 1851): 158–65.

15. Clare Anderson, *The Indian Uprising of 1857–8: Prisons, Prisoners and Rebellion* (London: Anthem, 2007, 2012), chapter 2.

16. W.H. Woodcock, *Report of the Inspector of Prisons on the Management of the Jails, from 1845 to 1851, and on the Present State of Prison Discipline in*

the North West Provinces (Agra: Secundra Orphan Press, 1852), pp. 3–10 (quote p. 9), India Office Records, British Library, London [henceforth IOR] V/24/2029.

17. Memorandum by W.H. Woodcock, inspector general of prisons NWP, Agra, 23 March 1851, North West Provinces Criminal and Judicial Consultations [henceforth NWPCJC], 1 April–19 May 1851, IOR P.233.24.

18. Woodcock to R. Thornton, officiating secretary to government, NWP, 6 April 1850, NWPCJC 13 April 1850, IOR P.233.12; J.W. Deane, officiating judge NWP, to Thornton, 27 April 1850, NWPCJC 13 April 1850, IOR P.233.12.

19. J. Murray, in charge Agra jail, to Woodcock, 17 December 1850, NWPCJC January–February 1851, IOR P.233.21. See Clare Anderson, 'The Transportation of Narain Sing: Punishment, Honour and Identity from the Anglo-Sikh Wars to the Great Revolt', *Modern Asian Studies* 44, no. 5 (2010): 1115–45 and Anderson, *Subaltern Lives*, chapter 4.

20. C.B. Thornhill, *Report of the Inspector General of Prisons, North Western Provinces, for the Year 1852* (Agra: Secundra Orphan Press, 1853), pp. 3–10 (quote p. 10).

21. Memorandum of good services of Surgeon Major J.P. Walker of the Bengal Medical Establishment, submitted to the Inspector General of Hospitals, Calcutta, in accordance with circular memorandum no. 58, 11 October 1867, with later additions to 1877, LMA H01/ST/NC/17/13; J.P. Walker, *Devanāgarī likhne kī kitāb* (Agra: Central Prison Sadar Jehalkhana Press, 1854); J.P. Walker, *Mubtadī kī pahilī kitāb* (Agra: Central Prison Sadar Jehalkhana Press, 1854).

22. J.P. Walker, 'On the Treatment of Hospital Gangrene' (read before the Agra Medical and Surgical Society, 7 November 1856), *Indian Annals of Medical Science, or Half-Yearly Journal of Practical Medicine and Surgery* 5, no. 9 (Calcutta: Lepage and Co., 1856): 83–7. I thank Anna Ryckbost for this reference.

23. Norman Chevers, 'A Brief Review of the Means of Preserving the Health of European Soldiers in India', *Indian Annals of Medical Science, or Half-Yearly Journal of Practical Medicine and Surgery* 7, no. 8 (Calcutta: Lepage and Co., 1860): 158–314.

24. Bivins, *Alternative Medicine?* p. 138.

25. Simons, 'Walker's Eclectic Collection', p. 8.

26. J.P. Walker to James Melville, secretary to the court of directors, 21 December 1856, letter book including diary of visits to prisons in Britain, Ireland and France, April–November 1855, LMA H01/ST/NC/17/1.

27. Walker to Melville, 30 April 1855; diary entry 14 June 1856, LMA H01/ST/NC/17/1.

28. Walker to East India Company's court of directors, 10 July 1856, LMA H01/ST/NC/17/1; Visit to Pankhurst Prison, 18 August 1856, LMA H01/ST/NC/17/1.
29. Walker to Melville, 21 December 1856, LMA H01/ST/NC/17/1.
30. C.B. Thornhill, officiating secretary to government NWP, to J. Murray, civil surgeon, Agra, 9 July 1856, LMA H01/ST/NC/17/1; D.G. Crawford, *Roll of the Indian Medical Service, 1615–1930* (London: W. Thacker, 1930), p. 128 (entry no. 1476); Simons, 'Walker's Eclectic Collection'; J.P. Walker's Obituary, *British Medical Journal* 2 (April 1906): 955.
31. Thornhill to Couper, 8 July 1859, NWPCJP, 1–18 October 1859, IOR P.235.7.
32. Unless indicated otherwise, this section is drawn from Anderson, *The Indian Uprising of 1857–8*, chapter 5.
33. 'Report on the Causes of the Severe Sickness and Great Mortality which Has Prevailed amongst the Convicts at Port Blair Penal Settlement, in the Andaman Islands, since the Formation of the Settlement on the 10th March, up to the 25th August 1858; [henceforth 1858 medical report], India Judicial Proceedings [henceforth IJP], 12 November 1858, IOR P.206.60.
34. Walker to C. Beadon, secretary to government of India, 4 September 1858, IJP, 12 November 1858, IOR P.206.60.
35. Report by G.G. Browne on the Sanitary State of the Andamans, March 1859 [henceforth Browne's report], IJP, 29 July 1859, IOR P.206.61.
36. Walker to Beadon, 4 September 1858, IJP 12 November 1858, IOR P.206.60; Browne's report, IJP, 29 July 1859, IOR P.206.61.
37. 1858 medical report, IJP, 12 November 1858, IOR P.206.60.
38. Browne's report, IJP, 29 July 1859, IOR P.206.61.
39. Extract from proceedings in foreign department, 10 January 1859, forwarding copy of the following dispatch from secretary of state for India, 30 November 1858, IJP, 29 July 1859, IOR P.206.61.
40. Extract from proceedings in foreign department, 10 January 1859, forwarding copy of the following dispatch from secretary of state for India, 30 November 1858, IJP, 29 July 1859, IOR P.206.61.
41. Memorandum of good services of Surgeon Major J.P. Walker of the Bengal Medical Establishment, submitted to the Inspector General of Hospitals, Calcutta, in accordance with circular memorandum no. 58, 11 October 1867, with later additions to 1877, LMA H01/ST/NC/17/13.
42. Philippa Levine, *Prostitution, Race and Politics: Policing Venereal Disease in the British Empire* (London: Routledge, 2003).
43. Statement of services of Dr J.P. Walker, Deputy Inspector General of Hospitals, Allahabad Circle 1845–1872, LMA H01/ST/NC/17/016; Grant

of honorary rank of Surgeon Major to James Pattison Walker, 1 October 1877, LMA H01/ST/NC/17/017.

44. Simons, 'Walker's Eclectic Collection', p. 10.

45. Lloyd Library, Walker's notebooks; Simons, 'Walker's Eclectic Collection', p. 12.

46. Felter published the famous dictionary *The Eclectic Materia Medica, Pharmacology and Therapeutics* in 1922.

47. C.G. Lloyd to Messrs Maddison, Stirling, Humm and Davies, 9 July 1906, Lloyd Library, Coll. 11, box 4, folder 40.

48. Testimony of Curtis Lloyd, 30 January 1907, High Court of Justice, in the matter of the estate of James Pattison Walker, deceased, Lloyd Library, Coll. 11, box 4, folder 40.

49. Lloyd Library, Walker's notebooks, L2, P26, S20.

50. J.P. Walker's Obituary, *British Medical Journal* (2 April 1906): 954–5.

7

ABSENCE, ABUNDANCE, AND EXCESS
Substances and Sowa Rigpa in Ladakh since the 1960s

CALUM BLAIKIE

Medicinal raw materials of many kinds have flowed into, around, and out of Asia throughout recorded history, involving extensive social networks that linked both contiguous zones and more distant regions to one another.[1] These networks and flows were crucial to the emergence of therapeutic systems, the invention of specific formulae, and the compilation of pharmacological texts, and were thus fundamental to the development of the medical traditions which became known as Ayurveda, Unani Tibb, Traditional Chinese Medicine, and Sowa Rigpa (*gso ba rig pa*—'the science of healing', otherwise known as Tibetan medicine).[2] Because histories of trade, colonialism, warfare, politics and medicine are so profoundly intertwined, the relationship between material flows and the evolution of medical knowledge, institutions, and practices demand careful scholarly attention.[3]

Recent anthropological and historical literature concerning Asian medical traditions has greatly expanded our knowledge of the relationship between textual sources and actual practice, the encounters between medical institutions, colonial and post-colonial states, biomedicine, 'modern science', and capitalism.[4] A further body of literature has taken important strides towards a clearer understanding of pharmaceuticals in terms of their production and marketing, social meanings, and consumption patterns in both 'traditional' and biomedical contexts.[5] There remains, however, a need to better account for the ways in which fluctuations in material availability effect medicine production, circulation, and the social dynamics of healing at various scales.

The current chapter examines the changing patterns of materia medica circulation in the Himalayan Indian region of Ladakh since the 1960s, and explores the effects these changes have had on Sowa Rigpa pharmacy and practice. I focus not only on macro-scale historical, political, and economic processes but also on much more localized networks of materia medica exchange, which involve complex and overlapping relations of gift-giving and barter, as well as monetary transactions. I trace the transition from widespread and chronic lack of raw materials in the period before Ladakh was connected by road to the outside world, through a period of unprecedented abundance once road transport was regularized, and into the present day, where despite the comparatively large quantities of these materials that are now available, inequalities of access remain prominent issues in pharmacy practice and in practitioners' narratives concerning it. I show how the sudden abundance of formerly limited raw materials was key to the emergence of larger scales of drug production and to the proliferation, complexification, and commodification of Sowa Rigpa medicines. These phenomena, in turn, allowed for the emergence of more professional forms of medical practice, the enfranchisement of certain groups, ideas and practices, and the marginalization of others. I argue that this was by no means a simple, unilinear progression, finding instead evidence of complex and uneven processes in which continuities have been maintained in the face of profound change and 'spaces of possibility',[6] for new material-social-practical-institutional configurations emerged and stabilized while others were closed off. The role that the changing economics of materia medica has played in the reconfiguration of medicine production and Sowa Rigpa knowledge and practice more broadly raises questions as to the boundaries of 'the medical' and its relationship to other realms which may, at first glance, appear unrelated.

Ladakh: From Independent, Trans-Himalayan Trading State to Indian Backwater

The trans-Himalayan region of Ladakh has been shaped throughout its history by the interplay of isolation and interconnectedness due to its remote geographical location and extreme topography, as well as its position at the meeting point of several great civilizations[7] and important long-distance trade routes.[8] A high-altitude cold desert region lying almost entirely above 3,000 m, Ladakh's low rainfall, cold winters, and poor soils present serious challenges to human habitation, which have kept the population low.[9] An independent kingdom from the tenth century onwards, Ladakh was forcibly incorporated into colonial India towards the end of the nineteenth century, and at Independence became roughly one third of the highly unstable state of Jammu and Kashmir. With Pakistan on one side and the Tibetan Autonomous Region of China on the other, Ladakh occupies a major geopolitical hotspot whose borders have been fought over several times since Independence and remain intensely disputed. Today, Ladakh's two districts of Leh and Kargil each have Autonomous Hill Development Councils, providing some degree of local power while remaining under the ultimate administrative control of the Srinagar government.[10]

The sealing of Ladakh's borders with Pakistan in the late 1940s and Tibet in the early 1960s destroyed formerly extensive long-distance and localized trade networks, halted the flow of goods and people, and interrupted the pilgrimage routes and deep religious links with Tibet.[11] In the space of thirty years, Ladakh's capital city of Leh ceased to be an important trading entrepot linking India, China, and Central Asia, and became instead an isolated backwater whose outward orientation pointed entirely to the south.[12]

The roads which today connect Leh to Srinagar to the southwest and Manali to the southeast were built in numerous phases throughout the second half of the twentieth century. Following ancient trade routes, the military road builders made slow progress through hostile terrain, with altitudes regularly exceeding 4,500 m, and in the face of severe cold and heavy snowfalls, as well as frequent border skirmishes and occasional full-scale wars. The most widely accepted completion dates are 1962 for the road to Srinagar and 1989 for the one to Manali, although both were prone to long closures well into the 1990s and remain blocked periodically in the present day.[13] Nevertheless, these two roads have been key to the profound transformation that has since affected almost every aspect of Ladakhi life, not least the economics of materia medica and the practice of Sowa Rigpa.

Making and Practising Medicine in the Pre-road Era

Ladakhi practitioners of Sowa Rigpa, known as *amchi*, historically found their place among a range of actors engaged in broadly health-related activities such as *lha pa* and *lha mo* (male and female oracles),[14] *onpo* (astrologers and ritual specialists), and certain Tibetan Buddhist monks. However, in many areas they were the only people practising a codified medical science[15] involving drug-based therapy until well into the final quarter of the twentieth century. Public biomedical services were extended throughout Ladakh from the 1960s onwards, but they remained patchy and of poor quality into the 1990s, and are still unreliable in many villages today.[16] For much of the twentieth century, therefore, amchi were the main actors providing physical diagnosis and medicines at the village level, and large numbers of people depended on them heavily in times of suffering. Although they were integral members of the community who enjoyed high social status, just below monks and nobles,[17] the actual standing, success, and reputation of individual amchi varied widely. This depended on the dynamic combination of numerous factors, some ascribed such as family background and medical lineage, others contingent such as perceived moral and religious qualities, past record of treating disease, and, crucially, the range and quantity of medicines at their disposal.[18]

Although traders, porters and certain monks were highly mobile prior to the adoption of motorized transport,[19] most ordinary people tended to move little from their villages and amchi primarily treated patients from their local areas. Therapeutic relationships took place at the meeting point of social, cultural, and economic matrices, with local *trims* (*khrims*—customary rules and institutional arrangements),[20] the ethical codes contained in the medical texts, and lay interpretations of Tibetan Buddhist philosophy all playing their part.[21] The time and resources that the amchi dedicated to medical practice were ideally balanced by the high status granted to them and by various forms of material and labour exchange, organized at village or individual levels, as well as by the religious merit accrued through compassionate service. The degree and form of material recompense varied considerably, but the following explanation of the arrangements in one western Ladakhi village in the 1950s provides an illustrative example:

> The people had great respect for the amchi at that time. Although amchi were not receiving *sod snyom* [*bsod snyoms*—alms][22] in my

village, they did not have to take part in the *tral* [*khral*—taxes and duties].[23] If the amchi had treated the patient for a long time or cured a serious disease, the people would thank him sincerely and invite him for a special meal. People also helped the amchi family, so they had much less work to do. In springtime, some people would always come to do the ploughing and in autumn people would come for harvest. This was how the amchi were able to practice: they had enough time and were not always busy with farming work.] Amchi did not take much money—only those whose family members were going to trade in Changthang could afford to be good amchi.[24]

Prior to the 1980s every amchi practised medicine alongside some combination of farming, trading, government employment and wage labour, or their duties as monks. Although it could bring considerable respect and status, offerings in kind, and the provision of agricultural labour, being an amchi was rarely lucrative and frequently loss-making in financial terms, and thus not a feasible full-time occupation.[25]

Before the opening of the roads, both medicinal raw materials and cash were scarce and there was little or no commercial production or sale of Sowa Rigpa drugs, requiring every amchi to make their own according to the resources, skills, and time available to them. Working alone or with family members, in their own homes, and using simple manual technology, they made small amounts of relatively simple formulae solely for their own patients. Tsewang Norphel, a well-known senior amchi, spoke of the early 1970s as follows:

> We had fewer kinds of medicine back then but we had very good knowledge of all the materials, how to do *sman jor* [*sman sbyor*—medicine production][26] and how to use the medicines that we did have. We would have 15 or 16 medicine bags and they were very small. We did not have much, but it was very effective.

Even practised in this simple way, sman jor demanded sound knowledge of the identification, collection, and preparation of numerous locally available medicinal plants and minerals, as well as the recognition, assessment, and use of a large number of substances with distant origins. It demanded practical knowledge of hundreds of individual processes of detoxification, compounding, and drug preparation, many of which are barely outlined in the texts and can only be learned through instruction from an experienced teacher.[27] Medicine making was thus an important part of amchi training and a continuous activity throughout every practitioner's life, representing a core element of their applied knowledge and daily practice, as well as an integral part of their identity and *habitus*.[28]

The resource limitations of the pre-road era required amchi to continuously adapt the ideal models of Sowa Rigpa pharmacology, as they appear in the main formulary texts, to suit the actual conditions in which they found themselves. Preparing the more complex 'ready-made'[29] medicines demanded reasonably large quantities of between ten and thirty-five raw materials to be available at one time for each individual formula. Because many amchi struggled to amass all that was needed to produce even a small selection of such medicines, they often resorted to the substitution or omission of unavailable ingredients. Several flexible and thrifty therapeutic modes were also popular, which enabled effective treatment to be given while reducing or avoiding reliance upon suboptimal readymade drugs.

In the mode referred to as *rjewo kor* (*rje bo*—master or principal; *skor*—surrounding), amchi produce a range of basic medicines using between two and six raw materials, according to formulations delineated in the texts and memorized in oral traditions.[30] These base preparations, the rjewo, contain the most therapeutically important materials for the disorder in question and can be used in their simplest form to restore equilibrium and prevent diseases from worsening or becoming more complex. They also provide the foundations upon which more complex drugs can be constructed according to the resources available to the amchi at the time, as well as the constitution of the patient and the exact nature and phase of their disease. Commonly amchi would add one to five kor ingredients to complete a single medicine and sometimes more than ten, allowing for each drug to be adapted on a case-by-case basis through principles known as *khatsar* (*kha tshar*) and *khagyur* (*kha 'gyur*). This is understood to be a precise and effective mode of treatment, yielding many highly specific permutations while being well adapted to conditions of material scarcity. Small amounts of several kor and khatsar materials could usually be added to the rjewo, according to availability and the circumstances of each case, while amchi who did not have access to such a wide array of components could give the patient the rjewo on its own, or with one or two appropriate additions.

Another important therapeutic mode is known as *sngonjor* (*sngo sbyor*—'herbal compounds'), which is described in chapter 12 of the final tantra of Sowa Rigpa's foundational texts, the *Gyushi* (*rgyud bzhi*).[31] These formulae are based on locally available high-altitude medicinal plants and are 'used when an easy-to-prepare medicament is needed, and this preparation is accessible to anyone, made of cheap ingredients and easy to get. The *sngon sbyor* is ideally opposed to precious medicaments, which mainly only wealthy people can afford'.[32] The *Gyushi* clearly states that medicinal plants are more potent than *rtsi sman* (essence medicines) and implies that sngonjor should not be considered inferior to medicines using imported materials.[33] Well adapted to conditions of resource limitation, this mode was widely used in former times by amchi with little money and weak supply networks, but was somewhat disparaged by wealthier and better-connected practitioners, who tended to see readymade or rjewo kor medicines, which included imported materials, as more powerful.

In summary, Sowa Rigpa medicines in the pre-road era were made individually within several therapeutic modes, selected according to personal preference and the availability of raw materials at the time. They circulated in regimes of value where money was not the main medium of exchange, nor financial profit the primary motivation. As I demonstrate in the following sections, the proliferation of medicinal substances that accompanied the advent of road transport links was a crucial element in the gradual (if partial) adoption of fee-for-service arrangements in place of reciprocal relations, in amchi speaking and behaving as members of a vestigial medical profession, and in the shifting of small-scale pharmacy from its former position at the core to the periphery of amchi training, practice, and identity.

Substance, Network, and Flow in the Pre-road Era

In this section I consider the sourcing and circulation of materia medica prior to Ladakh's road link to the outside world, before asking how and to what effect it changed following the completion of the roads. I am particularly interested in the networks facilitating flows of raw material, and in how larger-scale dynamics shaped practice at local and individual levels. Medicinal substances followed various routes into and around Ladakh, their flows channelled through relationships of lineage, locality, friendship, and mutual support, as well as commercial trade. As materia medica moved through physical space they also moved within and across socially constructed regimes of value and meaning which were by no means limited to a well-defined 'medical realm'.

Sowa Rigpa's numerous formulary texts list thousands of plant, mineral, metal, and animal materials originating in many ecological zones, from the high Himalayas to the equator and beyond.[34] This pharmacological diversity belies Sowa Rigpa's emergence from the folk traditions of the Tibetan plateau under the strong influence of classical Indian medical texts and, to a lesser extent, knowledge and substances of Chinese and Persian/Arabic/Greek origin.[35] The most popular formulae require between three and thirty-five components, of which generally less than half are endemic to the Himalayas, while the rest have much more distant origins. For example, the *zangpo dug* (*bzang po drug*—the 'excellent six') are crucial to almost every Sowa Rigpa formula and are primarily tropical or subtropical plants, including nutmeg, cardamom, and cloves. Although widely traded as spices in the region for many centuries,[36] these were expensive luxuries in Ladakh prior to road construction, beyond the reach of ordinary folk and difficult for most amchi to get hold of at all, let alone to amass in any great quantity. The range and quantity of medicines that individual practitioners were able to produce thus varied widely, and served as markers not only of an amchi's wealth and degree of connectedness but also of their achieved status, clinical prowess, and popularity with patients, or what Stephan Kloos refers to as their 'medical power'.[37]

The majority of amchi in today's Ladakh regularly rely upon 150 to 200 raw materials in order to make 50 to 100 different medicines.[38] Speaking to senior practitioners about the period before the roads were opened, it is clear that most had to make do with much smaller amounts of a comparatively limited range of ingredients. Although there were exceptions, the majority of amchi therefore depended upon a narrower range of relatively simple formulations, adapting them to resource restrictions and fluctuations through a flexible approach to pharmacy, as described earlier.

Although amchi were able to collect many useful plants and minerals from their native regions, a large number of therapeutically valuable materials had to be imported by horse, and access to them varied widely. Supply was insufficient to meet demand and enterprising amchi were prepared to go to great lengths to secure these materials, even in relatively small quantities. The following quote refers to a month-long trading mission made by Amchi Gurmet Namgyal in the late 1950s:

> At that time the lowland medicinal plants were very difficult to find, so I had to find a clever way to get hold of them. ... People told me that I should become a good amchi, but I asked them 'How can I become a good amchi if I cannot get the raw materials?' They told me I could find them in Kashmir and I had a strong intention to go there, but wondered how I could possibly do it. ... I borrowed 500 rupees from my grandfather Tashi Namgyal and walked to Kashmir to buy lowland plants. I thought I could take 20 kilograms on my back, because I was 20 years old and strong. I arrived there and met the right Pandit, as my grandfather had told me. ... I bought 20 kilograms and carried it back to Tingmosgang.

Here Amchi Gurmet underscores the scarcity of non-local raw materials and the high value attached to them at that time. He also directly connects access to such materials to the possibility of becoming a 'good amchi', supporting the view that the range, quantity, and quality of medicines that amchi had at their disposal was key to their status and popularity. Amchi Gurmet's words also hint towards his own hereditary medical lineage and wealthy household, which provided him with particular opportunities. Long periods away from home were problematic for those amchi deeply engaged in agriculture and Rs 500 was a vast sum of money at the time, far beyond the reach of those from more modest households. Practitioners from renowned lineages and wealthy landowning and trading households were at a huge advantage in this regard, although making something from such advantages demanded keen motivation and hard work, which not every lineage amchi was ready to invest.

Over the decades that followed, Gurmet Namgyal brought materia medica back to Ladakh from numerous trips across India and Nepal. A proportion of this he gave as gifts to his amchi teachers and members of his lineage, providing them with much-needed materials while cementing valued social connections. Some of it was exchanged for medicinal plants collected by other Ladakhi amchi in their local areas, further extending Gurmet's range of raw materials and reducing the time he needed to spend collecting plants himself. A small amount was also sold to other amchi, but the main part was kept for his own use. This enabled him to produce a wide range and large quantity of medicines, and thus to distinguish himself from his contemporaries and become, in his own words, a 'good amchi'. Through initiative and diligence, he made use of his ascribed position to develop a large and diverse network, which contributed to his reputation as a provider of good medicines, raised the respect people paid to him, and thus nourished his medical power.

While I know of several other amchi who made similar individual trading trips during this period, few were able to raise the capital and spare the time away from their farms. Most collected plants and minerals locally and sourced tiny amounts of imported materials from a handful of shopkeepers in Leh market with a sideline in materia medica. However, sold by the *thola* (10.5 gm), these tended to be expensive and of poor quality, so amchi sought other ways to access them, including through collective efforts. For example, several senior amchi from eastern Ladakh told me of the trips they made on foot to access materials before the completion of the road to Himachal Pradesh. Every few years, two or three amchi would set off with their donkeys on the twenty-day round trip south to collect lower-altitude medicinal plants, visit pilgrimage sites, and purchase lowland plants from the Himachali and Tibetan traders who gathered each summer near Keylong. The amchi carried with them as much cash as they could spare, as well as money to buy whatever items had been requested by the other amchi in the group who had stayed at home. Thus they collectively avoided the transportation charges and mark-ups that made buying these things in Leh so expensive. Although they were rarely able to bring back sufficient quantities to trade a surplus with others, each amchi saved money and secured better-quality medicines, while only needing to make the journey personally every five or six years.[39]

The contemporary recollections of senior amchi show that in the pre-road era materia medica circulated inside Ladakh through social ties and dynamics of various kinds, spanning several forms of exchange and regimes of value. For example, villagers frequently offered medicinal plants that they had collected to their local amchi, forming a part of multifaceted relationships between practitioners and patients within moral economies of healing. Valuable raw materials were regularly brought back by monks returning from Tibet or Nepal and were given as gifts to amchi friends and relatives, who may or may not have treated them as patients, or were sold for cash to more socially distant practitioners. Reciprocal exchange and gift-giving relationships also linked amchi from the same lineages and/or localities, improving access to raw materials while strengthening knowledge transmission, friendships, and regional solidarity.

Arguably the most important mode of materia medica exchange was known as *rdeb chas* (barter, exchange), which Gurmet Namgyal explained thus:

> We amchi collected many kinds of plant in large quantities, even if we didn't need them ourselves, so we could engage in rdeb chas. ... When we met, discussions about medicinal plants would always come up. For example, Urgyen—the most excellent amchi in all Ladakh—would bring whatever he had, including things that could only be found in Tibet. Others would come with things from Yarkhand. ... We would discuss what each needed and say 'next time you come you bring this and next time I come I will bring that'. It took time—it was three days to walk to my village from Leh and three days to come back, so it could take a month sometimes to complete an exchange, but it would happen eventually.

Such connections allowed for the flow of raw materials within and across ecological zones without any money changing hands. Estimates were used in place of exact weights and exchanges appear to have been based on trust, free of the haggling and brinkmanship usually associated with barter.[40] Although amchi certainly angled for the best outcomes to some degree, negotiations were tightly circumscribed by norms concerning fairness and good intention, Buddhist ideals of selflessness, and the amchi's ultimate aim of reducing suffering wherever it is manifest. As one senior amchi explained: 'We don't think about the price, the money, we just give what the other needs. Sowa Rigpa is for the benefit of others, for the patients, so we never compare the price, we just exchange.' Attempts to make a profit were considered unseemly and long-term mutual benefit was valued over short-term gain.

These examples illustrate how the circulation of materia medica in the pre-road era was intimately connected to social dynamics and processes both within and beyond the 'medical realm'. Ties of kinship, lineage, locality, and friendship coexisted with more obviously commercial relations between relative strangers. Pilgrimage and non-medical trade were combined with collective medicinal plant harvesting and purchasing trips; and locally available substances changed hands within the moral economies governing amchi–patient relationships.

1980–2000: Proliferation and Specialization

In this section I consider the role of increasingly abundant materia medica in the changing pattern, practice, and social significance of Sowa Rigpa medicine production during the final decades of the twentieth century. By the early 1980s the main external roads were open to civilian traffic. Buses, trucks, and jeeps cut travel times from the nearest major cities from a month to a few days, facilitating the greatly increased circulation of goods, people, and ideas. These freer flows were crucial to the mingling of Ladakhi and Tibetan exile 'currents of Sowa Rigpa tradition'[41] during this period, which was to have major effects on the former over the decades that followed. Several Ladakhi amchi studied under Tibetan exile teachers based in Dharamsala, either at the Men-Tsee-Khang medical college, which had been established in the early 1960s,[42] or privately under exiled Tibetan masters. Flows of materia medica invariably accompanied the transmission of knowledge. The Ladakhi students provided high-altitude plants that their refugee Tibetan masters lacked, receiving in return a high standard of education and exposure to a different medical model, as well as raw materials of lowland and tropical origins. Several of these Tibetan-trained Ladakhi amchi went on to become highly influential figures on their return home. I contend that these connections and exchanges combined material and non-material elements and played a key role in the reconfiguration of Ladakhi Sowa Rigpa during this period, notably by encouraging and enabling the emergence of commercial pharmacy.

The most famous Ladakh-based amchi pharmacist of recent times was Skalzang Norbu. He first visited Dharamsala in 1973 and then travelled back and forth for over a decade, exchanging medicinal plants collected in Ladakh in return for training and lodging, lowland plants, and readymade medicines. In the winter months he stayed in Dharamsala to study intensively under a renowned Tibetan pharmacist then working at the Men-Tsee-Khang. On his way back to Ladakh each spring, Skalzang sold pearls and turquoise bought in lowland India to villagers and traders in the foothills and mountains, using the profits to cover the cost of his ongoing medical education. He then spent the summers collecting alpine plants in Ladakh, ready to take back to his teacher in Dharamsala the following winter.

Skalzang Norbu explained to me that in Ladakh at that time there were no effective amchi associations;[43] pharmacology text books were scarce and most amchi practiced in a very simple way, relying on oral traditions and the most basic medicines. Despite being refugees, he saw how the Tibetans were much better organized, with a strong institute offering good training and a central pharmacy supplying a wide range of high-quality drugs to a network of subsidised clinics. All of this had a strong effect on Skalzang, who returned to Ladakh and steadily increased the quantity and range of medicines he produced through the 1980s and 1990s. He was the first to invest in electric grinding and pill-making machines, and among the first to order raw materials in bulk from the herb markets of Delhi and Amritsar. Not only was he inspired by what he had seen in Dharamsala, his activities were also directly enabled by the connections he had established there. They provided a reliable source of raw materials and also enabled him to sell his finished drugs outside of Ladakh, which in turn brought the income he needed to further invest in his medicine production.

Pioneered by Skalzang Norbu and several others who had trained in Dharamsala, a growing number of urban amchi pharmacists started to use grinding and pill-making machines, extensive supply networks, and financial capital to prepare medicines in quantities unimaginable using manual technology and largely non-monetary exchange. They were able to produce over 120 kinds of medicines compared to the 30 or 40 that were commonly being used before. This included more complex formulae, such as *Samphel Norbu* and *Agar 35*, which were difficult for ordinary amchi to assemble in any quantity, if at all, in former times.[44]

In the early days the medicines made by the pharmacists were purchased only by a very small number of Ladakhi amchi, largely working in urban areas or with non-governmental organizations. They either supplemented their homemade medicines in this way, or gave up pharmacy altogether and bought the full range in bulk from the pharmacists. Given the limited or negative cash flows that most rural amchi continued to face, however, it was simply too expensive for them to purchase medicines in any quantity. Most, therefore, continued to favour the home production of simpler formulae, which worked out considerably cheaper, and only to purchase the most difficult to prepare medicines in tiny amounts. Nevertheless, the growth of commercial pharmacy during the 1990s resulted in the proliferation of drugs, with larger quantities of a much wider range becoming available than ever before. This in turn enabled increasing numbers of amchi in urban and peri-urban locations to practice without making any of their own medicines, facilitated Sowa Rigpa's emergence as a full-time livelihood activity, and encouraged the division of the medical realm into special-ized subfields of pharmacy and clinical practice.

Exchange and Production in the Twenty-First Century

By the turn of the millennium, the vast majority of materia medica entering Ladakh was being imported by truck by a handful of amchi who were single-handedly running small pharmacies in the Leh area. Although they were making medicines primarily for use in their own clinics, the demand for readymade drugs continued to grow and the cottage industry mode of production continued to flourish. These pharmacists became major actors in the economy of materia medica, sitting at the centre of extensive networks, controlling the flow of large quantities of all kinds of raw materials, and thereby occupying positions of considerable influence. They largely replaced the shopkeepers and non-amchi traders who were formerly so important, rendered small-scale individual and collective trading missions obsolete, and, in theory at least, made formerly scarce imported materials and complex medi-cines easier for all amchi to source than ever before.

In contemporary practice, however, things are by no means simple. Although large quantities of materia medica are now being delivered directly from the major herb markets of India and Nepal, medicinal substances continue to flow through several coexisting modes of exchange and regimes of value, and according to logics other than short-term financial advantage. While cash has certainly become the predominant transactional mode, such transactions cannot be placed in a theoretical 'black box' without further need for explanation,[45] or assumed to possess a fixed set of properties based on universal prin-ciples of supply and demand, price and profit, as much recent literature suggests.[46] The maintenance of long-term and mutually beneficial ties, ethical precepts and social norms, and the generation of religious merit continuously interact with the exchange of materials and accumulation of money. Cash has been involved in materia medica flows for a very long time, and although it has become increasingly central, does not appear to act 'as a kind of acid which inexorably dissolves cherished cultural discriminations, eats away at qualitative difference and reduces personal relations to impersonality'.[47]

Neither has the increasing use of money entirely replaced other forms of exchange, which continue to play important roles in the present day. Alongside cash sales, most pharmacists also exchange imported raw materials and readymade medicines with rural amchi in return for medicinal plants collected from the mountains. They maintain long-term relationships based on mutual benefit, which are circumscribed by norms of fairness and unselfish motivation. Furthermore, gift-giving and horizontal rdeb chas linkages between rural amchi continue to allow them access to a wide range of materials without the use of money. Thus the exchange of materia medica remains embedded in social dynamics and relationships that are not reducible to profit-oriented commercial trade. Viewed through the ever-changing channels by which medicinal substances flow, the medical realm can be seen to have distinguished itself more clearly from other fields than in former times, yet remains connected to other logical frameworks and social dynamics which would be obscured by a myopic focus on monetary transactions and the quest for financial profit.

By the early 2000s, almost every Ladakhi amchi was sourcing at least some readymade medicine from the cottage industry pharmacists, but most still made the majority themselves due to a combination of financial imperative, personal preference, and greater perceived efficacy. However, as the decade progressed, the use of a wide range of commercially produced medicines became increasingly important to the mounting elite-driven efforts to professionalize Sowa Rigpa and gain long sought-after official recognition from the government of India.

When an amchi unit opened at Leh District Hospital in 2004 and a new generation of institutionally trained amchi were engaged in the state-backed 'mainstreaming' of Sowa Rigpa via the National Rural Health Mission (NRHM) in 2009, all were required to use centrally produced medicines from officially approved pharmacies. These developments further encouraged the scaling up of production, legitimized those pharmacists favoured by the local authorities, and strengthened the discourse of specialization so familiar from other Asian medical modernization efforts. At the same time, this increased the pressure on all Ladakhi amchi to stock a wider range of more complex drugs, irrespective of their actual ability and wish to do so.

Echoing developments which took place over a century ago in Ayurveda and Unani Tibb,[48] a model based on the separation of pharmacy and clinical practice as specialized professional domains has become increasingly dominant in contemporary Ladakh. However, despite this and the ongoing growth of the commercial pharmacy sector, there has been no simple transition from home to industrial production and no universal acceptance of the superiority of such a system. Of the fifty-eight amchi[49] I interviewed on the matter during my doctoral research (2006–9), thirty-three still made the majority of medicines themselves for a variety of compelling reasons. For example:

> The most important benefit of making your own medicine is confidence. I know exactly how much of which materials are in it. For example, *Agar 35*: if I make it myself I know which materials are in greater proportions, which are strong, and if some are missing. Secondly I have confidence that is has good potency. Thirdly, I can use khatsar,[50] which is dependent on knowing the exact constituents of the medicine. ... Doing sman jor also makes you more knowledgeable about the medicines and exactly how they work. Finally, it is better financially too—it is much cheaper to make your own than to buy from another.[51]

Because many raw materials can still be collected by oneself or obtained without the need for money through rdeb chas exchange, and because the pharmacists' mark-up can be avoided, making your own medicines remains significantly cheaper than buying them. Furthermore, only by making a medicine with one's own hands can one prescribe it and observe its effects with real confidence, as one rural practitioner underscored:

> Amchi must know precisely what quantities of the different materials are in the medicine—if you make them yourself then you know this. It is more difficult to use those medicines made in large quantities by others because you don't know exactly what is inside. It may be very strong, but on the other hand it may not have much of the powerful ingredients in it. ... Patients have different constitutions also: some are strong and others weak, so it also depends on the patient.[52]

If certain ingredients in a medicine are particularly strong, it will not be appropriate for some patients, and if others are weak or missing, the desired therapeutic effects will not occur. With one's own medicine, remedial action can be taken either through complementary prescriptions or via the admixture techniques outlined earlier. Medicines made by others remain widely seen as more difficult to prescribe, their effects harder to predict, and their inadequacies harder to compensate for.

There is a strong sense amongst older practitioners that foregoing sman jor altogether means losing a fundamental element of amchi knowledge, practice, and identity. Plenty of younger practitioners hold similar sentiments also, as the following quote from an urban amchi in his thirties, and a passionate advocate of small-scale production, illustrates:

> Many younger amchi have not taken time to learn sman jor and they are not taking proper interest in it. They are lazy and that is why they practise only through buying and giving, not through making. The problem is that they don't really understand which medicines will have benefits for which patient—they are not confident in their treatments. I go to the mountains and collect everything one by one—I know all the plants, which medicines to make from them and exactly which is good for what. If you buy, then you don't know the benefit of each plant, you forget, and this is simply laziness. Also the knowledge of the plants and of sman jor is lost.[53]

The abundance of materia medica has proved a crucial prerequisite to pharmaceutical proliferation, to specialization, and to the consolidation of a professional form of medical practice, but these have not completely superseded home production, which retains popularity for many reasons that continue to be valid, or have only become important in recent decades. A large number of amchi question the quality of medicines made industrially, often commenting along the following lines: 'The materials are all ground at the same time, which affects their properties, and they are often not mixed together properly. Also the heat, the metal and the electricity in the machines damages the potency of the medicine.' Such doubts provide another layer of resistance to the widespread adoption of mass production.

It does not appear accurate to portray the cottage industry pharmacists as following some pre-existing industrial teleology based upon inexorable expansion, mechanization, mass production, and the profit imperative. Many pharmacy processes are still carried out by hand, such as cleaning and detoxification, while understandings of quality and potency remain linked to the individual care and expertise directly invested in production, and are widely questioned in their absence. Pharmacists' narratives concerning their activities stress support for individual amchi with whom they have links and uplifting Ladakhi Sowa Rigpa as a whole, so that it can be on a par with the Tibetan exile current of tradition and hold its own when compared with Ayurveda. Providing a bigger selection of high-quality medicines at reasonable prices also appears as an important objective, with expansion and profit-making limited by ethical considerations as well as concerns over potency and efficacy, as Skalzang Norbu explained:

> I make my living from this, but what I really appreciate is when people tell me that the medicine works well for the patients. ... It is good that I can make money in the right way: if the medicine is working well, then it is alright to ask for money. I don't think 'Oh my medicine is working well, I am proud of this and I can earn money from others'—I never have this attitude.... The amchi is concerned with more important matters: he has to always keep in mind that his work is only to save the patients' lives. If you are doing this [pharmacy] with the wrong motivation, it is sinful: thinking only of money sows the seed of sin.

Complexity, Excess, and Therapeutic Strategy

As well as shaping the pattern and practice of medicine making, the growing abundance of raw materials has affected the kinds of drugs being made and the way that they are clinically deployed. Notable here is the increasing prescription of more potent and complex medicines, and the alteration of the ideal therapeutic order. Although accepted by most practitioners as inevitable and largely beneficial, some have also started expressing concern that these changes may not be entirely positive. Furthermore, it is also necessary to consider how the growing consumption of more complex medicines both within Ladakh and worldwide is affecting the availability of raw materials, the conservation status of certain species of medicinal plants and animals, and thus the long-term sustainability of the nascent Sowa Rigpa industry.

Sowa Rigpa's ideal therapeutic principles are delineated in chapters 27 to 30 of the Explanatory Tantra of the *Gyushi*.[54] Chapter 27 ends with the important statement that treatments should always be offered according to the level of the disorder, and 'like the load of a *dzo* [cow-yak hybrid] or the load of a sheep, these two should not be exchanged. In the same way a mild medicine should be administered for a mild disorder and a powerful medication for a serious one.'[55] In serious cases practitioners are advised to immediately resort to the full range of therapeutic options, including the most powerful medicines available. However, for minor disorders treatment should begin with dietary and behavioural advice and simple forms of medicine, which may be sufficient to restore equilibrium. If not, *chema* (powders) and *rilbu* (pills) of greater complexity are then prescribed, which should be of a *zhi* (calming) or *sbyang* (purgative) nature according to the disorder in question.[56] There is a further range of accessory therapies such as moxibustion, blood-letting, and hydrotherapy, which may be necessary in particular cases, or can be resorted to should the earlier phases of treatment prove ineffective. These stages are to be followed 'in the manner of one who climbs a staircase step by step'.[57]

Beyond its internal therapeutic logic, this ideal model is well suited to conditions of restricted access to material resources. The early stages require behavioural change and simple medicines which aim to reduce, or even avert, the need for more complex and difficult to source formulae. However, such a progression depends upon frequent contact between amchi and patient in order to assess the results of each stage and, if required, move on to the next. This was relatively easy in the static village settings of former times, but much less so in contemporary Ladakh where people often travel long distances to see the amchi, or lack the time in their busy lives for frequent consultations. Recent decades have seen the ideal therapeutic order widely truncated, often with the early stages such as the offering of advice and provision of simple drugs skipped altogether, and more powerful medicines given at the time of first diagnosis.[58] For patients, the prescription of powerful drugs has become the main symbol of medical treatment having been received, and these days amchi tend to prescribe them at an earlier stage than in former times. This pattern is consistent with the 'pharmaceuticalization' process, by which commodified drugs become the defining characteristic of medical intervention.[59]

A further effect of changes to the therapeutic order is well illustrated by the increasingly widespread use of *rinchen rilbu* (*rin chen ril bu*—'precious pills'). These are the most powerful and complex medicines known to Sowa Rigpa, containing a large number of ingredients such as precious metals and minerals, and require rituals and blessings which can only be bestowed by high religious figures who hold the right lineage.[60] Although most of the practitioners I have spoken to about it see no problem with the increasing use of rinchen rilbu, or see it as a positive development, this quote from a prominent Lhasa-based

professor of Sowa Rigpa highlights the changing use pattern of these
medicines and the unintended consequences that can be associated
with it:

> When you go to fight a war, you use ordinary weapons first and only
> gradually introduce more powerful weapons if necessary. In Tibet it was
> formerly very difficult to find rinchen rilbu, but today even those who
> are not rich can get them easily. Normally, *rinchen rilbu* should only
> be used after successful treatment: to prevent the disease from coming
> back again. They can also be used in very serious cases ... but the amchi
> must carefully establish how strong or weak the patient is and decide
> which medicines to use and when. We say that rinchen rilbu are the
> king of medicines, so ordinary medicines do not have anything like the
> same power. For those who have already taken a lot of rinchen rilbu,
> it is not so useful to give them other medicines—they do not make
> much difference. Thus these medicines must be used carefully—it is not
> a good idea to ignore the correct order of treatment.

Although they are not made in Ladakh, the increasing production of
rinchen rilbu in Dharamsala and the Tibetan areas of China is certainly facilitated by easier access to raw materials, financial capital, and
manufacturing technology. Demand is driven by the high material and
spiritual potency ascribed to them,[61] by their symbolic and political
association with Buddhism and the Tibetan cause,[62] as well as by economic development, which enables ordinary people to purchase them
on a regular basis. The alignment of these various forms of abundance is
seen by some to result in medically inappropriate patterns of consumption, characterized by overuse. This in turn reduces the effectiveness of
simpler medicines and forces continued reliance on the most powerful
and expensive drugs in order to achieve desired clinical outcomes.

Among Ladakhi amchi there is another sense in which abundance
can slip into excess, with ethical and spiritual as well as medical implications. The following quote from a senior rural practitioner illustrates
this well:

> Every amchi has more medicine now than before, but their knowledge is
> less and they do not have the right motivation. They only wish to make
> money. ... They don't think first of all how to cure the patient and this
> means they do not have *sems zangpo* ['good hearts']. Whenever patients
> come to me I only give them three or four doses of each medicine and
> if it is effective then they come back to get more. If it is not effective

then they don't waste their money. There is one amchi who has a clinic in Leh—he gives a lot of medicine every time, saying 'you should take this one and that one for this many weeks and give me that money', but if it is not effective then there is no good motivation, no sems zangpo.

This view was backed up by a much younger amchi practicing in Leh who is similarly critical of clinics which prescribe longer courses of medicine:

See how much medicine they give! This is only commercial—they take so much money, giving one month of medicine and this is not good. I only give a few days of medicine, even a few doses only, then the patient comes back and I find out if it is working or not and then give more, or change if it is not good for them.... I cannot take money for a month of medicine from the patients—they are poor, they cannot afford it—it is not good to do it like this.

As the early prescription of longer courses of more complex medicines becomes common practice in urban professional settings, poorer rural amchi face new dilemmas:

These days it is possible to make so many medicines, more than before. I learn how to make new medicines at the seminars; I can get plants more easily through rdeb chas and also I can buy expensive ingredients or medicines made with them from Leh, which were so hard to find before. Today I have more kinds of medicine than before, but I also have to spend much more money.

The proliferation of complex medicines raises expectations across the board, but the ability to produce and prescribe them is concentrated amongst the wealthier and better connected. By pushing themselves to keep up with the curve, rural amchi face even greater pressure on their scant financial resources, and thus on the moral economies within which their therapeutic relationships are embedded. This has become a divisive factor as elite and urban amchi frequently disparage their rural counterparts for relying on basic medicines or incomplete versions of complex formulae, while poorer village-based amchi are critical of what they see as self-interest and profiteering by the urban practitioners.

Finally, the scaling up of pharmaceutical production in an age of apparent abundance also has strong feedback effects on resource availability and the sustainability of the system as a whole. The recognition that was granted to Sowa Rigpa by the government of India in

2010 heralds a period of 'mainstreaming' into public healthcare and a strong push towards industrialization, aimed at securing higher profits by expanding further into national and global markets.[63] However, Ladakhi amchi are already reporting the depletion of many important local medicinal plant species, and the price of imported materials is rising steadily while their quality falls and adulteration becomes increasingly rife. Experiences in Ladakh and elsewhere show how easily the traditional medicine industry can become a victim of its own success, severely threatening wild plant resources while large-scale cultivation proves very difficult to achieve.[64] The recent abundance of raw materials thus appears to be but momentary; an impermanent state which is already leading to a new phase of unequally distributed shortage, widespread substitution, and reformulation in response to market-induced resource depletion.

* * *

A Ladakhi amchi once told me, 'Without plants there is no medicine, and without medicine I am nothing.' This simple statement serves as a reminder of the material basis of all medical activities which rely on drugs to effect change in suffering beings, and neatly summarizes the main argument of this chapter. The invention of formulae and their codification in formulary texts, the evolution of therapeutic systems, the emergence of medical professions and growth of pharmaceutical industries all depend on the sourcing, possession, manipulation, and deployment of substances. This point is often downplayed or overlooked in scholarly discussions of medical traditions in Asia and elsewhere, or is treated as somehow separate from the political, social, theoretical, and practical dimensions which attract the most attention. I hope that the examples discussed in this chapter, fragmentary as they are, contribute to correcting this common oversight, while shedding some light on the way that the 'medical realm', far from being self-evident, bounded, or stable, is perpetually emergent at the interface of many fields both material and social, human and non-human.

The vast number of formulae that reside in Sowa Rigpa texts, written from the tenth century onwards, reflects a hybrid pharmacology that calls upon knowledge and substances originating from numerous ecological and cultural zones. Making Sowa Rigpa medicines has always depended on complex actor-networks which involve ever-shifting combinations of wild plants, their habitats and collectors, farmers and their crops, traders and trade routes extending from Indonesia to Siberia and the Middle East, pilgrims, priests and tributary offerings, strangers, teachers and students, medical lineages, patients, kin, and friends. Prior to and throughout the half century covered by this chapter, these networks have been constantly shaped not only by warfare, colonialism, and state formation, socio-economic change, the opening and closing of borders and roads, but also by dynamics operating at much smaller scales. The substances in question have flowed and, although to a lesser extent, continue to flow through multiple exchange forms and regimes of value which cannot be sufficiently explained through orthodox economic theories or explained away through vague reference to 'market forces'.

Over fifty years the amchi of Ladakh have been engaged in the progression from chronic lack to unprecedented abundance of imported materia medica. I have shown how this development was crucial to the carving out of commercial pharmacy and clinical practice as specialized domains, and to the shift from individualized, flexible, and thrifty approaches to pharmacy, in which medicines existed in highly localized forms or as therapeutic entities in-the-making, to the proliferation of complex 'readymade' medicines with relatively fixed properties and numerous imported components. These transitions also enabled the emergence of a professional form of Sowa Rigpa, which played an important part in the national-level recognition that was granted in 2010 and in Sowa Rigpa's subsequent integration into Indian public healthcare and industrial strategy.

Through these interdependent processes the space of possibility in which Ladakhi Sowa Rigpa exists has been substantially reconfigured. Formerly central domains concerning knowledge of raw materials, the maintenance of extensive networks of raw material exchange and the techniques of small-scale production have become fragmented and increasingly confined to either specialized pharmacists or marginal practitioners. At the same time, new fields have opened up for amchi working in institutional settings, state-supported public health care facilities and profit-making private clinics, as well as for those supplying drugs in bulk to these emergent modes of Sowa Rigpa practice. Networks enabling the flow of plants, animal products, and minerals remain crucial for all Ladakhi amchi, but their shape and dynamics have altered significantly, and year by year fewer practitioners are directly engaged in the collection, trade, exchange, and transformation of substances.

I have also shown that while these general trends affect every Ladakhi amchi and are largely seen as positive by those involved, they are not without critics and not all the emergent elements have been universally accepted. As in the past, unequal access to medicines is a marker of differentiation amongst healers, and today this signifies the enfranchise- ment of the largely urban professionals and the marginalization of their 'traditional' rural counterparts. However, many amchi working in vil- lages and in towns still choose to produce their own medicines rather than purchase them from commercial pharmacists, thus maintaining Sowa Rigpa as a broad and heterogeneous field of knowledge and prac- tice which continues to incorporate objects, knowledge, techniques, people, social networks, and dynamics that many would locate outside the medical realm. In some cases, the pharmaceutical abundance of the present day can also be seen to tip over into a kind of excess, which has potentially negative implications for the efficacy of less-complex drugs and formerly valued therapeutic modes, while raising new questions of ethical, social, economic, and ecological, as well as clinical, import.

Notes

1. A. Akasoy, C. Burnett, and R. Yoeli-Tlalim, *Islam and Tibet: Interactions along the Musk Routes* (Farnham: Ashgate, 2010); A. Basham, 'The Practice of Medicine in Ancient and Medieval India', in *Asian Medical Systems: A Comparative Study* edited by C. Leslie (Berkeley: University of California Press, 1976).

2. Vernacular terms are rendered in simplified phonetic form based on Ladakhi pronunciation. On first usage of each term, in parentheses, I pro- vide an English definition and the standardized Tibetan spelling according to T. Wylie, 'A Standard System of Tibetan Transcription', *Harvard Journal of Asiatic Studies* 22 (1959): 261–7.

3. A. Akasoy and R. Yoeli-Tlalim, 'Along the Musk Routes: Exchanges between Tibet and the Islamic World', *Asian Medicine* 3 (2007): 217–40; P. Chakrabarti, *Materials and Medicine: Trade, Conquest and Therapeutics in the Eighteenth Century* (Manchester: Manchester University Press, 2010); M. Harrison, *Medicine in the Age of Commerce and Empire: Britain and Its*

Tropical Colonies 1660–1830 (Oxford: Oxford University Press, 2010); L. Schiebinger, *Plants and Empire: Colonial Bioprospecting in the Atlantic World* (London: Harvard University Press, 2004).

4. J. Alter, *Asian Medicine and Globalization* (Philadelphia: University of Pennsylvania Press, 2005); G. Attewell, *Refiguring Unani Tibb: Plural Healing in Late Colonial India* (New Delhi: Orient Longman, 2007); E. Hsu, *Innovation in Chinese Medicine* (Cambridge: Cambridge University Press, 2001); J. Langford, *Fluent Bodies: Recipes for Post-Colonial Imbalance* (London: Duke University Press, 2002); P. Mukharji, *Nationalizing the Body: The Market, Print and Healing in Colonial Bengal 1860–1930* (London: Anthem Press, 2009); K. Sivaramakrishnan, *Old Potions, New Bottles: Recasting Indigenous Medicine in Colonial Punjab 1850–1945* (Hyderabad: Orient Longman, 2006); P. Unschuld, *Medicine in China: A History of Ideas* (Berkeley: University of California Press, 1985); D. Wujastyk and F. Smith, *Modern and Global Ayurveda: Pluralism and Paradigms* (Albany: State University of New York Press, 2008).

5. M. Banerjee, *Power, Knowledge, Medicine: Ayurvedic Pharmaceuticals at Home and in the World* (Hyderabad: Orient BlackSwan, 2009); M. Bode, *Taking Traditional Knowledge to the Market: The Modern Image of the Ayurvedic and Unani Industry* (Hyderabad: Orient BlackSwan, 2008); L. Pordié and J-P. Gaudillière, 'The Reformulation Regime in Drug Discovery: Revisiting Polyherbals and Property Rights in the Ayurvedic Industry', *East Asian Science, Technology and Society* 8, no.1 (2014): 57–79; A. Petryna, A. Lakoff, and A. Kleinman, *Global Pharmaceuticals: Ethics, Markets and Practices* (London: Duke University Press, 2006); S. Whyte, S. van der Geest, and A. Hardon, *Social Lives of Medicines* (Cambridge: Cambridge University Press, 2002).

6. I. Hacking, *Historical Ontology* (London: Harvard University Press, 2002).

7. Ladakh has deep historical connections with Indian, Tibetan, and Central Asian socio-political, religious, and cultural configurations.

8. J. Fewkes, *Trade and Contemporary Society along the Silk Road: An Ethno-History of Ladakh* (London: Routledge, 2009); J. Fewkes and N. Khan, 'Social Networks and Transnational Trade in Early 20th Century Ladakh', in *Ladakhi Histories: Local and Regional Perspectives*, edited by J. Bray (Leiden: Brill, 2005); J. Rizvi, *Trans-Himalayan Caravans: Merchant Princes and Peasant Traders in Ladakh* (Oxford: Oxford University Press, 1999); J. Rizvi, 'Leh to Yarkand: Travelling the Trans-Karakoram Trade Route', in *Recent Research on Ladakh 7*, edited by T. Dodin and H. Räther (Ulm: Universität Ulm, 1997).

9. Ladakh's population was 232,924 according to the 2001 census, with the lowest density in the subcontinent.

10. R. Aggarwal, *Beyond Lines of Control: Performance and Politics on the Disputed Borders of Ladakh, India* (London: Duke University Press, 2004); S. Deboos, *Être musulman au Zanskar, Himalaya indien* (Editions Universitaires Européenne, 2010); M. van Beek, 'Beyond Identity Fetishism: "Communal" Conflict in Ladakh and the Limits of Autonomy', *Cultural Anthropology* 15, no. 4 (2001): 525–69; M. van Beek, 'The Art of Representation: Domesticating Ladakhi Identity', in *Ethnic Revival and Religious Turmoil: Identities and Representations in the Himalayas*, edited by M. Lecomte-Tilouine and P. Dollfuss (New Delhi: Oxford University Press, 2003).

11. J. Rizvi, *Ladakh: Crossroads of High Asia* (Oxford: Oxford University Press, 1996).

12. Fewkes and Khan, *Social Networks and Transnational Trade*.

13. J. Demenge, *Living on the Road, Waiting for the Road: The Political Ecology of Road Construction in Ladakh* (PhD diss., University of Sussex, 2011).

14. F. Kressing, 'The Increase of Shamans in Contemporary Ladakh: Some Preliminary Observations', *Asian Folklore Studies* 62, no. 1 (2003): 1–23.

15. J. Gyatso, *Being Human in a Buddhist World: An Intellectual History of Medicine in Early Modern Tibet* (New York: Columbia University Press, 2015); V. Adams, M. Schrempf, and S. Craig, *Medicine between Science and Religion: Explorations on Tibetan Grounds* (New York: Berghahn, 2011); G. Samuel, 'Tibetan Medicine in Contemporary India: Theory and Practice', in *Healing Powers in Contemporary Asia: Traditional Medicine, Shamanism and Science in Asia Societies*, edited by L. Connor and G. Samuel (Westport: Bergin and Garvey, 2001), pp. 247–68.

16. K. Ball and J. Elford, 'Health in Zangskar', in *Himalayan Buddhist Villages: Environment, Resources, Society and Religious Life in Zangskar, Ladakh*, edited by J. Crook and H. Osmaston (Bristol: University of Bristol, 1994); C. Blaikie, 'Where There Is No *Amchi*: Tibetan Medicine and Rural–Urban Migration amongst Nomadic Pastoralists', in *Healing at the Periphery: Ethnographies of Tibetan Medicine in India*, edited by S. Kloos and L. Pordié (Durham: Duke University Press, in press); K. Gutschow, 'From Home to Hospital: The Extension of Obstetrics in Ladakh', in *Medicine between Science and Religion*, edited by V. Adams, M. Schrempf and S. Craig (London: Berghahn Books, 2010), pp. 185–213; T. Norboo and T. Morup, 'Culture, Health and Illness in Ladakh', in *Recent Research on Ladakh 6*, edited by H. Osmaston and N. Tsering (New Delhi: Motilal Banardsidass Publishers, 1997).

17. A. Heber and K. Heber, *Himalayan Tibet and Ladakh: A Description of Its Cheery Folk, Their Ways and Religion* (New Delhi: Ess Publications, 1976 [1926]); A. Kuhn, 'Ladakh: A Pluralistic Medical System under

Acculturation and Domination', in *Acculturation and Domination in Traditional Asian Medical Systems*, edited by D. Sich and W. Gottschalk (Stuttgart: F. Steiner Verlag, 1994), pp. 61–73.

18. S. Kloos, *Tibetan Medicine amongst the Buddhist Dards of Ladakh* (Vienna: ATBS, 2004); L. Pordié, 'La pharmacopée comme expression de société: Une étude himalayenne', in *Des sources du savoir aux médicaments du future*, edited by J. Fleurentin, G. Mazars, and J. Pelt (Paris: Editions IRD–SFE, 2002).

19. J. Rizvi, 'Trade and Migrant Labour: Inflow of Resources at the Grassroots', in *Ladakhi Histories: Local and Regional Perspectives*, edited by J. Bray (Leiden: Brill, 2005).

20. 'Trims' are rules established at the village level which provide the normative foundations of the social order. They govern relationships between human inhabitants and local deities, the agricultural cycle, and many localized institutions, including Sowa Rigpa practice. See F. Pirie, *Peace and Conflict in Ladakh: The Construction of a Fragile Web of Order* (Leiden: Brill, 2007), pp. 55–8.

21. B. Clark, *The Quintessence Tantras of Tibetan Medicine* (Ithaca: Snow Lion Publications, 1995); F. Meyer, 'La médecine tibétaine: Tradition ancienne et nouveaux enjeux', in *Tibet: l'envers du décor*, edited by O. Moulin (Geneva: Olizane, 1993), pp. 89–95; S. Kloos, 'Good Medicines, Bad Hearts: The Social Role of the Amchi in a Buddhist Dard Community', in Pordié, *Healing at the Periphery*; L. Pordié, 'Buddhism in the Everyday Medical Practice of the Ladakhi *Amchi*', *Indian Anthropologist* 37, no. 1 (2007): 93–116.

22. These are offerings which bring merit to the giver. Through instituted sod snyom arrangements, amchi were given a fixed amount of produce (usually barley) annually by every household in the village, in return for providing their services.

23. Under locally specific tral arrangements, every household must contribute produce, labour, and/or money towards events such as village festivals and the visit of dignitaries. See Pirie, *Peace and Conflict in Ladakh*, pp. 53–5.

24. Unless otherwise stated, all the quotes that appear in this chapter are extracts from interviews and discussions that took place during my doctoral (2006–9) and post-doctoral (2011–15) fieldwork.

25. Kloos, *Tibetan Medicine among the Buddhist Dards*; Kuhn, *Ladakh: A Pluralistic Medical System*; Pordié, *La pharmacopée comme expression de société*.

26. The term 'sman jor' is used as shorthand for the entire process of Sowa Rigpa medicine making, although it also refers to a specific stage within that process, in which the materials needed for each formula are measured out and

compounded. I use the term 'amchi pharmacist' to specify those engaged in commercial Sowa Rigpa medicine production, but clearly distinguish them from biomedical pharmacists.

27. C. Blaikie, 'Currents of Tradition in Sowa Rigpa Pharmacy', *East Asian Science, Technology and Society* 7 (2013): 425–451; F. Cardi, 'Principles and Methods of Assembling Tibetan Medicaments", *Tibet Journal* 30, no. 4 (2005); T. Hofer, 'Foundations of Pharmacology and the Compounding of Tibetan Medicines', in *Bodies in Balance: The Art of Tibetan Medicine*, edited by T. Hofer (Seattle: University of Washington Press, 2014), p. 52; F. Meyer, *Le système médical Tibétain Gso-Ba-Rig-Pa* (Paris: CNRS Editions, 1981).

28. L. Pordié and C. Blaikie, 'Knowledge and Skill in Motion: Layers of Tibetan Medical Education in India', *Culture, Medicine and Psychiatry* 38, no. 3 (2014): 340–68.

29. I use 'readymade' to refer to those medicines prepared in their complete form, according to well-known textual formulations. Once compounded, these are ready to give to patients, with no further additions required. This contrasts with the other modes described in this section, in which base compounds are prepared for subsequent case-by-case adjustment, or drugs are made in the absence of imported raw materials.

30. Printed pharmacology texts were rare and valuable items in the pre-road era. Although the more established medical lineages passed such books down through the generations, many amchi were forced to rely on hand-copied versions, or to learn the main formulations by heart within oral traditions.

31. Hofer, 'Foundations of Pharmacology and the Compounding of Tibetan Medicines', p. 52.

32. Cardi, 'Principles and Methods of Assembling Tibetan Medicaments', p. 95.

33. Men-Tsee-Khang, *The Subsequent Tantra from the Four Tantras of Tibetan Medicine* (Dharamsala: Men-Tsee-Khang, 2011), p. 135.

34. For example, the *Shel Gong Shel Phreng* (Crystal Orb and Crystal Rosary), a widely used eighteenth-century formulary, lists 2,294 medicinal sub-stances of highly varied origin, although considerably fewer have come into common usage (C. Millard, 'The Integration of Tibetan Medicine in the United Kingdom: The Clinics of the Tara Institute of Medicine', in *Tibetan Medicine in the Contemporary World: Global Politics of Medical Knowledge and Practice*, edited by L. Pordié [Abingdon: Routledge, 2008], p. 191).

35. Akasoy and Yoeli-Tlalim 'Along the Musk Routes'; D. Damdul, 'History of Tibetan Medicine', in *Sowa Rigpa and Ayurveda*, edited by P. Roy (Varanasi: Central Institute for Higher Tibetan Studies, 2008), pp. 25–50; D. Martin, 'An Early Tibetan History of Indian Medicine', in *Soundings in Tibetan Medicine: Anthropological and Historical Perspectives*, edited by M. Schrempf (Leiden: Brill, 2007), pp. 307–27.

36. Nutmeg, for example, has been in global trade for millennia, despite only growing on a handful of Indonesian islands. See L. Andaya, *The World of Maluku: Eastern Indonesia in the Early Modern Period* (Honolulu: University of Hawaii Press, 1993); and R. Ellen, *On the Edge of the Banda Zone: Past and Present in the Social Organisation of a Moluccan Trading Network* (Honolulu: University of Hawaii Press, 2003).

37. Kloos, *Tibetan Medicine among the Buddhist Dards*.

38. This is comparable with the 138 raw materials required to produce the 71 most widely used Sowa Rigpa medicines in contemporary Nepal (C. Witt, N. Berling, Ngari Thingo Rinpoche, M. Cuomo, and S. Willich, 'Evaluation of Medicinal Plants as Part of Tibetan Medicine Prospective Observational Study in Sikkim and Nepal', *Journal of Complementary and Alternative Medicine* 15, no. 1, [2009]: 59–65). It also compares well with the 229 plant species regularly used in the Bhutanese Sowa Rigpa industry (P. Wangchuk, S. Pyne, and P. Keller, 'An Assessment of the Bhutanese Traditional Medicine for Its Ethnopharmacology, Ethnobotany and Ethnoquality: Textual Understanding and the Current Practices', *Journal of Ethnopharmacology* 138, no. 1 [2013]: 305–10).

39. I have also heard of similar collective trips being made by Zanskari amchi during this period.

40. Ellen, *On the Edge of the Banda Zone*, and C. Humphrey and S. Hugh-Jones, *Barter, Exchange and Value: An Anthropological Approach* (Cambridge: Cambridge University Press, 1992).

41. V. Scheid, *Currents of Tradition in Chinese Medicine 1626–2006* (Seattle: Eastland Press, 2007); Blaikie, 'Currents of Tradition in Sowa Rigpa Pharmacy'.

42. For a detailed history of this institution, see S. Kloos, 'The Politics of Preservation and Loss: Tibetan Medical Knowledge in Exile', *East Asian Science, Technology and Society* 11, no. 2 (2016): 135–59.

43. Ladakh Amchi Sabha, the largest association of its kind in the region, was founded in 1978 but its activities were extremely limited until the late 1990s.

44. These two classical formulae are widely understood to be highly powerful and effective, but require upwards of thirty components, including several rare and expensive materials, making them awkward to prepare for the majority of amchi. See C. Blaikie, 'Wish-Fulfilling Jewel Pills: Tibetan Medicines from Exclusivity to Ubiquity', *Anthropology and Medicine* 22, no. 1 (2015): 7–22.

45. M. Serres, *Genèse* (Paris: Grasset, 1982); R. Wilk, *Economies and Cultures: Foundations of Economic Anthropology* (Oxford: Westview Press, 1996).

46. C. Olsen and H. Larsen, 'Alpine Medicinal Plant Trade and Himalayan Mountain Livelihood Strategies', *Geographical Journal* 169 (2003): 243–54;

C. Olsen and N. Bhattarai, 'A Typology of Economic Agents in the Himalayan Plant Trade', *Mountain Research and Development* 25, no. 1 (2005): 37–43; Y. Thomas, M. Karki, K. Gurung, and D. Parajuli, *Himalayan Medicinal and Aromatic Plants: Balancing Use and Conservation* (Kathmandu: Government of Nepal Ministry of Forests and Soil Conservation, 2005).

47. M. Bloch and J. Parry, *Money and the Morality of Exchange* (Cambridge: Cambridge University Press, 1989), p. 3.

48. Attewell, *Refiguring Unani Tibb*; Banerjee, *Power, Knowledge, Medicine*; Bode, *Taking Traditional Knowledge to the Market*.

49. Of these fifty-eight amchi, twelve were women, twenty-three were under forty years of age, and almost half had some form of institutional training. The sample comprised thirty-three amchi practising predominantly in rural areas and twenty-five based in towns, and included both private individuals and those working in institutional settings. See C. Blaikie, *Making Medicine: Materia Medica, Pharmacy and the Production of Sowa Rigpa in Ladakh* (PhD diss., University of Kent, 2013).

50. As explained earlier, 'khatsar' involves the addition of extra ingredients to a basic medicinal compound, tailoring it to the precise nature and phase of an individual's disorder, as well as to the availability of raw materials.

51. Interview with Amchi Karma Chodon.

52. Interview with Amchi Jigmet Singe.

53. Interview with Amchi Sonam Tondup.

54. Clark, *The Quintessence Tantras of Tibetan Medicine*, pp. 205–22; Men-Tsee-Khang, *The Basic Tantra and the Explanatory Tantra from the Secret Quintessential Instructions on the Eight Branches of the Ambrosia Essence Tantra* (Dharamsala: Men-Tsee-Khang, 2008), pp. 259–86.

55. Clark, *The Quintessence Tantras of Tibetan Medicine*, p. 209.

56. Y. Donden, *Health through Balance: An Introduction to Tibetan Medicine* (Ithaca, New York: Snow Lion Publications, 1986); T. Dummer, *Tibetan Medicine and Other Holistic Healthcare Systems* (New Delhi: Paljor Publications, 1988); Meyer, *La médecine tibétaine*.

57. Clark, *The Quintessence Tantras of Tibetan Medicine*, p. 209.

58. S. Craig, *Healing Elements: Efficacy and the Social Ecologies of Tibetan Medicine* (Berkeley: University of California Press, 2012); Samuel, 'Tibetan Medicine in Contemporary India: Theory and Practice'.

59. J. Abraham, 'Pharmaceuticalization of Society in Context: Theoretical, Empirical and Health Dimensions', *Sociology* 44, no. 4 (2010): 603–22; M. Nichter and M. Nichter, *Anthropology and International Health: South Asian Case Studies* (Amsterdam: OPA, 1997), pp. 271–2.

60. J. Aschoff and T. Tashigang, *Tibetan Jewel Pills: With Some Remarks on Consecration (Byin rlabs) of the Medicines* (Ulm: Fabri Verlag, 2009);

M. Saxer, *Manufacturing Tibetan Medicine: The Creation of an Industry and the Moral Economy of Tibetanness* (Oxford: Berghahn Books, 2013).

61. Saxer, *Manufacturing Tibetan Medicine*, p. 72.

62. A. Prost, *Precious Pills: Medicine and Social Change among Tibetan Refugees in India* (Oxford: Berghahn, 2009).

63. Government of India (Planning Commission), *Eleventh Five Year Plan (2007–2012)* (New Delhi: Government of India, 2007); Government of India, *Department-related Parliamentary Standing Committee on Health and Family Welfare: Forty-Sixth Report on the Indian Medical Council (Amendment) Bill 2010* (New Delhi: Government of India, 2010).

64. S. Craig and D. Glover, 'Conservation, Cultivation, and Commodification of Medicinal Plants in the Greater Himalayan-Tibetan Plateau', *Asian Medicine* 5 (2011): 219–42; W. Law and J. Salick, 'Comparing Conservation Priorities for Useful Plants among Botanists and Tibetan Doctors', *Biodiversity and Conservation* 16, no. 6 (2006): 1747–59; Saxer, *Manufacturing Tibetan Medicine*; D. Shankar and B. Majumdar, 'Beyond the Biodiversity Convention: The Challenges Facing the Biocultural Heritage of India's Medicinal Plants', in *Medicinal Plants for Forest Conservation and Health Care*, by G. Bodeker, K. Bhat, J. Burley, and P. Vantomme (Rome: FAO, 1997), pp. 100–8; D. Tewari, *Report of the Task Force on Conservation and Sustainable Use of Medicinal Plants* (New Delhi: Government of India Planning Commission, 2000); Thomas, Karki, Gurung, and Parajuli, *Himalayan Medicinal Plants*.

8

COLONIZING CANNABIS
Medication, Taxation, Intoxication, and Oblivion, c. 1839–1955

JAMES H. MILLS

As the editors of this volume make clear in their introduction, the question 'what is colonial about colonial medicine' has stimulated a range of fresh approaches to the issues it raises. Among these approaches has been a focus on substances considered to be medical and the production of detailed accounts of their histories and the ways in which they came to feature in British scientific and medical circles. After briefly considering the rewards to be had from such an approach, this chapter will look at cannabis products and their history in the nineteenth and twentieth centuries. In part this story is about the entry of preparations of the plant into Western medical knowledge and practice. However, the chapter also demonstrates that cannabis was not simply constructed as a medicine in Western circles in this period. The ways in which competing understandings emerged of the plant and the substances that could be manufactured from it will also be explored. The purpose of doing this is twofold. In the first instance the chapter begins to provide some answers to the question related to the one of 'what is medical about colonial medicine?' In addressing this question the chapter also addresses its second concern, which is to put the plants back into the picture of the history of medicine in the colonial period.

'Colonial' Medicines and Their Histories

Two recent papers provide fine examples of the benefits of considering the history of medicinal substances rather than practitioners, institutions, or programmes in colonial South Asia. Markku Hokkanen's article on *Strophanthus kombe* shows how an African substance became a 'medicine' in Western systems during the colonial period.[1] Extracts from the plant were used in poison arrows in various parts of Africa including Malawi and also featured in local medical systems, although the extent to which this was the case could vary considerably. Interest in the nature of the poisons used ensured that British botanical explorers in the region worked hard to trace their sources with the help of local chiefs and guides. Once *Strophanthus kombe* was 'discovered', samples were sourced and regularly sent back through commercial and missionary networks to Edinburgh University's laboratories. There the important work was done in translating an African substance into a Western medicine through the medium of experimentation and eventually through the publication of results in scientific journals; work which caught the eye of representatives of the British pharmaceutical sector. A market for the substance already existed as its properties were thought to make it useful for the treatment of cardiac conditions, which were routinely treated with digitalis. The Burroughs Wellcome & Company set about funding facilities to perfect the process of producing 'Tincture of Strophanthus' for commercial purposes. The company's marketing campaigns and free samples served to establish its product in the Victorian doctor's medicine chest by 1887. Hokkanen's paper is an excellent study of the processes and actors involved in producing a Western 'medicine' from an African plant. The story features African leaders, locals, and their knowledge, 'bio-prospectors', colonial governments, missionary organizations, private companies, and university laboratories. Warfare, diplomacy, exploration, colonialism, investment, experimentation, commercialization, and validation by 'science' are among the processes that shaped the trajectory. It has been recently observed that movement and circulation between locales is crucial for the production of scientific knowledge. Hokkanen's paper is a reminder of the importance of looking for who and what drives that travel.[2]

Guy Attewell's longue durée perspective on tiryaq faruq, a concoction used to treat beriberi, offers other important conclusions. It shows how British doctors grappling with the condition in the 1830s failed to successfully deploy their own medicines and reluctantly turned to the local remedy. They had initially viewed this with some reservation as it was an unfamiliar substance recommended by both Muslim and Hindu medical practitioners. Yet its provenance was more complex, as the drug was in fact an import to local medicines, delivered by Indian Ocean traders at the end of a journey from Venice, where the substance had originally been prepared by Jewish physicians using Greek-inspired Arabic medical texts. Attewell concludes that 'Tiryaq meets criteria for being western, colonial, Islamic and Indian medicine at the same time—and it therefore highlights the problem with using these very terms to describe and analyse complex intercrossings and encounters'.[3] In his account the history of the substance's mobility renders unstable any effort to locate it in the categories that dominated the historiography until recently, and therefore similarly renders those categories unstable.

Cannabis and Colonial Medicine

Before the nineteenth century the cannabis plant and its preparations sometimes featured as entries in medical and botanical dictionaries but were little known or discussed in practice in the United Kingdom.[4] It was not until the nineteenth century that accounts began to appear in British medical circles of preparations of cannabis, and it was the efforts of one scientist that lay behind their emergence in Victorian medicine in the 1840s. William Brooke O'Shaughnessy was born in Limerick in 1809 and graduated as an MD from Edinburgh University when only twenty-one. Just three years later he was on his way to India as an assistant surgeon.[5] On arrival in India he eagerly conducted experiments with local drugs and medicines and published the results of these in journals such as the *Transactions of the Medical and Physical Society of Bengal*, eventually collecting his conclusions and observations together in *The Bengal Dispensatory, and Companion to the Pharmacopoeia* in 1842 and *The Bengal Pharmacopeia* in 1844.[6] In 1842 he also found time to publish *A Manual of Chemistry Arranged for Native, General and Medical Students*,[7] and by then had been made a Professor of Chemistry and Medicine in the Medical College of Calcutta.

His entry on cannabis in the *Bengal Dispensatory and Companion to the Pharmacopoeia* spanned twenty-five pages and had already been partially published as 'On the Preparations of the Indian Hemp or Gunjah (*Cannabis Indica*)' in the *Transactions of the Medical and Physical Society of Bengal* of 1839. What set his work apart from the entries on cannabis in earlier medical and botanical dictionaries was the evidence provided from O'Shaughnessy's close personal work with the substance. He was careful to refer to the 'several experiments which we have instituted on animals, with the view to ascertain its effects on the healthy system; and lastly, we submit an abstract of the clinical details of the treatment of several patients afflicted ... in which a preparation of hemp was employed'.[8] His first test subject was a 'middling sized dog' that 'became stupid and sleepy' for six hours on being fed a cannabis sample. Further experiments revealed that 'while carnivorous animals and fish, dogs, cats, swine, vultures, crows and adjutants, invariably and speedily exhibited the intoxicating influence of the drug, the graminivorous, such as the horse, deer, monkey, goat, sheep and cow experienced but trivial effects from any dose we administered'.[9]

Human trials were hastily arranged as a result of these animal experiments. One patient who was suffering from severe rheumatism was given a cannabis substance and became 'very talkative ... singing songs, calling loudly for an extra supply of food, and declaring himself in perfect health'. Once awake, the patient declared himself to be much improved and he was discharged three days later. O'Shaughnessy concluded that the substance had been an effective sedative and pain-killer. A case of rabies was treated with cannabis and while it did not cure the disease, it allowed the patient constant relief from the horrendous hydrophobia of the condition to the extent that he could drink water, eat fruit, and swallow rice. O'Shaughnessy included this example in his account of the drug as he was impressed by the power of hemp to alleviate the hydrophobia. Cannabis tincture was also administered to cholera victims and it seemed to have the effect of controlling diarrhoea and vomiting and of inducing rest. A case of 'infantile convulsions' was similarly treated, and although the child was at one point 'in a sinking state' it survived not only the illness but a range of treatments that included 'two leeches ... to the head', 'a few doses of calomel and chalk', and a mouthful of opiates.[10] O'Shaughnessy also reported that considerable improvement could be effected in cases of delirium tremens through the administration of cannabis preparations.

O'Shaughnessy's conclusions were clear. He recorded in his 1839 paper that 'the results seem to me to warrant our anticipating from its more extensive and impartial use no inconsiderable addition to the resources of the physician'.[11] Indeed, in his subsequent guide to the Bengal Pharmacopoeia of 1844 he described it as a 'powerful and valuable remedy in hydrophobia, tetanus, cholera and many convulsive disorders'[12] and as 'narcotic, stimulant and anti-convulsive, given in cholera, delirium tremens, tetanus and other convulsive diseases, also in neuralgia, in tic doloroux etc'. He outlined the treatment to be used and advocated twenty minims and upwards, administered in syrup. He even helpfully included the recipe for the tincture of hemp—'ganja tops two pounds, rectified spirit one gallon. Macerate for two days, then boil for twenty minutes in a distilling apparatus, strain while hot'.[13]

O'Shaughnessy looms large in the story of the introduction of cannabis substances into Victorian medicine because he took on so many of the roles in it. In Hokkanen's account of Strophanthin, different individuals and institutions acted in various capacities. John Kirk was the 'bio-prospector' who sought out the plant and liaised with locals about its identity and potential and he was in Malawi as a member of David Livingstone's Zambezi expedition. It was John Buchanan, a former missionary and settler there, who began to supply it to the UK, and Thomas Fraser, professor of materia medica at Edinburgh University, who used these supplies to conduct experiments. On delivering his conclusions from these experiments in an academic paper to the annual meeting of the British Medical Association in 1885, Fraser inspired Burroughs Wellcome & Co. to see the potential for profit in the concoction and to seek to develop it for commercial purposes.

By contrast, O'Shaughnessy does not appear to have been a man given to delegation. That he took on the task of working with locals to establish the uses of cannabis preparations was obvious in his acknowledgements, as he thanked both Muslim and Hindu acquaintances for their help in providing information. Syed Keramut Ali was a trustee of the local Imambarrah and Hakim Mirza Abdul Rhazes was credited as coming from Teheran and providing O'Shaughnessy with information on cannabis in the countries between the Indus and Herat. Modoosudun Goopto came from a family of Ayurvedic practitioners and he studied at the Sanskrit College in Calcutta before teaching at the British Medical College,[14] while Kamalakantha Vidyadanka was identified by O'Shaughnessy as 'celebrated Pundit of the Asiatic Society'. Not that all of his contacts were elite scholars or practitioners, as he was careful to note when outlining a particular method of preparing cannabis that 'the process has been repeatedly performed before me by Ameer, the proprietor of a celebrated place of resort for Hemp devotees in Calcutta, and who is considered the best artist in his profession'.[15] If he was the 'bio-prospector' in the story then he also took on the task of translating this local substance into a Western medicine through the process of experimentation and publication in scientific media. While his earliest work appeared in books and journals published in India, the *Provincial Medical and Surgical Journal* back in the UK was quick to pick up on it. In 1843 it devoted the front page of two consecutive editions to updated versions of O'Shaughnessy's earlier papers[16] and published an additional letter from him recommending cannabis for its 'extraordinary anticonvulsive power'.[17] Indeed, it was O'Shaughnessy who took on the job of promoting the drug to British audiences, as he was invited to present to the Royal Medico-Botanical Society for which 'the meeting room of the society was exceedingly crowded throughout the evening, the gentlemen present manifesting the most lively interest in the discussion'. His paper went down well and he was presented with the diploma of a corresponding member of the society.[18] Finally, it was O'Shaughnessy who was behind the commercialization of the substance as he supplied Peter Squire, a pharmacist on Oxford Street in London, with a sample from which was produced a tincture that was marketed as Squire's Extract.[19] If Hokkanen's account of Strophanthin is one of a drug's trajectory through professional and commercial networks, this glimpse of the route for cannabis from Asian substance to Western medicine adds the picture of the determined entrepreneur who drives it through such professional and commercial networks.[20]

Once established as a remedy available to Victorian doctors, cannabis went on to enjoy a modest career in British medicine from the 1840s until the 1890s.[21] O'Shaughnessy lost interest in it once he secured more profitable work, and the difficulties in isolating the active ingredient in order to produce standardized medicines from cannabis meant that tinctures prepared from it remained unpredictable in practice. But to leave the story here would be to tell only part of it. While O'Shaughnessy and his contacts in Calcutta and London succeeded in deploying the processes and language of contemporary science to establish value for cannabis as a medicine, other British doctors used

similar techniques to create for the plant and its preparations a reputation as a dangerous intoxicant.

Throughout the nineteenth century the British set up a network of
lunatic asylums across colonial India. At first these had been established
to separate out Indian soldiers who had gone mad from the rest of the
regiment, and later on the British found that they were useful places
in which to place those who they found dangerous and disruptive in
the local population. As the colonial superintendents at these asylums
kept increasingly detailed records of their charges and began to collate
these into statistical tables in end-of-year reports for their superiors,
an alarming conclusion began to emerge. The preponderance of hemp
narcotics in the statistical tables on causes of mental illness among
inpatients was regularly commented upon in the statements of those
in charge of the hospitals. For example, the superintendent of the
Dullunda Asylum near Calcutta commented in 1867:

> Among the causes of admissions, there appear nothing of novelty or
> special interest. The fact which each succeeding year brings prominently
> forward, of the prevalence of ganja smoking as a fertile source of insanity,
> is as prominent as ever in the records of 1867.[22]

Similarly, in 1871, Surgeon Cutcliffe pointed out in his report on the
asylum at Dacca that 'Table no. 4 shows the causes to which the insanity of the patients has been attributed. 33 percent of all the cases are
attributed to gunja smoking and 7.18 to spirit drinking'.[23] In 1875 the
officer in charge of the asylum in Cuttack pointed out that 'Ganja is
reputed as the cause of the majority of the admissions and nearly half of
the admissions during the past ten years into this asylum are attributed
to its abuse'.[24] Throughout the 1860s and into the 1870s the statistical
evidence emerging from India's mental hospitals pointed to the conclusion that the largest single cause of the problems experienced by their
patients was cannabis use.[25]

By 1871 these statistics had alarmed the Government of India
(GOI). The colonial administration ordered an enquiry into cannabis
use in its South Asian empire with the following remit:

> It has been frequently alleged that the abuse of ganja produces insanity
> and other dangerous effects.
>
> The information available in support of these allegations is avowedly
> imperfect, and it does not appear that the attention of the officers in

charge of lunatic asylums has been systematically directed to ascertain the extent to which the use of the drug produces insanity.

But as it is desirable to make a complete and careful enquiry into the matter, the Governor-General in Council requests that Madras, Bombay etc. will be so good as to cause such investigations as are feasible to be carried out in regard to the effects of the use or abuse of the several preparations of hemp.[26]

In 1873 the resolution of the GOI at the end of the enquiry stated of cannabis that 'there can ... be no doubt that its habitual use does tend to produce insanity'.[27] The administration was so confident of this assertion about the link between use of hemp substances and mental illness because it had been persuaded by the numbers. In its resolution, figures were produced from asylums in the Central Provinces, Mysore, the Punjab, and Bengal and a statistical table from the Delhi institution was reproduced as was its superintendent's observation:

> Of 317 lunatics received into the Nagpur Asylum since 1864, there were 61 in whom insanity had been occasioned by an immoderate use of ganja. ... From this result it is inferred that excess in ganja-smoking does produce an insanity which is transient.[28]

The colonial officials in the GOI had been convinced by the science of the statistic. It acted upon its conclusion by prohibiting the cultivation and consumption of ganja in Burma and urging other parts of British India to 'discourage the consumption of ganja and bhang by placing restrictions on their cultivation, preparation and retail, and imposing on their use as high a rate of duty as can be levied without inducing illicit practices'.[29]

It has been argued that these statistics were deeply flawed, as they were shaped by cultural misunderstandings, bureaucratic shortcomings, and the assumptions of the psychiatry of the period.[30] However, these flaws were deemed unimportant at the time because statistical data was highly regarded in colonial India. It lent authority to the efforts of colonizers in comprehending and managing a context that they often found bewilderingly complex.[31] In this case the statistical data acted much as the experiments had in the tale told in Hokkanen's paper and in the story of O'Shaughnessy.[32] They rendered impressions formed in South Asia into scientific conclusions for circulation amongst Westerners. But, in this case, the production of scientific data on cannabis consumption gave rise to a conclusion that challenged existing understandings

and practices. In the 1860s, ideas about the dangers of using preparations of the plant emerged that countered therapeutic assessments
of the substance.

Cannabis and the Anti-opium Campaigners

Yet cannabis was also given further meanings elsewhere in colonial
networks that linked South Asia and Britain. The GOI had first shown
an interest in the substance not as a medicine or as a cause of disease
but as a commodity. Preparations of the plant had been commercially
traded across South Asia long before the arrival of the British and the
cultivated form was prized as the key ingredient in a range of intoxicating
products.[33] As early as 1793 East India Company officials at the
Bengal Board of Revenue had recognized this and sought to derive
income from the trade by including cannabis products in their lists of
excise items to be subjected to government duties. The system that
they devised demanded that the retailer of the drug, before approaching the peasant producers, had to turn up at the office of the local
colonial official and pay for a licence that would grant him permission
to proceed and buy his stock of the drugs. Having done this, he was free
to head on to meet his supplier and to purchase as much as he wanted,
after which he was equally free to go and sell it wherever he wanted.
In other words, the government was simply concerned to guarantee
that the licences were bought and they cared little about how much of
the drugs were being produced or consumed. It was decided by the
middle of the century that there was more money to be had from the
trade as the scheme was changed in 1854 to tax the wholesaler in his
place of business rather than at the point of purchase or production. In
other words, once the stock of ganja was in the wholesaler's warehouse,
the district collector there would be able to assess his approximate
holdings and to maintain surveillance of how much the retail buyers
were taking from the wholesaler. The amount sold by the wholesaler
to the retailer was therefore taxed. The British gradually realized that
the key to the success of levying this duty was an accurate knowledge
of the amount of ganja in the system. To this end the board of revenue
introduced a series of additional licences in 1876. The peasant pro-
ducer of the hemp plant had to approach the authorities to obtain a
licence to cultivate the crop. When the crop was ready and the ganja

had been processed, the cultivator had to apply for a licence to store the drug. To be granted this licence he stated how much of the drug he intended to store and the permit was made out to cover this amount. The wholesaler meanwhile needed to apply for a permit to collect supplies from the cultivators which stated how much he intended to purchase.[34] By the 1880s levies on cannabis products were worth almost Rs 200,000 in Bengal alone. This made tax on preparations of the plant in the Presidency a more important source of revenue than tax on opium sold in the region.[35]

Various constructions of cannabis existed by the 1880s: the useful medicine, the cause of mental illness, the product on the excise list. As the 1880s progressed another version emerged, one that drew on these previous ideas but which recast them within the political and cultural tensions of late Victorian Britain. Mark Stewart, member of parliament, stood up in the House of Commons on 16 July of that year 'to ask the Under-Secretary of State for India whether his attention has been called to the statement in the Allahabad Pioneer of the 10th May last that ganja 'which is grown, sold and excised under much the same conditions as opium', is far more harmful than opium, and that 'the lunatic asylums of India are filled with ganja smokers'. He pressed his point, asking further of the secretary of state 'whether he is aware that the possession and sale of ganja has been prohibited for many years past in Lower Burma and that the exclusion of the drug was stated in the Excise Report of that province for 1881–2 to have been 'of immense benefit to the people'. The reason for his curiosity was that he wanted to know 'whether he [the secretary of state] will call the attention of the Government of India to the desirability of extending the same prohibition to the other Provinces of India?'[36]

The figures generated by India's mental hospitals had finally arrived back in the UK, and the conclusion that they had generated, that cannabis was a source of ill health, had been used in parliament to challenge the idea that it was simply an article of excise. The multiple constructions of cannabis no longer existed apart from one another, but were now in direct conflict with one another. While Stewart initiated the campaign against cannabis, it was his colleague, William Caine, who took it forward. A founder member of the Anglo-Indian Temperance Association, he had visited India in 1888 to promote that organization through the missionary networks there.[37] Accompanied on his trip by

the experienced Baptist missionary Thomas Evans, who had over thirty
years of service in India to his name, Caine had his attention drawn to
cannabis:

> Here and there throughout the bazar are little shops whose entire stock
> consists of a small lump of greenish pudding, which is being retailed out
> in tiny cubes. This is another 'Government monopoly' and is majoon,
> a preparation of the deadly bhang or Indian hemp known in Turkey
> and Egypt as Haseesh, the most horrible intoxicant the world has yet
> produced. In Egypt, its importation and sale is absolutely forbidden
> and a costly preventive service is maintained to suppress smuggling
> of it by Greek adventurers; but a Christian Government is wiser in
> its generation and gets a comfortable income out of its sale. When an
> Indian wants to commit some horrible crime, such as murder or wife
> mutilation, he prepares himself for it with two anna's worth of bhang
> from a government majoon shop. The little rooms, open to the street, of
> which the sole furniture is some matting and a few Hukas, are churras
> or Chandu shops, farmed out by the government of India to provide
> another form of Indian hemp intoxication which is smoked instead of
> eaten.[38]

Caine and Stewart were not simply veteran temperance campaigners
but also active members of the anti-opium movement, which was
gathering pace in the 1890s and which was to lead to the Royal Opium
Commission of 1895. They drew on Caine's networking in India to
cast existing discourses on cannabis within the ideas that drove these
campaigns, in which intoxication was self-evidently immoral and those
that enabled it were wrong. Cannabis as a source of excise, and cannabis as a source of mental health problems, was rewoven by these
campaigners to produce the conclusion that cannabis was 'the most
horrible intoxicant the world has yet produced'.

By the 1890s cannabis had multiple meanings in different discursive
systems. In the medical world there were those that saw its positive values, and there was a revival of interest in British pharmacology towards
the end of that decade in isolating its active ingredient. However, there
were also those that saw it as a cause of mental health problems and,
despite detailed investigation into the reliability of the statistics from
Indian asylums in the 1890s, that data continued to stimulate debate
into the twentieth century. For those at the board of revenue in Bengal,
cannabis was simply a source of revenue to be managed and augmented.

For the anti-opium campaigners it had a deliciously negative value in their moral system, its consumption for intoxication making it an evil and the GOI's revenue from it providing evidence of its failure to live by high standards. Such was the force of the recasting of cannabis as a moral issue that the GOI was compelled to appoint the Indian Hemp Drugs Commission (IHDC) in 1893 to investigate it. The task of the IHDC was to test the various discursive representations and to see how far they could be reconciled. It opted to privilege the version of cannabis that held it to be the source of useful medicines, and to destabilize the notion that it was a dangerous intoxicant by promoting the idea that it was a harmless one. The IHDC stood accused by its critics of really seeking to privilege the discourse that simply saw cannabis as a lucrative excise item. Its conclusions, and the controversies surrounding them, are dealt with more fully elsewhere.[39]

* * *

The conclusions to be drawn from these stories for the purposes of this volume are various. Much good work has been done recently to respond to the question 'what is colonial about colonial medicine?' and if this chapter sheds light in that direction it is in order to draw further attention to the unstable nature of the 'colonial' in the question. After all, in the stories the 'colonial' is fractured and incoherent, with Western doctors using different methodologies and samples to reach conflicting conclusions about the nature of preparations of the plant, British administrators framing the drug simply as an excise item to be carefully managed to maximize revenues, and Victorian moralists condemning cannabis substances as perilous intoxicants. Hokkanen's paper on Strophanthus is an excellent account of the way in which an African plant acquired technical meaning as it travelled along the scientific network that linked Malawi and Britain. This chapter has shown how an Asian plant similarly travelled along the scientific network that linked the empire with the UK, but that it did this in multiple ways, and at the same time was propelled along some of the many other networks linking south Asia with Britain in this period.

The editors of this volume are right that 'medicine [is] an important organizing concept, which is historically produced, and yet shapes discourses, practices, and subjectivities'. This chapter suggests that

cannabis is only one such organizing system in this period and that
as it travelled along the various networks mentioned earlier in the
chapter it acquired multiple meanings. The outcome was that the
status of cannabis as a therapeutic substance in this context was a
contested one, so the eye is drawn to the question of 'what is "medical"
about colonial medicine?' The account given here of cannabis shows
how difficult it is to fix that plant and its preparations in a medical
system at all. Its history since the British arrived in south Asia has been
one where efforts to establish cannabis as a medicine were constantly
contested by its other associations and meanings attached to it outside
of medical circles. Indeed, this chapter has not had the space to dwell
on a further set of meanings established for cannabis once news of
it arrived back in Britain, where at various times it was recast as an
exotic source of delightful oblivion or even 'astral travel' in literary
and occultist circles.[40] It seems that cannabis was sometimes, and in
some places, a medicine, but that often it was not seen as medical at
all, but rather it was viewed as a moral concern, an excise problem,
or even a spiritual opportunity. The story of cannabis and the various
ways in which it was imagined as it was encountered in colonial India
and made its way to Britain point to the instability of the notion of
'medicine', and how historically contingent the award of that label
can be.

While the chapter has traced the competing agendas and systems of
meaning that framed cannabis and produced so many different versions
of it in British culture, it has not fully addressed a final reason that cannabis was imagined or constructed in so many different ways. It seems
important to consider the plant itself in trying to explain why cannabis
has not been fixed in any one particular discursive context or by any
one agenda, be it scientific, economic, or moral. Cannabis is a bewilderingly complex plant, with over a hundred active ingredients, which
have multiple effects (only some of which are psychoactive) on human
bodies, which are mediated by individual constitutions.[41] One of the
key reasons—perhaps the most significant of them—why cannabis has
defied efforts to lodge it within moral, medical, or economic systems of
meaning is the plant itself, as its complicated nature defies generalization and easy categorization. In this case at least, a 'biological turn'
seems important in understanding why a set of plant substances first
encountered by the British in a colonial context has enjoyed such an

unstable and contested career as a medicine. It will be interesting to see if such a 'biological turn' is of wider use to those seeking to rethink the nature of the notion of the 'medical'.

Notes

1. M. Hokkanen, 'Imperial Networks, Colonial Bioprospecting and Burroughs Wellcome & Co.: The Case of *Strophanthus Kombe* from Malawi (1859–1915)', *Social History of Medicine* 25, no. 3 (2012): 589–607. Additional information on the plant and the colonial history of its extracts can be found in A. Osseo-Asare, 'Bioprospecting and Resistance: Transforming Poisoned Arrows into Strophanthin Pills in Colonial Gold Coast, 1885–1922', *Social History of Medicine* 21 (2008): 269–90.

2. K. Raj, *Relocating Modern Science: Circulation and the Constitution of Scientific Knowledge in South Asia and Europe, 1650–1900* (Palgrave: Basingstoke, 2007); C. Hayden, *When Nature Goes Public: The Making and Unmaking of Bioprospecting in Mexico* (Princeton: Princeton University Press, 2003).

3. G. Attewell, 'Interweaving Substance Trajectories: Tiryaq, Circulation and Therapeutic Transformation in the Nineteenth Century', in *Crossing Colonial Historiographies: Histories of Colonial and Indigenous Medicines in Transnational Perspective*, edited by A. Digby, W. Ernst, and P. Muhkarji (Newcastle: Cambridge Scholars, 2010), p. 14.

4. J. Mills, *Cannabis Britannica: Empire, Trade and Prohibition, c. 1800–1928* (Oxford: Oxford University Press, 2003), pp. 17–39.

5. Assistant Surgeon's Papers, India Office Library L/Mil/9/383/124.

6. W. O'Shaughnessy, *The Bengal Dispensatory and Companion to the Pharmacopoeia* (London: Allen, 1842); *The Bengal Pharmacopoeia and General Conspectus of Medicinal Plants* (Calcutta: Bishops College Press, 1844).

7. W. O'Shaughnessy, *A Manual of Chemistry Arranged for Native, General and Medical Students and the Subordinate Medical Department of the Service* (Ostell and Lepage: Calcutta, 1842).

8. O'Shaughnessy, *Bengal Dispensatory*, pp. 579–604.

9. O'Shaughnessy, *Bengal Dispensatory*, pp. 579–604.

10. O'Shaughnessy, *Bengal Dispensatory*, pp. 579–604.

11. W.B. O'Shaughnessy, 'On the Preparations of the Indian Hemp or Gunjah', *The Provincial Medical Journal* 5 no.123 (1843): 368. The journal acknowledged that this article had originally been published in the *Transactions of the Medical and Physical Society of Bengal* for 1839, and that this was a revised version by the author.

12. O'Shaughnessy, *The Bengal Pharmacopoeia*, p. 91.

13. O'Shaughnessy, *The Bengal Pharmacopoeia*, p. 428.

14. D. Bose, 'Madhusudan Gupta', *Indian Journal of the History of Science* 29, no. 1 (1994): 31–40.

15. O'Shaughnessy, *Bengal Dispensatory*, p. 583.

16. *Provincial Medical and Surgical Journal* 5, no. 122: 343–47 and *Provincial Medical and Surgical Journal* 5, no.123: 363–9.

17. *Provincial Medical and Surgical Journal* 5: 397.

18. 'Royal Medico-Botanical Society February 22 1843', in *Provincial Medical and Surgical Journal* 5 (1842–3): 436–8.

19. M. Booth, *Cannabis: A History* (Doubleday: London, 2003), p. 138.

20. I have argued elsewhere that O'Shaughnessy's personal circumstances and life story suggest that he always had one eye on personal advancement and his income. From an Irish Catholic landed family on hard times, he sought employment in the East India Company after his father's death. He rose rapidly through the ranks, and while his interest in cannabis flared early in the 1840s, he soon abandoned it when he secured lucrative posts at the Calcutta Mint and eventually as Superintendent of Electric Telegraphs in 1853 ('Irishman, Scottish Doctor, British Knight: The Career of William O'Shaughnessy of Curragh, 1808–1889', unpublished paper at Ireland and India, and presented at Education: Colonial Connections Conference, Trinity College, Dublin, October 2008).

21. See Mills (2003), pp. 49–81; S. Snelders, C. Kaplan, and T. Pieters, 'On Cannabis, Chloral Hydrate, and Career Cycles of Psychotropic Drugs in Medicine', *Bulletin of the History of Medicine* 80, no. 1 (2006): 95–114.

22. *Asylums in Bengal for the Year 1867* (Calcutta: Thacker and Spink, 1868), p. 10.

23. *Asylums in Bengal for the Year 1870* (Calcutta: Thacker and Spink, 1868), p. 35.

24. *Asylums in Bengal for the Year 1875* (Calcutta: Thacker and Spink, 1868), p. 24.

25. For more on this network and for the details of the argument of this section, see …

26. 'Papers Relating to the Consumption of Ganja and Other Drugs in India', in *British Parliamentary Papers*, volume 66 (London: Hansard, 1891), pp. 7–8.

27. 'Papers Relating to the Consumption of Ganja', p. 92.

28. 'Papers Relating to the Consumption of Ganja, p. 88.

29. 'Papers Relating to the Consumption of Ganja, p. 92.

30. Mills (2000).

31. This argument draws on A. Appadurai, 'Number in the Colonial Imagination', in *Orientalism and the Postcolonial Predicament: Perspectives*

on South Asia, edited by C.A. Breckenridge and Peter van der Veer (Philadelphia: University of Pennsylvania Press, 1993); and B. Cohn, 'The Census, Social Structure and Objectification in South Asia', in *An Anthropologist among the Historians and Other Essays*, by B. Cohn (New Delhi: Oxford University Press, 1987).

32. For more on the competing types of evidence that were established as valid for scientific enquiry, see J. Pickstone, *Ways of Knowing: A New History of Science, Technology and Medicine* (Manchester: Manchester University Press, 2000), pp. 135–61.

33. For more on uses for cannabis products in South Asia in this period, see Mills (2003), pp. 47–51.

34. This summary of the evolution of the ganja excise system is compiled from Hem Chunder Kerr, 'Report of the Cultivation of and Trade in Ganja in Bengal', in British Parliamentary Papers, volume 66 (London: Hansard,1891); G. Rainy, 'Report on the Manufacture and Smuggling of Ganja' (Calcutta: Bengal Sec Press, 1904).

35. G. Watt, *Hemp or Cannabis Sativa (Being an Enlargement of the Article in the 'Dictionary of Economic Products of India')* (Calcutta, 1887), p. 21.

36. Hansard's Parliamentary Debates, vol. 355 (3rd series), 16 July 1891, pp. 1395–412.

37. J. Mills, 'Cannabis in the Commons: Colonial Networks, Missionary Politics and the Origins of the Indian Hemp Drugs Commission 1893–4', *Journal of Colonialism and Colonial History* 6, no. 1 (2005).

38. W.S. Caine, *Picturesque India: A Handbook for European Travellers* (London: Routledge, 1890), p. 292.

39. For more on attitudes towards cannabis in the 1890s and the origins and outcomes of the IHDC, see Mills (2003), pp. 93–151.

40. See Mills (2003), pp. 149–51; V. Berridge, 'The Origins of the English Drug "Scene" 1890–1930', *Medical History* 32, no. 1 (1988): 51–64.

41. R. Pertwee, 'The Pharmacology of Cannabis: New Discoveries and Therapeutic Possibilities', unpublished paper presented at The Royal College of Psychiatrists in Scotland Addictions Faculty Annual Residential Meeting, 2012.

IV

CONTOURS OF THE MEDICAL

9

RE-THINKING THE 'MEDICAL' THROUGH THE LENS OF THE 'INDIGENOUS'
Narratives from Mahanubhav Healing Shrines in Maharashtra, India

SHUBHA RANGANATHAN

Medical Systems in India: The Dialectic between the Indigenous and the Biomedical

The last few decades have seen a proliferation of scholarship on medical pluralism in India.[1] In writing about the parallel existence of various indigenous healing practices in India, much of the literature has differentiated between two broad categories: biomedicine/'modern medicine'/ Western medicine/'cosmopolitan medicine', as Dunn terms it,[2] on the one hand, and 'Indian medicine'/'indigenous medicine'/'traditional medicine' on the other hand.[3] While such categorizations have enabled the understanding of the diverse ways by which different modes of healing function, they have also led to the setting up of a range of binaries along the traditional/modern dichotomy. In such a discourse indigenous medicine is largely conceptualized in terms of its relation to biomedicine: it is constructed either as the *opposite* of biomedicine or as another *kind* of medicine. At the same time, it is increasingly recognized that these binaries—local and Western, indigenous and biomedical, traditional and modern—are no longer tenable,[4] with indigenous medicine responding to market forces by recasting itself in a modern avatar, whether in the case of herbal medicine, Unani, or Ayurveda.[5]

This chapter draws on the healing narratives of women experiencing spirit possession to reflect on how the 'medical' is constituted in the 'indigenous'. It is not the study of the 'medical' as a system, as if it were a reified and naturalized object, but an exploration of how the 'medical' is invoked in narratives of indigenous healing. What thereby emerges is a picture of the 'medical' from the vantage point of the 'indigenous'. Ultimately, the chapter hopes to illustrate that the conceptual differentiation between 'biomedical' and 'indigenous' healing systems is in fact at odds with people's everyday lived experiences of illness and healing.

This chapter is based on a contemporary anthropological study of spirit possession and healing in Mahanubhav temples in Maharashtra. Persons staying in Mahanubhav healing temples to deal with the experience of persistent illness were interviewed about their experiences of temple healing and modern medicine, which were the two primary modes of healing accessed by them. In their narratives, the 'biomedical' and the 'indigenous' are not two separate worlds but come together and move apart in various ways, thereby calling for a re-imagining of our understanding of 'healing systems'.

The Mahanubhav Healing Shrines

The Mahanubhav shrines in this study are situated in Maharashtra, a large state (comprising a total area of 307,690 square kilometres) in western India, identified as the Marathi-speaking region of India. The Mahanubhav sect is one of the many 'Little Traditions' of folk movements and cults.[6] The thirteenth century saw the rise and growth of various devotional sectarian movements which worked to challenge the orthodox Brahmanical religion.[7] One of the most well known of these, the Varkari sect, went on to become a central part of popular Hinduism at the time.[8] In contrast, the Mahanubhav *panth*, founded in the thirteenth century by Chakradhar (approximately AD 1194–1274), during the rule of the Yadava kings, was less well known.[9] The Mahanubhavs have a monotheistic belief in one God incarnated in five avatars, the Panchakrishna or the 'five Krishnas'. According to

Raeside's account, Chakradhar, known as Haripaldev, was the son of Vishaldev, a Gujarati Brahmin minister from Bharuch. Haripaldev died at an early age but his body was reanimated by the soul of Chang Dev Raul, the third avatar (incarnation) of Parameshwar. He later became the disciple of Gundam Raul (Govindaprabhu), the fourth incarnation of God. Chakradhar's open opposition to the Brahmin orthodoxy earned him the hatred of the Brahman ministers of king Ramdevraja Yadava. He was eventually arrested and beheaded by them. His death is estimated to have occurred in A.D. 1274. After Chakradhar's death, the followers gathered around Gundam Raul, till his death. When he died, the leadership of the sect was taken over by an ardent devotee of Chakradhar, Nagdev. After Nagdev's death, the sect became a scriptural tradition, with devotees basically following the sacred texts rather than any person or guru.[10]

The Mahanubhav sect has a long tradition of providing succour to and healing people suffering from various kinds of afflictions, particularly spirit-related afflictions.[11] The local term for spirit-related affliction is *baher cha dukkha*, meaning affliction that is caused by forces that are 'outside' the natural world. These forces of the supernatural or spirit realm are believed to cause afflictions that are understood as part of one's 'dukkha'. The term 'dukkha' is a multilayered word with several meanings in different contexts. Most generally, dukkha means 'suffering'. However, it can also refer to 'illness', 'pain', 'unhappiness', or 'distress'.

Thus, spirit possession was understood as a particular kind of affliction caused by cosmic forces that do not belong to this world (hence 'outside'). Afflicted persons visited the temple at the point when they sensed that their affliction was spirit-related. In order to be healed of the affliction, they stayed as 'patients'[12] in the temple for a ritual period of forty days (preferably) or ten days. Most of the visitors who chose to stay in the temples came from lower-income groups and belonged to the lower castes. They were daily wage earners, or worked in factories, or as labourers. Devotees were predominantly Hindu, with the occasional Dalit Buddhist. While most of the visitors came from the state of Maharashtra, there were a few from adjoining states such as Gujarat and Karnataka.

During their stay in the temple, 'patients' participated in the temple activities and rituals, such as *seva*,[13] *smaran*,[14] and *ārati*. The most important ritual is the ārati (sessions involving the singing of devotional songs to the sound of the *dhol*, kettledrums, and cymbals). It is expected that the ārati will induce afflicted persons to go into a trance, an event that serves as proof of the spirit-related cause of the affliction. Most people then continued to experience trances regularly during the worship sessions, a process that is regarded as crucial in drawing out the illness from within the person and thereby moving the person towards healing.

Healing Trajectories: Complexities and Complications

In trying to understand people's healing trajectories, a number of complexities and contradictions emerge through what often appear to be straightforward accounts of 'pathways'. People's treatment trajectories cannot be reduced to managerial factors such as the accessibility, availability, and feasibility of options. Although their descriptions of past healing trajectories sought to construct a coherent and linear narrative of their healing pathways, a closer look suggests far more variation and complexity in these trajectories. Two important 'events' emerged prominently in their narratives: one, the failure of biomedical treatment, and two, the emergence of the temple as the last resort when all other treatment options had failed them. Thus, they generally spoke of having visited doctors first and then having turned to other informal sources such as healers and healing shrines after no relief was obtained from medical treatment.

At the same time, these narratives about 'medical failure' and the 'last resort' were complicated by other narratives describing a back and forth movement across various healing systems. Most pilgrims spoke of alternation between biomedical and indigenous systems of healing, depending on various factors and circumstances, not all of which could be articulated clearly. These narratives complicate the understanding of 'healing pathways', bringing out a greater complexity in health-seeking than is often acknowledged in the social scientific literature on 'medical pluralism'.

Narratives of 'Medical Failure' and Indigenous 'Efficacy'

In describing their healing trajectories, pilgrims often complained of having spent considerable money on diagnostic tests and medicines but having obtained neither a clear picture about the illness that they were suffering from nor relief from their symptoms. They spoke of turning to the Mahanubhav temple as the last resort after all other options had failed them.

For instance, Sharada complained that medicines had only a temporary effect in relieving her symptoms of body aches, vomiting, and fever.

> I would be well as long as I took the medicines but after I stopped them, the same problems would start again. This happened repeatedly. That was because it was a baher cha problem [interviewed on 20 May 2007].[15]

Eventually, Sharada said, she went to the temple and then felt better.

Similarly, Shanta complained that medicines provided only temporary relief and sometimes even worsened her illness.

> I went to doctors once or twice but it was of no use. The power of the medicines lasts for about two days. After that the problems start again. So there is no point. Now, I do not go to doctors at all. I have stopped it. It only gets worse when I go to a doctor.

In some cases, even expensive medical treatment provided only temporary relief from symptoms, as attested by Suresh, who had spent 100,000 rupees on medical treatment and diagnostic tests over a period of a year and a half.

> I took medicines for about a year and a half but did not feel better. I was taking about twenty-five pills each day. After one week, they would do an X-ray and again prescribe medicines. This went on for a long time. Then I went to a private doctor and took his treatment for about six months. But I did not feel any better and so I started coming here.[16]

Not experiencing relief, pilgrims often decided to discontinue the expensive medical treatment and approach the temple, as Sunanda's narrative illustrates.

> I had been to a doctor in Nasik who had said that I had a *maansik* [mental] illness caused by tension. He gave me medicines which cost Rs 450 per week. I was not able to continue the treatment as I couldn't afford it. So I discontinued it. Then, I went to several local healers, but did not feel better. I came to this temple after failing to find any relief from doctors and *bhagats* [local healers]. Someone told me about the temple and then I came and stayed for one and a quarter months. I felt better and then went back home.[17]

Narratives of medical failure were typically accompanied by character-
izations of biomedicine as ineffective in healing spirit-related afflictions
as seen in Suresh's conclusion:

> Doctors are useful only for medical illnesses. They are of no use in baher
> cha problems that are related to spirits. Mine is not a medical illness; it
> is caused by people who know how to work black magic and sorcery.[18]

Similarly, Shobha said:

> Doctors do not understand anything about *bhutache traas* [ghost
> illnesses]. They will say that this is because of weakness, BP [blood pres-
> sure], less blood. They don't know that it's a ghost illness and not a
> medical illness. I have stopped going to doctors now. I only go for the
> pain in my neck.[19]

Doctors were often characterized as having no knowledge or expertise
in matters of spirit possession, as reflected in Lankabai's narrative about
her consultations with doctors.

> [Showing me her palm] Look at my hand. Does it look like I have less
> blood? The doctor recently told me that I have less blood. He said that
> my blood was very thin. Another doctor said that I have too much blood;
> that it is too *thick*. Blood should be *thin*, he said. I don't understand what
> these doctors say! They don't know *anything*![20]

Nanda, too, described how doctors had not only failed to cure her
symptoms of mental illness, but had also been clearly wrong in their
estimate of her condition. 'The doctors there predicted that I would
live for only one hour', she said. 'Instead, I lived for twenty years!' She
concluded:

> Doctors do not really know anything about my illness; they do not
> understand baher cha illnesses. I did not experience any improvement
> with their treatment.[21]

Some pilgrims described biomedical treatment as not simply expensive
and ineffective, but also dangerous. Indubai explained, 'If I went to a
hospital, doctors who do not know me, who are strangers, might *kill* me
with their treatment!' she said, adding, 'I know my illness; it is not of
that [medical] type. It is a baher cha illness.'

These narratives about medical failure seem to suggest a more or
less linear healing pathway in which pilgrims 'first' seek medical treatment and 'then' turn to the temple as a 'last resort'. Similar findings

have been reported by other scholars of healing shrines.[22] Sébastia too found that pilgrims arrive at the shrine of Saint Anthony of Padua in Puliyampatti, Tamil Nadu, after biomedical treatments were found to be expensive and ineffective. Describing the shrine as 'the last resort' for pilgrims, she argued for an improvement in the quality of psychiatric facilities in the area.[23] In such analyses, the efficacy of indigenous healing is explained with reference to the failure of the biomedical.

At the same time, pilgrims' narratives about medical failure also proposed distinctions between medical illnesses and spirit-related (baher cha) illnesses. An explicit contrast was drawn up between medical illnesses on the one hand (which were caused by known natural forces and could be treated by modern medicine) and spirit-related afflictions (which could only be cured at the temple) on the other. These narratives seemed to construct two distinct worlds of the 'biomedical' and the 'indigenous'. At the same time, this separation of the indigenous and the biomedical was complicated by other narratives of simultaneously engaging in both modern medical treatment and indigenous healing. Pilgrims often described healing shrines as 'hospitals', thus drawing parallels between modern medicine and indigenous healing. These narratives brought out the fluidity in the temple discourses of healing, which made space for the biomedical, even while possession was framed as a non-medical baher cha illness.

Complexities in Healing Trajectories

In contrast to the linear healing trajectories (from biomedical to the indigenous) described in the previous section, a number of counter-narratives provided a more complex picture of healing pathways. Pilgrims often spoke of moving back and forth between various treatment approaches. For instance, Sakubai said, 'I go to both the temple and to doctors. Sometimes when I am ill I go to doctors, while at other times I come to the temple.' Similarly, Sangeeta's father explained the need to make use of both medical treatment and temple healing, saying, 'We do both—we go to doctors as well as worship God. We need to do both.'[24]

Particularly when the nature of the illness was not evident, pilgrims often sought both biomedical and alternative treatments. For instance, Jayashree wondered whether she should take medicines for her dizziness or restrict herself to temple healing, saying, 'I don't know what this problem is—whether it is dizziness, or possession, or black magic.'[25] She eventually resorted to both, visiting the temple regularly as well as occasionally visiting a doctor.

Clearly, pilgrims did not see any contradiction in seeking temple healing and medical treatment simultaneously. Thus, after staying in the temple for forty days and having experienced little relief, Manisha planned to visit a psychiatrist. Her father explained the importance of using medical treatment along with temple healing, explaining that while temple healing might deal with the underlying (supernatural) cause of the illness, medicines might calm Manisha and thereby help her. Medicines, by inducing sleep in her, might reduce her tension, he said.

Thus, doctors were described as basically dealing with the 'medical' aspects of the problem, while the temple was seen as dealing with the possessing ghost. As a monk explained:

> Doctors don't really give medicines for the illness as such. They give medicines for appetite and sleep. They deal with pilgrims as 'mentally affected' and give them medicines to calm them down. For the *illness*, pilgrims can only get well at the temple.[26]

Another monk reiterated:

> Doctors can treat medical illnesses; temples heal ghost illnesses. Doctors can treat the illness if it is a medical illness. But when they cannot even diagnose the illness, when they carry out tests and discover new symptoms each time, then they realize that it's a baher cha illness or an illness caused by *karni* [sorcery]. These people would only get well through worshipping God.[27]

At the same time, the monks were not averse to pilgrims seeking medical treatment. They acknowledged that this was often required if the problem was a physical or a mental illness. It was often not possible to discriminate between 'medical illnesses' and 'spirit afflictions'. In some Mahanubhav temples, allopathic doctors made visits to the temples on specific days of the week, much like medical consultations. For the monks, such arrangements worked to prove the 'modern' and 'rationalist' temper of the shrines.

In any case, the understanding about medical treatment as dealing with 'superficial symptoms' and temple healing as dealing with the 'root cause' of the problem (the ghost) allowed people to approach both systems of healing simultaneously. Long-term fieldwork in the temples indicated that pilgrims often alternated between allopathic and spiritual treatments, while still being convinced about the efficacy of the temple in healing spirit afflictions.

In some cases pilgrims' choices about treatment were related to pragmatic considerations such as what was accessible and what worked best in the specific situation. Particularly when distressing symptoms persisted, pilgrims were ready to try anything, as seen in the case of Vaishali. Her mother expressed their desperate search for treatment:

> We have been all over and have tried everything—doctors, temples. ... She [Vaishali] even took shock treatment [electroconvulsive therapy]. The doctors had told her that she had a mental illness. Then we brought her to this temple earlier this year. She stayed for three months. She was also taking medicines during that time. I don't know what it was that made her well—the medicines or the temple. Whatever it was, she became well.[28]

A host of contingencies appeared to operate in pilgrims' trajectories in healing. Pilgrims did not have fixed notions about what kinds of treatment to avail of but drew from diverse options. Moreover, people's narratives of their engagement with the biomedical and the indigenous often called into question the assumption of two distinctly different worlds or systems of healing. This was particularly evident when the language of biomedicine was invoked to describe the indigenous.

Healing Temples as 'Hospitals'

When describing the curing function of the Mahanubhav shrines, pilgrims and monks often used the English word 'hospital'. They described the temple as another *kind* of hospital, for another *kind* of illness (the baher cha illness). Thus, Satyabhama described the temple as 'basically a temple for ill and afflicted people', particularly those affected by spirit-related problems. Her mother described the temple as 'God's hospital', using the Marathi word *davākhāna*.[29] While elaborating on the expenditure incurred on Satyabhama's treatment and her frequent stays in the temple, her mother said: 'We spent about a hundred thousand rupees on her treatment.' When I asked her if she had spent that amount of money on hospital treatment she retorted vehemently: 'Not *those* [allopathic] hospitals—*this* hospital! *God's*

hospital!' She then explained that they often referred to the temple as
devāchā davākhāna: 'God's hospital'.[30] Similarly, Mainabai explained:
'This [temple] is nothing but a hospital! We all call this a hospital,
God's hospital.'

Pilgrims also drew comparisons between the use of medicinal
substances in allopathic treatment and the use of rituals in the healing
temple. They referred to the rituals of smaran and seva as analogous
to medicines. Pramila explained what made her recover in the temple:

> When you go to a doctor, how do you get well? You have to take medi-
> cines, right? In the same way, here, you have to do seva and smaran to
> get well.[31]

Similarly, Satyabhama compared the rituals of the temple to medical
treatment.

> We get well here because of God. He makes us well. Just like when you
> go to a hospital, you get well by taking medicines, in the same way when
> you come here and do smaran, *paaraayan* [prayer readings], and seva,
> you get well.[32]

One of the monks described the seva in the temple as analogous to
medicine.

> People get well through doing seva. They get the fruit of their seva. Just
> like a doctor gives medicines which have the power to cure, the seva
> cures the person. So people stay here for one and a quarter months and
> do seva.[33]

Another monk compared the deity in the temple to 'a doctor who
understands the dukkha and removes it'. Every illness had its own
specified period, he said, which one has to endure.

> One has to endure the illness till it lasts. Just like doctors carry out tests
> and then give the prescription that one has to follow for ten or fifteen
> days, in the same way, one has to endure the illness for the period that
> it lasts.[34]

These narratives clearly illustrate that the Mahanubhav temples
were regarded as not just sacred spaces but also as curing institutions
analogous to hospitals. In fact, in the Mahanubhav temple complex at
Phaltan (which is an important pilgrimage centre for the Mahanubhavs
as it is considered the birthplace of one of the five incarnations), there
were even formal procedures for the admission of pilgrims into the

temple. Every person who wanted to stay in the temple for healing was first 'interviewed' by the monks and the head of the temple trust to determine that he or she satisfied the criteria to be 'admitted' as a 'patient' into the temple. Only those who suffered from 'unidentified' symptoms and had been found to be free from HIV/AIDS and cancer were 'admitted'. One of the monks explained this process:

> We do not accept those patients who are very sick and for whom there is no cure. We only accept those patients who do not have any identified physical illness but are still ill. Those patients with doubtful symptoms, who have been having serious physical symptoms since a long time, have to show a certificate from a doctor testifying that they are free from HIV/AIDS, cancer, and other such serious illnesses.[35]

He also added that it was mandatory for 'patients' to have someone stay with them at the temple. Clearly, there were specific rules about who could be 'admitted' into the temple, indicating the extent to which the temples had become medicalized into treatment centres.

However, apart from medicalization, what was also noted was the characterization of the shrine as a different *kind* of hospital/clinic. The healing shrine was constructed, not so much in opposition to the biomedical clinic, but rather as parallel to it. The implication was that just as there are allopathic hospitals which cure people, these temples work accordingly. These narratives appear to be in contradiction to other narratives about the inefficacy of medical treatment and the difference between medical illnesses on the one hand and baher cha illnesses on the other. How do we make sense of these contradictions?

In studying people's health-seeking pathways, much of the research on medical pluralism has interpreted people's resort to healing shrines with respect to the availability and 'efficacy' of various treatment options. Such an inference characterizes people as either passively determined by external circumstances (such as availability of medical services) or actively choosing certain treatment options for their efficacy or pragmatic value. Yet, Kalpana Ram has pointed out that the logic of pragmatism is based more on notions of rational choice and economic utilitarianism.

> Many of the characteristics of the pragmatic choosing and strategic subject of medical pluralism are in fact also the characteristics of the bourgeois subject of liberal pluralism and economic utilitarianism. The sufferer weighs up the options with impeccable utilitarian logic and,

with goals clearly in sight, sets about pursuing them with a pragmatic zeal worthy of a neo-liberal subject. Villagers are turned into individual choosers, busy constructing 'hierarchies of resort for curative practices' and assigning complementary functions to 'scientific' and 'folk' medicine on the basis of illness typologies which they construct for themselves.[36]

However, my study found that while on many occasions pilgrims made a clear decision to visit either biomedical practitioners, or indigenous practitioners, or both, on other occasions, their healing trajectories were guided by other contingencies. While various concerns including, but not restricted to, pragmatism, 'efficacy', and accessibility worked to determine whether and when pilgrims approached the temple, they were not simply passive receptors of systems of health care but actively engaged with both biomedical and indigenous healing systems.

More importantly, the temple discourses illustrated that the alternation between the biomedical and the indigenous was allowed for in the very conceptualization of possession. The temple discourses characterized the baher cha illness as consisting of various kinds of symptoms that might be similar to the symptoms of medical illnesses, even while the underlying causes are sorcery and ghost possession. There was therefore no contradiction in receiving medical treatment for the symptoms and temple healing to remove the possessing ghost. Thus, the engagement between the biomedical and the indigenous was allowed for in the very conceptualization of possession and healing.

Re-thinking the Medical

The practices and discourses around healing in the Mahanubhav temples illuminate the complex ways by which indigenous healing was conceptualized. The temple narratives blurred the distinction between the religious and the medical, between science and superstition. Thus, the temple was not just a spiritual shrine, but also a medical institution with bureaucratic procedures and systems. As a 'hospital' the temple became transformed into a modern, scientific, faith-based spiritual site for which the term 'indigenous shrine' is no longer meaningful.

At the same time, it was not just the 'indigenous' that was transformed but also the 'medical', as seen in the conceptualization of illness and healing in the Mahanubhav temples. Thus, the illness of possession was understood not just in terms of medical symptoms but as part of a broader experience of suffering. The 'symptoms' of possession might be physical ailments, mental distress, financial crises, or family disturbances. Clearly, 'illness' was understood differently from biomedical discourses, which focus on symptoms as the identifying feature of illness. Moreover, the temple's theories about illness causation allowed for movement between both biomedical treatment and indigenous healing, since both natural and spirit-related causes were implicated in the baher cha illness.

The idea that people can receive medical treatment to deal with the symptoms and temple healing to remove the possessing ghost also means that healing was understood more in terms of recovery than cure. For ghost afflictions, it was no longer sufficient to reduce the symptoms; the spiritual dimensions of the sickness had to be addressed by dealing with the ghost. This conceptualization of healing as being beyond cure of symptoms brings a new spiritual dimension to the medical.

These complexities and crossovers suggest that neither the indigenous nor the biomedical can no longer be understood in terms of alternate 'medical systems'. Following Dunn's categorization of medical systems into 'local', 'regional', and 'cosmopolitan' medicine, scholars have identified medical systems as watertight compartments (despite the fact that Dunn pointed out that local systems are always in contact with other systems).[37] The literature on medical pluralism reflects the same notion of medical systems: there *are* references to cross-fertilization and cross-prescribing across medical traditions;[38] it *is* acknowledged that 'traditional systems' are increasingly becoming modernized and commercialized; and it *is* recognized that people adopt a pragmatic approach in their use of pluralistic therapies. Yet, the literature on medical pluralism maintains the existence of independent, autonomous systems of knowledge and practice.

This chapter has shown that in actual practice there is much more heterogeneity and variation than allowed for in the term 'system'. Pilgrims' healing trajectories are marked by oscillation between biomedical treatment and temple healing, which are presumed to work in different ways to heal the affliction. People do not have preconceived beliefs about the causes of illnesses. Rather, as Das and Das point out in their study of the illness experiences of the urban poor in Delhi, people deploy various kinds of languages and, correspondingly, make use of various types of therapies.[39]

I suggest, therefore, that instead of speaking of *medical systems*, which, as Attewell points out, implies homogenous, universal, static, and systematized knowledge systems, it might be more useful to focus on *medical practices*, which are dynamic and diverse. The focus in the latter shifts to what these practices *do*. When studying the medical in terms of practices rather than systems, one might find that Ayurvedic practices have more in common with biomedicine than with faith-healing practices. The temple discourses of healing thus illustrate the tenuousness of these binary categories of biomedical and indigenous: although these categories are maintained in theory, in actual practice, they are often blurred.

Notes

1. See, for example, V. Sujatha and Leena Abraham, eds, *Medical Pluralism in Contemporary India* (Delhi: Orient BlackSwan, 2012) and Arima Mishra, ed., *Health, Illness, and Medicine: Ethnographic Readings* (Delhi: Orient BlackSwan, 2010).
2. F.L. Dunn, 'Traditional Asian Medicine and Cosmopolitan Medicine as Adaptive Systems', in *Asian Medical Systems: A Comparative Study*, edited by C. Leslie (Berkeley: University of California Press, 1976), pp. 133–58.
3. The terms 'Indian' and 'indigenous' continue to be retained despite various difficulties. For instance, while Unani and homoeopathy fall under the rubric of 'Indian systems of medicine', Unani actually has Graeco-Arabic origins and homoeopathy originated in Germany. Further, as Projit Mukharji pointed out, the ambiguous phrase 'indigenous drugs' does not recognize the plurality of botanical traditions involved and could refer to drugs available in India, drugs grown in India, or drugs used in indigenous pharmacopoeias. See Projit Mukharji, 'Pharmacology, "Indigenous Knowledge", Nationalism: A Few Words from the Epitaph of Subaltern Science', in *The Social History of Health and Medicine in Colonial India*, edited by Biswamoy Pati and Mark Harrison (New Delhi: Primus Books, 2009), pp. 195–212.
4. See Biswamoy Pati and Mark Harrison, eds, *Health, Medicine, and Empire: Perspectives on Colonial India* (Hyderabad: Orient Longman, 2001); and Guy Attewell, *Refiguring Unani Tibb: Plural Healing in Late Colonial India* (Hyderabad: Orient Longman, 2007).
5. See Maarten Bode, *Taking Traditional Knowledge to the Market: The Modern Image of the Ayurvedic and Unani Industry 1980–2000* (Hyderabad: Orient Longman, 2008).

6. See Meera Kosambi, ed., *Intersections: Socio-cultural Trends in Maharashtra* (New Delhi: Orient Longman, 2000).

7. Anne Feldhaus and Eleanor Zelliot, *The Deeds of God in Rddhipur* (New Delhi: Oxford University Press, 1984).

8. The Varkari sect, founded by saint Dnyaneshwar, is characterized by the worship of the deity Vitthal (or Vithoba) of Pandharpur. A central part of this sect is pilgrimage to the holy site of Pandharpur, with the term 'Varkari' translating as 'those who perform the tour'. For more details, see Gérard Colas, 'History of Vaisnava Traditions: An Esquisse', in *The Blackwell Companion to Hinduism*, edited by Gavin Flood (New York: Blackwell Publishing Ltd, 2003), pp. 229–70.

9. See Anne Feldhaus, 'Maharashtra as a Holy Land: A Sectarian Tradition', *Bulletin of the School of Oriental and African Studies* 49, no. 3 (1986): 532–48 and Anne Feldhaus, 'The Orthodoxy of the Mahanubhavs', in *The Experience of Hinduism: Essays on Religion in Maharashtra*, edited by Eleanor Zelliot and Maxine Berntsen (Albany: State University of New York Press, 1988), pp. 264–79.

10. See M.P. Raeside, 'The Mahanubhavas', *Bulletin of the School of Oriental and African Studies* 39, no. 3 (1976): 585–600.

11. Others have also recounted this. See Eleanor Zelliot, 'Introduction', in *The Experience of Hinduism: Essays on Religion in Maharashtra*, edited by Eleanor Zelliot and Maxine Berntsen (Albany: State University of New York Press, 1988), pp. xv–xx and Vieda Skultans, 'Women and Affliction in Maharashtra: A Hydraulic Model of Health and Illness', *Culture, Medicine, and Psychiatry* 15 (1991): 321–59.

12. In the Mahanubhav temples, the term 'patient' is used by healers, monks, and the suffering to refer to afflicted persons staying in the temples for 'treatment', as distinguished from those who make a day trip to the temple for worship.

13. *Seva* (literally 'service') refers to the performance of various actions that indicate an attitude of 'service' towards the deity. It includes various kinds of activities such as participating in the ritual bathing of the deity, sweeping the temple, and assisting the monks during temple festivals.

14. *Smaran* refers to worship and prayer through recitation of the name of God.

15. Interviewed on 2 April 2008. All quotes in this chapter are drawn from interviews conducted by the author during ethnographic research in Mahanubhav healing temples.

16. Interviewed on 18 May 2007 and 26 May 2007.

17. Interviewed on 7 July 2007.

18. Interviewed on 27 April 2007.

19. Interviewed on 31 March 2008.

20. Interviewed 21 August 2007.

21. Interviewed on 20 July 2007.

22. See, for example, the work of Vieda Skultans on the Mahanubhav temple at Phaltan ('Trance and the Management of Mental Illness: Among Maharashtrian Families', *Anthropology Today* 3, no. 1 [1987]: 2–4) and Graham Dwyer's work on the Balaji temple in Rajasthan (*The Divine and the Demonic: Supernatural Affliction and Its Treatment in North India* [London: RoutledgeCurzon, 2003]).

23. Brigitte Sébastia, 'The Last Resort: Why Patients with Severe Mental Disorders Go to Therapeutic Shrines in India', in *Restoring Mental Health in India: Pluralistic Therapies and Concepts*, edited by Brigitte Sébastia (New Delhi: Oxford University Press, 2009), pp. 184–209. Also see, B. Sébastia, 'A Protective Fortress: Psychic Disorders and Therapy at the Catholic Shrine of Puliyampatti (South India)', *Indian Anthropologist* 37, no. 1: 67–92.

24. Interviewed on 1 April 2008.

25. Interviewed on 22 September 2007.

26. Interviewed on 2 April 2008.

27. Interviewed on 31 March 2008.

28. Interviewed on 29 March 2008.

29. *Davākhāna* could be translated as clinic, medical dispensary, or hospital. I prefer the meaning of hospital here as in this context patients are referring to the temple not simply as a dispensary of medicines but as a place that one goes to when one is sick; therefore, 'hospital' would be more appropriate.

30. Interviewed on 24 April 2008.

31. Interviewed on 26 may 2007.

32. Interviewed on 24 April 2008.

33. Interviewed 8 August 2007.

34. Interviewed on 8 August 2007.

35. Interviewed on 31 March 2008.

36. Kalpana Ram, 'Class and the Clinic: The Subject of Medical Pluralism and the Transmission of Inequality', in *Health, Culture, and Religion in South Asia: Critical Perspectives*, edited by Assa Doron and Alex Broom (Routledge, 2010), pp. 15–34.

37. Dunn, 'Traditional Asian Medicine'.

38. Bode, in *Taking Traditional Knowledge to the Market*, refers to allopathic doctors prescribing Ayurvedic tonics such as Septilin and Ayurvedic doctors prescribing antibiotics.

39. Veena Das and Ranendra Das, 'How the Body Speaks: Illness and the Lifeworld among the Urban Poor', in *Subjectivity: Ethnographic Investigations*, edited by João Biehl, Byron Good, and Arthur Kleinman (Berkeley: University of California Press, 2007), pp. 66–97.

10

VERNACULARIZING POLITICAL MEDICINE

Locating the Medical betwixt the Literal
and the Literary in Two Texts on the
Burdwan Fever, Bengal c. 1870s

PROJIT BIHARI MUKHARJI[*]

Locating the medical was an intensely political question in the first
half of the nineteenth century in Great Britain. Especially in Ireland
and Scotland, many doctors and a significant part of the public pushed
for a more expansive understanding of health that would take account
of both poverty and dearth as well as a diverse array of mental anxieties. These expansive visions of the medical had particularly important
consequences for public health. By contrast, in England, led by the
sanitarian Edwin Chadwick, a much narrower view of the medical was
promoted. This latter view sought to exclude issues such as poverty
and mental anxiety from the domain of the medical and refocus public
health more narrowly on impure water and accumulated urban filth.
Christopher Hamlin calls the more expansive view of the medical
available in Ireland and Scotland 'political medicine'.[1]

* I would like to thank Manjita Mukharji for her help in developing the
argument I make in this chapter. I am also indebted to Christopher Hamlin for
reading and commenting on an earlier draft. The editors of this volume also
deserve my gratitude for their patience and understanding. Naturally, I alone
am to blame for whatever inadequacies remain.

Chadwick's legislative success, it is largely believed, operated to effectively shut down 'political medicine' as a viable alternative and propel public health in a direction that was progressively more reductionist and narrowly medical. William Pulteney Alison, the charismatic Edinburgh doctor and teacher who had begrudgingly participated in Chadwick's legislative campaign while seeking to push the campaign towards more capacious visions of health, is generally seen to be the last great exponent of 'political medicine'. In this chapter I want to qualify this view. I will argue that 'political medicine' survived Alison's death in 1859 and was relocated to Bengal, via Bengalis with strong connections to Scotland and Ireland, in the 1860s and 1870s.

It is this act of relocation that I describe as 'vernacularization'. As I have pointed out elsewhere, vernacularization for me is not a mere linguistic process of translation.[2] While the term 'vernacularization' clearly suggests a linguistic model, actual linguistic translation is incidental and in the present case almost entirely redundant. It is instead a creative and agential process of refiguration whereby an idea or practice is relocalized in a new historical context by subordinated agents. In this article I shall focus on two such agents, namely Rev. Lal Behari Dey (1824–1892) and Dr Gopaul Chunder Roy (1844–1887).

Rev. Dey was a Bengali Hindu convert to Christianity and a pastor in the Free Church of Scotland. He was also an educator, an ethnographer-folklorist, and possibly the first South Asian to write a full-length English novel. Dr Roy was one of the first South Asians to successfully enter the Indian Medical Service (IMS). He held an MD from the University of Glasgow and was a Fellow of the Royal College of Surgeons. He is perhaps best remembered for his treatise on the Burdwan Fever of the late 1860s and early 1870s.

Considering Rev. Dey and Dr Roy side by side also raises the old question of the relationship between the literary and the literal. After all, Rev. Dey's writings on the Burdwan Fever were within the fictional context of the novel he wrote while Dr Roy wrote a medical work on the subject. Though they appeared in the same year, that is 1874, there is little to suggest that there was any direct connection between the two. Yet, both authors were part of the Bengali elite and came from the same part of Bengal. Moreover, they both had strong connections to Scotland. They almost certainly knew of each other and most likely had also met each other, though unfortunately no record of such a meeting has survived. Looking at them side by side provides us then with yet another way of determining the ambit of the medical.

Political Medicine

Before going any further it would be cogent to understand exactly what was 'political medicine'. At its most basic level, political medicine rejected monocausal etiologies of disease in favour of multicausal explanations, which gave space to dearth and debility as key factors in human health. As a result it generally eschewed the notion of disease specificity in favour of patient specificity.

At a time when political economy was emerging as the supreme arbitrator of state policy, 'political medicine' sought to intervene in policy-making circles by claiming to speak of basic human health. Hence, as Hamlin points out, 'political medicine' was often directly orthogonal to the tenets of political economy. It advocated active state and community intervention to ensure the amelioration of poverty and dearth, which in turn it understood to be putatively connected to health and mortality. Indeed, Friedrich Engels drew directly upon the writings of Alisonian 'political medicine' and Karl Marx's formulations too showed similarities with it.[3] Its claims of speaking for the common basic 'necessaries of life' impelled it to reject relativism and insist upon a common baseline without which any human health was bound to be impaired.[4]

For 'political medicine', 'health' meant more than simply the absence of disease understood in a narrow reductionist sense. Disease existed somewhere along a continuum of health and ill health and was always utterly individualized in the sense that the concrete circumstances of the patient was what brought it on. It did not exist as an abstract entity, but was always already inflected by the particularities of the conditions of individual sufferers. Disease was understood as resulting from the integration of the entirety of the negative biological, social, and emotional experiences of the patient. Summing up 'political medicine', Ian Burney describes it as 'the broadly humanitarian paradigm of a traditional, holistic and person-centred approach to medicine—and the political implications entailed by it'. This medical imaginary stood in bitter contrast to the paradigm that superseded it by the middle of the nineteenth century. This latter operationalized a 'model of public health dominated by the highly abstracted and analytical calculus of political economy'.[5]

What allowed this broadly social and expansive 'political medicine' to operate was a threefold notion of causality. A basic distinction was made between 'proximate' and 'remote' causes. While the former was what we would today call the most narrowly anatomical or physiological cause, the latter was much broader in its ambit. The remote causes were themselves divided into 'exciting' and 'predisposing' causes. Of these the latter was the most expansive and could include anything that could be seen to be diminishing an individual's constitutional strength.[6] The site upon which the environment, the body, and the mind were integrated in 'political medicine' was the nervous system. It was here, in the nervous system, that all the different causes found their shared media of operation. Be they emotional stresses or environmental pressures, or indeed physical injuries, their ultimate action on the person who suffers them is mediated by the nervous system.[7]

This already complex idea of causality was further complicated by the multiple senses in which the very question of 'what is the cause of disease?' could be interpreted. As Hamlin points out, physicians in the early nineteenth century could still interpret this question in at least four ways. First: what is the cause behind this person, rather than another, taking on this disease now? Second: what is the cause behind the course the disease has taken in this person, whilst it has taken a different course in another? Third: what is the cause of the general epidemic in this time and place? Finally: what is the cause of the spread of this epidemic?[8] Each of these ways of understanding the question of causality led in turn to its own multi-causal answers. Some of the rich diversity that could follow from the complexity of the causal question can be glimpsed in Sir Thomas Watson's mid-nineteenth-century comment:

> Of a score of persons exposed to the same noxious influence—to the combined influence of wet and cold during a shipwreck, for example— one shall have catarrh, another rheumatism, a third pleurisy, a fourth ophthalmia, a fifth inflammation of the bowels, and fifteen shall escape without any illness at all. A man shall do that with impunity to day, which shall put his life in jeopardy when he repeats it next week.[9]

What this rich and multilayered understanding of causality did was to accommodate a variety of social and personal factors into considerations of health and disease. It also remained flexible as to the ways in which these social and personal factors might affect the health of concrete individuals. Such an accommodating and flexible framework resisted the kind of causal reductionism that would progressively dominate public health after Chadwick. Eschewing such reductionism also meant resisting narrow technocratic solutions for the amelioration of public health problems.

'Political medicine' was particularly prominent in Ireland and Scotland since the poor in these countries did not have recourse to welfare entitlements that the English poor could access through the church.[10] In Ireland, many doctors in the wake of the disastrous fever epidemic of 1816–19 came to view poverty as a predisposing cause for ill health and while not all of them actually practised 'political medicine' and recommended direct intervention into poverty, practically all acknowledged its connection to illness.[11] In Scotland on the other hand, the embracing of 'political medicine' by influential medical professors gave it an even greater prominence. Andrew Buchanan, a professor at the Andersonian University in Glasgow, explicitly connected hunger, poverty, and health in the 1830s.[12] In the following decades, Alison at Edinburgh would become the most prominent and vocal exponent of 'political medicine'.

It would be wrong, however, to mistake political medicine's diagnosis of poverty and want as a key factor in the maintenance of human health for political radicalism. Most exponents of political medicine, including such champions as Alison, were deeply paternalistic. They did not seek a social revolution, merely an amelioration of the extreme physical hardships that the poor had to labour under in industrial Britain. Of course their paternalism found echoes in the demands of the poor themselves, but that partial overlap between paternalistic concern and the demands of the poor is precisely what constituted the moral economy that was being attenuated and discredited by the new political economy. As E.P. Thompson has told us, the English crowds rioting for food in the eighteenth century 'derived [their] sense of legitimation, in fact, from the [pre-existing] paternalist model'.[13] The hungry crowds 're-echoed so loudly' what was largely already accepted in the paternalist tradition.[14] Hamlin builds on this. He writes of Alison's 'highly paternalist' views on the plight of the Scottish highlands. For Alison, '[l]iberty, prosperity, and progress were secondary; the maximization of capital was not a goal, nor was the betterment of the individual. The doctor's job was to produce healthy survival'.[15] Yet, the production of health engendered a congruence between the demands of the poor and the advice of the paternalist doctor to policy-makers. This medico-moral congruence was enabled at least partially, no doubt, by the simple fact that in the first half of the nineteenth century medical and lay views of disease causation were still fairly close to each other. The 'key to understanding therapeutics at the beginning of the nineteenth century', writes Charles Rosenberg, 'lies in seeing it as part of a system of belief and behavior participated in by physician and layman alike'.[16] Though Rosenberg made his comments mainly about American medicine, they are certainly equally applicable to British medicine. The complex world of research, laboratories, and pathological tests that would make the physician's understanding of pathogenesis almost entirely unintelligible to the layman was still at least half a century in the future. And, it was this mutually intelligible view of pathogenesis that, at least partially, created the grounds for a convergence between a paternalist tradition of political medicine and the demands of the poor themselves.

Gopaul Chunder Roy's Political Medicine

Rohan Deb Roy points out that Gopaul Chunder Roy's treatise on Burdwan Fever 'was widely circulated and reviewed' and 'extensively cited'.[17] Elsewhere he clarifies further that Roy's work was 'the most extensively cited English book on malaria written by a Bengali in the nineteenth century'.[18] David Arnold adds that beyond strictly medical circles, Roy's 'mournful account' had resonated with Bengalis over the next fifty years.[19] Historians of medicine too have thus continued to cite Roy's treatise. Yet, unfortunately, so far as I am aware there exists no close study of the text or the man who wrote it.

In the absence of such studies, his views are often abstracted out of their larger narrative context and redeployed in historical accounts. Thus, Arnold, for instance, emphasizes his 'funereal images'. Deb Roy focuses on the symptomatology described by Roy. Mark Harrison cites Roy as a defender of 'medical registration'.[20] But we remain largely ignorant of Roy's larger views on medicine in general or even Burdwan Fever for that matter. What, we are left to speculate, were the actual medical views of the author of the 'most cited English work on malaria by a Bengali author'? What did the author think caused disease and how did he advocate its cure?

Roy's treatise was originally written as an entry into an essay competition organized by the viceroy. Roy did not win the prize, but the work was serialized in the *Calcutta Medical Journal* along with some additional material. This serialized version was published in pamphlet form in July 1874. Two years later, in 1876, an expanded version of this pamphlet appeared as the treatise proper. Yet, even as the essay gradually changed form and evolved into the treatise, some of Roy's core concerns remained the same. In the preface to the pamphlet, Roy had stated that his object in the essay had in the main been to investigate the 'mysterious subject of the etiology of the [Burdwan] fever' by surveying those causes which were known to be patent violations of 'sanitary principles'.[21] In other words, Roy sought to test through personal experience to what extent the violation of 'sanitary principles' could be held responsible for Burdwan Fever.

His answer to this basic question could not have been clearer: 'Poverty, over-crowding and deficient vital energy ... it implies that endemic disease has become general not from any increased potency of "malaria" but from diminished power of resistance in the constitution of the people, brought on by over-crowding, insufficient food and general poverty.'[22] Poverty, Roy clarified, did not create disease, but once disease had set in, poverty played 'a very important part in retarding convalescence, bringing on repeated relapses after fatigue and exertion, and hurrying on those sequelae, from the complication of which the patient finds himself impossible to extricate'. As a result, 'the greatest mortality has been amongst the poor working classes, whilst the rich have escaped with very little suffering, but no party have [*sic*] enjoyed absolute immunity'.[23]

Clearly the model of causation Roy was working with was a complex and multilayered one. When he said poverty did not 'create' disease but shaped the course the disease was to take in the patient, he was plainly interpreting the causal question at multiple levels. Likewise, his invocation of the impact of poverty, over-crowding, and so on, upon the body's powers of resistance resonated with discussions about 'predisposing causes'. Indeed, in introducing the discussion on poverty, he explicitly said:

> The general causes of dampness have slowly and gradually increased and the increasing rice cultivation in Lower Bengal has added still more to exaggerate the evil. Yet something more is wanting to explain the

explosive way in which the disease showed itself. This will lead us to the consideration of those causes which we have termed as immediate or exciting.[24]

Elsewhere I have shown that there is a long history of *daktar*s (doctors) using the doctrine of 'predisposing' or 'exciting' causes to vernacularize 'Western' medical theory.[25] In Roy's case, he was not only vernacular-izing medical theory, but also the political impulse that was constitu-tive of political medicine. Thus, whereas many other Bengali daktars in the late nineteenth century used notions of predisposition to develop nationalist and proto-nationalist programmes for social reform, Roy's programme had little that was nationalist. Instead it remained much closer to the paternalistic Scottish 'political medicine' which sought state intervention in ensuring a healthy life for the working poor.

Writing just over a decade after the death of Alison, when political medicine was hardly a powerful force in Britain any longer, Roy still sought to deploy it against the hegemonic vision of political economy. Explicitly taking on John Stuart Mill, he quoted the latter at length before dismissing his theory of population growth with almost a touch of contempt. Having stated Mill's Malthusian premise in detail, he asked just how could 'pauperism'—that favourite term of the Malthusians—be taken to be a natural fact related to overpopulation? 'Do the Zamindars feed less than before?' Are the 'European officers with their princely incomes' any worse off for the overpopulation? No. For Roy, pauperism was not a natural consequence of the growth of population. Some fared worse than others when the population grew and it was the poor that fared the worst. It was their poverty that laid them low and brought about their ill health and death, not the number of children.

Roy's use of Mill is noteworthy and distinctive, especially when we compare it to other contemporary writers. Jessica Baron's excellent study of Florence Nightingale's views on public health in India has pointed out that she too came, late in life, to occupy views remarkably reminiscent of Alisonian political medicine.[26] Nightingale, however, drew explicitly on John Stuart Mill's notion of 'peasant proprietorship' to make her case.[27] By contrast, though Roy quoted Mill at great length—nearly two whole pages of direct quotation—it was not his ideas about peasant proprietorship that Roy emphasized. Rather it was entirely the Malthusian elements about population growth and its links to pauperism that held Roy's attention.[28] As a result, far from finding inspiration in Mill, Roy builds his case through a critique of Mill's views on population. This is slightly perplexing since there is much in Mill's critique of the rent system and his advocacy of peasant tenure that would have fitted snugly into Roy's programme. The reasons for such divergent readings of Mill are beyond the scope of this chapter but would be a worthy project in itself.

Yet, having dismissed overpopulation as the pre-eminent cause of the disease, he did not then proceed to ignore it altogether. Instead, he turned the overpopulation question into a locally redolent one about the age of marriage. He spoke of the custom of 'early marriage' that was seen as a 'necessary institution of Hindu Society both amongst the high and the low classes' and the 'animal instinct of propagation with which the Hindus look upon the multiplication of species' as being the chief causes for the unhealthy increase in the population of Burdwan and other areas of Bengal.[29] It was but natural for Roy to bring up the age of marriage. The first civil marriage act, Act III of 1872, had only been passed two years ago.[30] Moreover, Keshab Chandra Sen, the religious reformer who led the agitation for the promulgation of the Act in order to gather support for it, had circulated a letter to the leading local doctors of the time asking about what should be the appropriate age of marriage. Most of those consulted such as Mahendralal Sircar, Charles Day, Armaram Pandurang, decided against the prevailing custom of child marriage. Sen summarized their view by stating, 'The medical authorities in Calcutta almost unanimously declared that 16 is the minimum marriageable age of girls in this country.'[31] But most significantly, Sen was Roy's cousin. Furthermore, during Roy's stay in Britain, he and Sen, who too was in Britain on a lecturing tour at the time, had jointly addressed public meetings such as one at the Hunterian Society.[32] Roy thus incorporated marriage reform into his version of political medicine. But it remained rather awkwardly poised as the main thrust of his medical argument remained focused on dearth and distress.

In a move that would be familiar to anyone who had read the works of Buchanan or Alison, Roy invoked the 'necessaries of life'—that favoured yardstick of the exponents of political medicine—to connect the economic plight of the poor to their diminished health. He argued that it was the absence of rent control that was at the root of rural poverty. Zamindars, he pointed out, tended to rack-rent every piece of land, thus squeezing the peasantry so hard that very little money was left in the hands of the cultivators. Together with the rising prices, this ever-shrinking income meant that the peasants could no longer afford the 'domestic necessaries'.[33]

But it was not the rapacious zamindars alone who had pauperized the peasants. Roy mentioned the 'superseding of some native manufactures, such as cloth &c., by foreign supply', the introduction of industrial manufacture at jails that then competed for the local market, and finally, the introduction of the railways that had adversely effected local markets by raising prices.[34] While the gains that accrued by technologies like the railways had had only a 'trifling effect' on the 'working classes', the prices of all the 'domestic necessaries' had risen sharply.

The staple diet of the 'working classes', as he called the rural poor, remained largely as before, that is, rice, salt, and vegetables. But fish and milk, which previously they had been able to occasionally consume, had now become completely unaffordable. At the same time, the 'wear and tear' to which the bodies of the poor were now liable had also become greater owing to the greater amount of labour that was now required to produce for both domestic and foreign consumption. All this had 'induced a failing stamina of health'. 'A weak fortress', Roy asserted, 'gives way at the first assault, and a weak constitution succumbs under the presence of a poison against which a stronger one maintains its ground for some time with success.'[35]

But it was not food alone that made up the 'domestic necessaries'. Commenting on the want of adequate clothing, Roy wrote, 'His poverty does not allow him to clothe himself sufficiently, and thus scantily clad, he is exposed to all variations of temperature.'[36] Later, commenting on the complications that might arise on top of the fever, he wrote that 'dysentery is sometimes an attendant complication of malarious fever. It is most frequent in the month of December and January, when increased cold, greater ranges of variation in hygrometry and temperature render the badly clothed peasants more liable to such attacks'.[37] Adequate food and clothing were therefore both thought to be crucial. Even when, on occasions, Roy seemed to superficially conform to Chadwickian public health and insist that the proximate

cause be related to some kind of 'poison' in the air or soil, he immediately added that had the peasants been well clothed such poison's
impact would have been reduced.

Roy was also clear that the government had a responsibility to
these starving, toiling, rural workers. It was, according to him, pitiable
to observe the condition of 'honest bod[ies] of workmen' such as the
weavers of Jehanabad, and Government ought to put a stop to 'unfair
competition'. Here clearly we see the paternalist moral economy at
work. Roy is appalled by the misery brought about by the laissez faire
practices, and considered any competition which pauperized honest
local workers as unfair. As Thompson had said, 'It is not easy for us to
conceive that there may have been a time ... when it appeared to be
"unnatural" that any man should profit from the necessities of others.'.
yet, there had been such times and men such as Roy had believed that
political economy was an unfair and unnatural apparatus.[38] What was
'natural' was that good, honest, and hardworking men should be able
to consume the 'domestic necessaries' of life.

In the final reckoning, while repeating the usual post-Chadwickian
sanitary homilies about drainage and water, he added that 'a better
standard of living is an indispensable necessity. Better clothing and
better food will enable them to bear against malaria or any vicissitude
of temperature with greater power of resistance than before'.[39] Beneath
this rather bland statement there was the entire complex system of
exploitation that he had outlined. Conservancy, drainage, and government intervention to control the rapaciousness of the free market
had to work together to stop the Burdwan Fever. But alongside it, the
people also needed to change one crucial aspect of their lives, and that
was their marital practices. 'The custom of early marriage giving rise
to a generation of paupers, whom their parents are not able to sustain,
should be discouraged as much as possible', he concluded.[40]

Lal Behari Dey's Political Medicine

Whereas Roy's treatise is well known and widely cited in histories
of medicine, the Rev. Lal Behari Day's novel, *Govinda Samanta, or
the History of the Bengal Raiyat*, has rarely featured on radar of the
historian of medicine.[41] Yet, not only is it one of the earliest South
Asian novels in English and contains a wealth of ethnographic data

about the Burdwan region, it, in fact, also devotes two complete chapters to fever. Moreover, it appeared in the same year as Roy's pamphlet, 1874.[42]

Day wrote the novel two years earlier, in 1872, as an entry into a competition sponsored by the improving zamindar of Uttarpara, Joykrishna Mukherjee. Unlike Roy, Day actually won the prize and bagged a then princely sum of £50. Day's intention had been to write a novel that would also accurately depict the everyday life of a typical Bengali peasant or *raiyat* in the Burdwan region.[43]

Day, interestingly, made a clear distinction between two types of fever in his novel. The two chapters that are exclusively about fever are therefore not about the same type of fever. The first such chapter, Chapter XXXVII in the novel, was titled *Bengal Fever and the Village Leech*. The chapter describes the febrile illness of Badan the father of the hero, Govinda. The bulk of the chapter is devoted to the description and sarcastic denunciation of the village *kaviraj*, practitioner of traditional medicine, named Mrityunjaya and his therapeutics.[44] Day was utterly dismissive of the typical rural kavirajes and depicted Mrityunjaya in an extremely poor light. As for the fever, however, there was nowhere any suggestion of it being anything out of the ordinary. Day was clear that such fevers are common and there is a clear way of dealing with it. Most people of the Burdwan region, he said, allowed the fever three days before calling in the physician. In this time, the patient was generally made to fast and given very little water.[45] Badan was an old man and Mrityunjaya's therapeutics are described as having made the situation worse. The chapter closes with the death and funeral of Badan, but it is unclear as to whether it was the fever or the quackery attributed to the kaviraj that killed him. Describing the consequences of the therapy, Day wrote that '[a]ll these poisons, instead of contributing to Badan's recovery, only made him worse. He became delirious. It was evident he was fast sinking, and there was not the remotest chance of his recovery'.[46]

The second chapter devoted to fever, Chapter LX, was titled *The Epidemic*, and stood in stark contrast to the former.[47] There was very little discussion of therapeutics in this chapter. Moreover, it was clear that this fever was entirely distinct from the regular fever we had met in the previous febrile chapter. Like the many official reports on the Burdwan Fever, Day commenced the chapter by giving readers a brief history of the disease, which immediately served to distinguish it from the regular Bengal Fever he had earlier spoken of. He wrote:

> In the year 1870, Kanchanpur was visited by a terrible epidemic. That dreadful plague had years before manifested itself amid the marshes of the district of Jessore; and year after year it had been marching westwards, not only decimating the population, but depopulating entire villages and reducing them to jungles, the abode of the hyena and the tiger.[48]

This attribution of the origin of the Burdwan Fever to Jessore in the 1820s was almost universal in the official reports. The very first official report on the Burdwan Fever by John Elliot, for instance, had commenced with the lines, 'a peculiar type of fever, called by Natives 'Jur Beekar', of the same nature as that now prevalent in many of the large Villages of the Burdwan and Nuddea Divisions'.[49]

It was clear that Day had actually read some of the medical reports on the fever, but it was equally clear that he did not find their causal explanations entirely satisfactory. On the cause of the epidemic, he wrote,

> Of the origin of this 'scourge of God' no rational account could be given. Some people ascribed it to the rank vegetation with which the villages had been covered; others to the accumulated filth of centuries; and others still, to the checking of drainage by the laying on of the iron road. But, whatever the cause, there could be no question but that the epidemic carried off a large percentage of the population.[50]

Both the listing of an entire litany of alternate causes as well as the phrase 'whatever the cause', I will argue, strongly suggests Day's lack of conviction about any one or all of them.

If I am correct in assuming Day to have been agnostic to the prevalent medical theories about the origin of the Burdwan Fever, we might conjecture that Day had some theory of his own. As a man who was virulently opposed to quackery, he may not have felt confident to articulate this theory clearly enough, but as a widely read thinking man, I feel, he was bound to have had some personal opinion—if not theory—about the genesis of the dreaded disease. Studying the architecture of the novel itself, I would suggest, might then illuminate Day's opinion.

The chapter on the epidemic came immediately after a long series of chapters where Govinda is locked in an epic battle with the local zamindar. The latter, a picture of unreformed feudal oppressiveness, tries everything to undermine Govinda's independence. Through a series of blatantly oppressive actions, the zamindar, Jaya Chand Raya Chaudhuri, beat Govinda with his shoes, abused him, had his henchmen set fire to Govinda's house, and eventually demanded rents that had already been paid. Day wrote, 'It mattered nothing to Jaya Chand, though a tenant whom he wanted to ruin had paid up his rent; it was not difficult for him to make the tenant out to be a defaulter by the arts of chicanery, perjury, and forgery, in which he was so great an adept.'[51] Having thus made Govinda out to be a defaulter, the zamindar invoked the law and had the sale commissioner sell everything Govinda owned—his stock of paddy and sugarcane, his cows, the few possessions of the women of his house, and even the brass vessels—by public auction. When the commissioner finished the auction, Day wrote that the 'man of the law was now satisfied and our hero was completely ruined'.[52]

Besides being deprived of everything of value, Govinda was also left with a very sizeable debt to the moneylender from whom he had borrowed heavily as a consequence of his confrontation with the zamindar.[53] With a large debt to repay, a fairly large joint family still to feed, and nothing left at home, the future seemed bleak for Govinda.

All this happened around 1858. In 1859 the new government of Queen Victoria brought in what Day described as the Bengal peasant's Magna Carta: Act X of 1859, which put a stop to the zamindar's ability to charge countless additional cesses over and above the rent.[54] It also disallowed the zamindar his powers to arbitrarily raise rents of old, long-established tenants. Govinda's conflict with Chaudhuri had commenced over his initial refusal to pay a cess for the zamindar's son's marriage. It was precisely these additional cesses or *abwabs* that Act X attempted to stop.

The Magna Carta came, however, a little too late for Govinda. Already pauperized and in debt, it took him a full ten years to pay off his debts and regain a semblance of the lifestyle his family had had before the zamindar reduced him to penury. Day's closing paragraph in the chapter just before the chapter on the epidemic states, 'The history of those ten years, as it was a history of silent suffering and self-denial, I shall not here recount.'[55]

Day may not have recounted it for us, but the structure of his novel made it amply clear that it was the 'history of silent suffering and self-denial' that led putatively up to the epidemic. The epidemic may have arrived in Burdwan from Jessore, but it seems but natural to assume that what made both Govinda and his family vulnerable to the deadly epidemic was the long history of privations and poverty that had been ushered in by the oppressive cesses of the zamindar.

Day was clear that the fever affected different people differently and there was a sense in which physical weakness might be said to have contributed to the outcome. When the epidemic entered Govinda's village, Day tells us that it 'went from one end of the village to the other, killing some people and reducing others to skeletons'.[56] When the disease finally entered Govinda's home, though it affected him first and gradually the rest of the family, his mother, the eldest and there-fore one might safely presume physically the most frail, was the only one to die.

The chapter on the epidemic is the penultimate one in the novel. The final chapter is set in 1873. The famine that year once more reduced Govinda to penury. After a lifetime of struggle to clutch on to his ancestral freehold, he is finally forced to become a coolie and go to work in the famine relief camps opened by the Maharaja of Burdwan. Here we get another and possibly the clearest state-ment of Day's theory of health and disease. With utmost pathos Day wrote:

> It was with a heavy heart, and with tears in his eyes, that Govinda left his home, and wended his way towards Burdwan. He had never in his life hired himself out as a day-labourer. He had always tilled his paternal acres, and lived upon their produce. But now, in mature life, he had to stoop to the degradation of becoming a coolie. This thought dried up his life's blood. ... It preyed upon his spirits. He wept day and night over his wretched lot. His health visibly declined. He was reduced to a skeleton. His heart was broken. And one morning he was found dead in his miserable hovel, far from his home and from those he loved.[57]

Poverty, want, and degradation were more than simply peripheral appendages to human health. They directly contributed to health and mortality. It is clear from the passage that what killed Govinda finally was not a specific disease but the fact that he was a broken man. If we reflect back from the end of the novel then, we might be even surer that the ten years of silent suffering and self-denial had taken its toll on both Govinda's and his mother's health. It was this poverty that had made the epidemic a killer, and the root of the poverty was the zamindari system.

The Act of 1859 might have been the Magna Carta of the Bengal raiyat, but Day was also clear that half a century of systematic oppression had left an indelible mark on the bodies of the peasantry. What was more, Day held the government directly responsible for the situation. He wrote,

> The object which Government had in giving such extraordinary powers to landholders was to enable them to realise their rents regularly, and transmit them punctually to the public exchequer; but, in consulting its own interest, the Government virtually consigned the entire peasantry of Bengal to the tender mercies of a most cruel and rapacious aristocracy. Happily, a more enlightened and humane legislation has taken away from the code those iniquitous regulations; but it is worthy of note that, for half-a-century those horrible engines of oppression were allowed, by a Government calling itself Christian, to grind to the dust many millions of probably the most peaceful people upon earth.[58]

Betwixt the Literal and the Literary

I have argued that both Roy and Day had vernacularized Scottish political medicine in writing about the Burdwan Fever. But what is the relationship between these two texts? Are they exactly the same? What might the historian gain from reading them side by side?

To answer these questions, I would begin by first comparing Roy's treatise to the mainstream medical opinion within the IMS, before moving on to a comparison of his text with that of Day's. For the purposes of comparison, I shall take two texts written by British medical officers to be representative of mainstream IMS thinking: John Elliot's 1863 report and Surgeon-Major John Gay French's 1875 tract on the subject.[59] I choose these two texts as representative texts because Elliot's 1863 report was the very first official account of the fever and French's was the one most proximate in time to the works of Roy and Day. French, moreover, had been the civil surgeon of the district of Burdwan during much of the duration of the outbreak.

The first thing that would strike any reader reading Elliot, French, and Roy side by side is the brevity of the two former texts. Elliot's text was only 32 pages long and French's was 69 pages. By contrast, Roy's 1874 text was already 99 pages in length and this increased to 124 pages (plus two tangentially related appendices of about 40 pages) at the time of its second issue in 1876. This additional girth was not simply verbosity. While Elliot and French both seem closely focused upon isolating a specific set of causes, Roy gives us something of a scattershot. Despite pursuing the same ends as Elliot and French, Roy's work provides a much thicker description of average village life in Burdwan. His particular focus, as we have already seen earlier, is the poverty of the average villager and the causes behind it. By contrast, neither Elliot nor French mention rural poverty at all. Their focus is on the soil, on drainage, on temperature, and not so much on human beings at all. The rural people feature in their texts only incidentally as they by their allegedly 'insanitary habits' aggravated pre-existing pathogenic conditions. There was no account in their texts of how life in Bengali villages had changed for the worse through zamindari rack-renting, railway-enabled dumping of Manchester-made goods, and so on. Nothing political or economic appeared in their treatises.

In this regard it would be pertinent to recognize that while Roy's broader vision was distinctive in the context of Burdwan Fever, there were others within the IMS, and the medical establishment more generally, in different parts of the Raj who shared his view that poverty and deprivation needed to be a part of the thinking about public health. I have already noted Baron's observation that Florence Nightingale's views came to resemble 'political medicine' towards the end of her life.[60] Similarly, without drawing an explicit connection, Leela Sami describes Dr William Robert Cornish's efforts to connect poverty and starvation to famine mortality in Madras Presidency in the 1870s.[61] A broader, social framework for understanding disease and mortality were therefore not completely absent within the medical circles in British India. Yet, there were clearly distinctive elements about Roy's framework. In Cornish, for instance, there is a tendency to reduce poverty to nutrition alone.[62] For Nightingale, by comparison, peasant education was a key component in her 'biomedical liberalism'. It was through education that she sought to produce healthy peasants who would be 'precursors to a liberal, democratic, citizen'.[63] Neither of these two elements features in Roy's programme. Peasant education is not something Roy comments on and he does not necessarily wish to transform peasants into proto-citizens. Likewise, his critique of poverty does not get reduced to dietary measurements alone. Clothing and over-crowding, for instance, are also mentioned as the negative consequences of poverty. Indeed, there is a long tradition of colonial attempts to compute adequate dietaries; that Roy chose not to pin his critique of poverty to this tradition and retain a fairly broad attack on poverty per se is in itself worth noting.[64]

This broader canvas upon which Roy sketches his account of the Burdwan Fever often overwhelms the reader. Whereas Elliot or French evince a clear sense of purpose that allows them to ignore the messiness of life around them and focus on a small set of issues they felt were possible causes, Roy constantly got sucked into the minutiae of that very mess. As a result there is a lot of detail that is better suited to an in-depth, immersive ethnography of rural change than a simple medical treatise.

Despite this expansive and generous framework, Roy failed to accommodate certain aspects of the patient's being. Particularly absent was any consideration of the emotional state of the patient. This is particularly significant given what Surgeon-Captain Baman Das Basu, a junior colleague, had to say of Roy's own health. Towards the middle of 1886, Roy applied for medical leave for himself. According to Basu, 'For some time past he had suspected that he was suffering from albuminuria and the condition of his heart was also unsatisfactory. The anxiety and worry of the last few months had considerably accelerated the progress of the disease.'[65] While the statement is not clear as to whether Roy himself thought that the 'anxiety and worry of the last few months' had accelerated the disease or Basu was adding this to Roy's self-diagnosis, it is clear that there were at least colleagues in Roy's circle who were willing to see a connection between emotional strain and ill health. Yet, this does not feature at all in Roy's account of Burdwan Fever.

The absence is made more conspicuous still by Elliot's brief comment on the role of fear in the epidemic. Though otherwise disinterested in the lives and sufferings of the peasants, Elliot mentioned,

The influence of fear and depression on the minds of the people during epidemic periods is well known to exercise a prejudicial effect on the body in rendering it less able to oppose and withstand disease.

The minds of many of the people at the present time are filled with anxiety and alarm, dreading a fresh outbreak of the epidemic during the approaching rainy season.[66]

Notwithstanding the narrow and circular cause Elliot attributed to the 'fear and depression', he did at least acknowledge the role of psychological strain in the disease.

The absence of any discussion of the emotional life of patients in Roy's treatise begs explanation. Emotional health was well established within the tradition of political medicine. It was also clearly something Roy's peers such as Basu—and possibly Roy himself—looked at while making specific diagnosis. It was also something that had already been connected by Elliot, in however inadequate a fashion, to the Burdwan Fever. So why did Roy eschew any discussion of it?

In order to answer this question we must look closer, I will argue, at Day's narrative framework. In connecting Gobinda's humiliation and the depth of his sorrow to his eventual death, Day wrote, 'But the thought of his degradation haunted him day and night. It preyed upon his spirits.'[67] It is these 'spirits' which I believe hold the clue to Roy's inability to include the patient's emotional world in his framework. It is also my belief that it is this very 'spirit' that distinguishes Roy from Day. The word 'spirit' appears frequently in the novel, but not once in Roy's medical essay.

The phrase 'preyed on his spirits' appears frequently in nineteenth-century discussions of health, but seldom in the writings of doctors. John Clark Marshman's history of the pioneering Baptist missionaries of Serampore, for instance, in discussing the health of his father, Joshua Marshman, wrote, 'It was the effect of this continued opposition to the interests of the mission, and the dread of its extinction under the pressure of embarrassments, which preyed on his spirits. He experienced the first attack of melancholy about nine months after his return from England, when the prospect of support for "the cause" appeared desperate.'[68] A biography of the famous English admiral Robert Blake similarly said of Blake's father, 'His troubles preyed on his spirits, and with the increasing darkness of his fortunes his health began to fail.'[69] Similarly, of the eminent French mathematician, Gaspard Monge, it was said that following the second Bourbon restoration in 1815 and their suppression of his Polytechnic (as vengeance for his proximity to Napoleon), the 'sad reverse preyed on his spirits and produced an alienation of the mind; in which melancholy state he languished for sometime, and expired on the 28th July 1816'.[70] Likewise, of the electrician Alexander Volta it was said, 'During the fervour of reform and revolution, he laid aside the ecclesiastical habits, and married; but, in the decline of his life the early impressions regained their ascendancy, and compunction for the breach of the vow of celibacy, preyed on his spirits and undermined his health. He died on the 6th March 1826.'[71]

The sort of 'anxiety and worry' that Basu spoke of was easily reminiscent of these descriptions of 'preying on the spirits'. What I alluded to as the 'emotional world' of the patient is thus perhaps more accurately framed as the state of her spirits in the idiom of the nineteenth century.

The word spirit is, however, much more capacious than simply a basis for emotions and is rich in allusions. In the nineteenth century it could have meant a vital principle, the immaterial aspects of a person's being, such as emotions, as also his or her soul.[72] Day used the full range of meanings of the word in his novel. He made, for instance, several references to the 'spiritual guidance' that was provided by the guru to average Hindu householders like Gobinda.[73] He also described at length average Bengali beliefs in 'spirits' or ghosts that gestured towards the departed immortal soul.[74] He described the funerary rituals of villagers in terms of rites to enable the smooth departure of the 'spirit', thus hinting again at the immortal soul.[75] Finally, he described the 'spirit' of the Bengali peasants as something akin to a shared vital principle or chutzpah.[76] There were also several references to drinkable spirits, but these latter, though originally related to the soul till the eighteenth century,[77] by Day's time were clearly distinguished from the immortal soul.[78]

By the 1870s, it was much less likely to find a discussion of the immortal soul directly in medical works. As a result, Roy's medical essay was naturally hesitant to venture into the spiritual domain. That he was a practicing Hindu and his views on the soul may not have matched the dominant Christian beliefs of his fellow medical men may also have made him reticent to bring up the topic. As both a Christian pastor and a novelist, Day did not have such hesitation. In the very last line of his novel—wherein he described the cremation of Gobinda's dead body by his son—when he finished by saying, 'thus was Gobinda delivered from all his troubles', it was for him almost certainly not just a metaphoric allusion to deliverance. As a deeply religious man, he did believe that at last Gobinda, in spirit, had entered a better world. The emotional depth that we find lacking in Roy and present in Day is, therefore, attached to a deeper absence, that of the immortal soul, in Roy's medical essay.

What is remarkable is how lightly Day introduces this immortal soul. He does not write like a preacher, but like an ethnographer-turned-novelist. It is perhaps his deep empathy for his overwhelmingly non-Christian neighbours whose lives he narrates as well as the novel form that forestalls his expounding more fully upon Christian ideas of the soul. In the absence of such fulsome exposition, the spiritual dimension of his writings is articulated in the liminal space between ethnographic description and the narrator's introspection into the subjectivity and emotional depth of the characters.

Not only did Day's choice of a bildungsroman format enable him to deftly integrate ethnographic insight with emotional depth, but his allusive language also allowed him certain communicative licence that Roy could not access from within the generic structure of his medical essay. When Day wrote, for instance, of the 'heavy heart' and 'tearful eyes' of Gobinda alongside his failing health and eventual death within the context of the final ignominy of having to work as a hired coolie, he did not need to specify exactly what was meant by a 'heavy heart' or how this 'heavy heart' mediated between his social abjection and his deteriorating health. He could simply allude to them, bring them together in a single sentence or paragraph and then allow the reader to make the connections. The 'spirit' shimmered somewhere betwixt and between literal descriptions and the literary allusions. But Roy, of course, could not do this in his medical essay. Were he to speak of a 'heavy heart', one would expect of him a clearer physiological exposition. Likewise, were he to posit this 'heart' as the mediator between poverty and ill health, he would be required to develop a much more precise language to spell out the connections.

Political medicine worked with what one critic called a 'fluffy sort of generalization' at its core.[79] The 'soul' or 'spirit' was perhaps the fluffiest of all generalizations. In a multi-religious context, where much had to be left allusive and imprecise in order to be communicated beyond theological boundaries, this already extant fluffiness was further exacerbated. It was this 'fluff' that was relatively easily accessible to a literary author than a literal one. For Day, a novelist, the 'fluff' could be adequately and effectively conveyed by allusions and suggestions. For Roy, a medical essayist, the 'fluff' was often incommunicable without being reduced to a false precision. This is where the literal and the literary attempts to describe a political medicine, notwithstanding their shared ambitions, parted ways.

It is perhaps tragic to recall that Roy too had aspired to a literary style. Recall Arnold's comment about the resonances of his 'funereal images'. In fact, several contemporary reviewers reproduced some of these images in their reviews. The anonymous reviewer of the book in *The Medical Times and Gazette* of London quoted him as saying that, villages in 'countries that once smiled with peace, health and prosperity, have been turned into hot-beds of disease, misery and death'.[80] Another reviewer, writing in the *Journal of the National Indian Association*, reproduced the same quotation at greater length, recalling with Roy how 'skulls of human beings now strew the fields' where once happy infants played.[81] Both these reviewers, one British and one Indian, also commended Roy's writing. Thus, the reviewer for the *Medical Times* stated that the book was 'very well written', whilst the Indian reviewer spoke of Roy's eloquence. Yet—and here is the tragedy—neither they nor any other reviewer I have read commented on Roy's political critique of poverty and its connection to health. The reviewer for the *Medical Times* elaborated on the deltaic geography of Bengal and the 'filthy habits of the Hindus' at length and even quoted Roy on these matters, but glossed over insufficient clothing, food, and so on without a single comment that framed these within a Malthusian framework of overpopulation. The Indian reviewer was hardly any different and focused again on largely the same set combination of geography and overpopulation. The anonymous reviewer for *The Doctor* by contrast focused on Roy's views on contagion, but once again completely eschewed any mention of his political critique. This latter reviewer did, however, state that 'in point of literary style and medical value it is far above the ordinary standard of many European works'.[82] In short, while most reviewers explicitly appreciated Roy's literary style and prose, they distilled it from his medical arguments and completely misread the thrust of his larger framework. His political medicine was thus buried within a deluge of reviews that read into his work a tame and standard, anti-contagionist, pro-miasmatic, and pro-Malthusian position. Given this reception, we can easily imagine why Roy may not have pushed his literary style even further to accommodate the complex 'spiritual' dimensions of political medicine.

In sharp contrast to Roy's reception, and despite the persistent neglect of the medical dimensions of Day's novel, the latter's work has generally been remembered for its poignant socio-economic descriptions. So much so that in the twentieth century, two statistical surveys of village life, in 1933 and 1958, were undertaken in the real village upon which Day's novel was allegedly based upon. It was felt that the details in Day's novel were accurate enough to be used to gauge socio-economic change in the village over the decades since Day's publication.[83]

* * *

Burdwan Fever remains a popular topic for social historians of medicine. Many of them cite Roy and, more rarely, Day, and occasionally both of them. Yet, the political medicine that these authors espoused continues to be ignored. Social historians usually mine Day for pithy descriptions of 'the social context', while Roy is generally excavated to retrodiagnostically identify 'Burdwan Fever'.[84] As a result, not only are the 'social' and the 'medical' clearly divorced, but the 'medical' is located squarely in an etiological space where it is pliable to technoscientific manipulation.

Once rendered into such an object of technoscientific manipulation, medical problems are no longer putatively tied up with the politics of poverty alleviation and social justice. All that matters for the control of ill health are sufficient trained personnel, proper diagnostic technology, and adequate medicines. Hashim Amir Ali, who presided over the two statistical surveys of Day's 'fictional' village could thus fondly reminisce in the 1950s that 'malaria which was the bane of Bengal villages in those days had completely disappeared and, thanks to antibiotics and the increase in the number of doctors per thousand of the population, there were only 1.3 deaths as against 3.0 births in 100 of the population'.[85] In Ali's framework, this picture of healthfulness was an issue entirely distinct from the growing income disparity and pauperization of the working classes in the village. By 1958, therefore, 60 per cent of the agricultural land in the same village had become the property of investors and only a mere 10 per cent remained in the hands of agrarian castes such as the Aguris, the peasant caste to which Day's fictional yeoman hero, Gobinda, had belonged.[86] In fact, statistically, the Aguris had ceased to be considered a 'landholding caste' at all and the vast majority of agricultural land had passed onto the hands of upper-caste absentee landlords who lived in cities.[87] Yet, none of this was any longer connected to the issue of health. The 'medical' and the 'political economic' were distinct and independent entities. It is this distinctiveness that social histories such as that by Binata Sarkar naturalize.

But this was not the framework that informed the works of Roy and Day. Borrowing from the 'fluffy generalizations' of Scottish political medicine, they had located the 'medical' betwixt the literary and the literal. Healthfulness, to them, had meant much more than being free of the 'malarial poison' in one's blood. In fact, in Day's writings, where I believe we find the fullest—if fluffiest—image of vernacularized political medicine, we can discern a capacious notion of health which went much beyond the purely somatic and included within it the economic, social, moral, and even spiritual aspects of a patient's being. For Roy and for Day, I will argue, tackling Burdwan Fever was not simply about reducing mortality statistics, but of addressing their more general plight under colonial capitalism. Their aim, unlike Ali's, was not to simply foster biological life without any reference to the quality of that life, or indeed, the spirit.[88] The enemies of public health, in the eyes of Roy and Day, were not mere miasmas and poor drains, but also rack-renting zamindars, callous government legislation, capitalist markets, and much else. Health for them was not simply a somatic ideal of a disease-free body, but a moral economic ideal in which the hardworking poor had an inalienable political right to the basic necessaries of life that included, food, clothing, shelter, and, perhaps above all, dignity.

In relocating the 'medical' betwixt the literal and the literary, as Roy and Day had done, my ambition then is not merely to arrive at a more accurate reading of these two early Bengali authors. Instead, I hope such a reappraisal of their vision of a political medicine might help us craft a contemporary politics of health that goes beyond both a mere politics of audit devoted to the enumeration of 'trained doctors' and antibiotics and a reductionist and enumerative 'social determinants of health' approach. My hope is that in revisiting the forgotten political medicine of Roy and Day we might glimpse a way of insisting that the politics of life itself ought not to be limited to the reduction of mortality and the enhancement of productive capacities alone. Keeping a man alive and working, despite crushing poverty and its attendant psychic injuries, so that he may produce wealth for others, as far as I am concerned, cannot be the goal of medicine. It is akin to a form of torture. If medicine is to have a goal at all, it must address itself to questions about the quality of life. Its ideal of 'health' must include a consideration of what is the life worth living and not just the fact of continuing to be biologically alive.

Notes

1. Christopher Hamlin, *Public Health and Social Justice in the Age of Chadwick: Britain, 1800–1854* (London: Cambridge University Press, 1998).
2. Projit Bihari Mukharji, 'Vernacularizing the Body: Informational Egalitarianism, Hindu Divine Design and Race in Physiology Schoolbooks, Bengal 1859–77', *Bulletin of the History of Medicine* 91, no. 3 (forthcoming).
3. Christopher Hamlin, 'William Pulteney Alison, the Scottish Philosophy, and the Making of a Political Medicine', *Journal of the History of Medicine and Allied Sciences* 61, no. 2 (2006): 144–86.
4. Christopher Hamlin, 'The "Necessaries of Life" in British Political Medicine, 1750–1850', *Journal of Consumer Policy* 29, no. 4 (2006): 373–97.
5. Ian Burney, *Bodies of Evidence: Medicine and the Politics of the English Inquest, 1830–1926* (Baltimore: Johns Hopkins University Press, 2000), p. 198.
6. Hamlin, *Public Health*, pp. 55–6.
7. Hamlin, 'William Pulteney Alison': 163–4.
8. Christopher Hamlin, 'Predisposing Causes and Public Health in Early Nineteenth-Century Medical Thought', *Social History of Medicine* 5, no. 1 (1992): 43–70, discussion on p. 52.
9. T. Watson, *Lectures on the Principles and Practice of Physic*, vol. 1 (Philadelphia: Henry C. Lea, 1872), p. 101.
10. Hamlin, 'William Pulteney Alison': 157.
11. Christopher Hamlin and Kathleen Gallagher-Kamper, 'Malthus and the Doctors: Political Economy, Medicine, and the State in England, Ireland, and Scotland, 1800–1840', *Clio Medica/The Wellcome Series in the History of Medicine* 59, no. 1 (2000): 115–40, 123–8.
12. Hamlin, *Public Health*, p. 59.

13. Edward P. Thompson, 'The Moral Economy of the English Crowd in the Eighteenth Century', *Past and Present* 50 (1971): 76–136, 95.

14. Thompson, 'Moral Economy', p. 79.

15. Hamlin, 'William Pulteney Alison': 177.

16. Charles E. Rosenberg, 'The Therapeutic Revolution: Medicine, Meaning, and Social Change in Nineteenth-Century America', *Perspectives in Biology and Medicine* 20, no. 4 (1977): 485–506, 487.

17. Rohan Deb Roy, 'Malarial Connections: Diagnostic Categories, Medical Authorities and Market Situations in British India and Beyond, 1820–1912' (unpublished PhD diss., University College London, 2009), p. 167.

18. Deb Roy, 'Malarial Connections', p. 158.

19. David Arnold, *Science, Technology and Medicine in Colonial India*, vol. 5 (Cambridge: Cambridge University Press, 2000), p. 80.

20. Mark Harrison, *Public Health in British India: Anglo-Indian Preventive Medicine 1859–1914* (Cambridge: Cambridge University Press, 1994), p. 17.

21. G.C. Roy, preface of *An Essay on the Causes, Symptoms and Treatment of the Burdwan Fever* (Calcutta: Anglo-Sanskrit Press, 1874).

22. Roy, *An Essay*, p. 37.

23. Roy, *An Essay*, p. 42.

24. Roy, *An Essay*, p. 37.

25. Projit Bihari Mukharji, *Nationalizing the Body: The Medical Market, Print and Daktari Medicine* (London: Anthem Press, 2009), pp. 98, 114–16.

26. Jessica L. Baron, 'Reforming the Raj: Florence Nightingale's Biomedical Liberalism in British India' (unpublished PhD diss., University of Notre Dame, 2013), p. 209.

27. Baron, 'Reforming the Raj', p. 211.

28. Roy, *An Essay*, pp. 37–9.

29. Roy, *An Essay*, p. 39.

30. Rochona Majumdar, *Marriage and Modernity: Family Values in Colonial Bengal* (Durham: Duke University Press, 2009), pp. 167–204.

31. Cited in Majumdar, *Marriage and Modernity*, p. 180.

32. Anon., 'Baboo Gopaul Chunder Roy on Indian Medicine', *Medical Times and Gazette*, 30 July 1870, p. 142.

33. Roy, *An Essay*, p. 40.

34. Roy, *An Essay*, pp. 40–1.

35. Roy, *An Essay*, p. 41.

36. Roy, *An Essay*, p. 13.

37. Roy, *An Essay*, p. 73.

38. Thompson, 'Moral Economy': 131.

39. Roy, *An Essay*, p. 92.

40. Roy, *An Essay*, p. 92.

41. Some exceptions to this are Achintya Kumar Dutta, *Economy and Ecology in a Bengal District: Burdwan 1880–1947* (Calcutta: Firma KLM, 1958); Arabinda Samanta, *Malarial Fever in Colonial Bengal, 1820–1939: Social History of an Epidemic* (Firma KLM: Calcutta, 2002); Binata Sarkar, 'Malaria and Medical Intervention, Burdwan 1870–1947' (unpublished PhD diss., University of Burdwan, 2010), p. 54.

42. Lal Behari Day, *Govinda Samanta or The History of a Bengal Raiyat* (London: Macmillan & Co., 1874).

43. Tara Krishna Basu, *The Bengal Peasant from Time to Time* (Calcutta: ISI, 1962), p. 1.

44. Day, *Govinda*, pp. 247–51.

45. This belief and practice seem to be in agreement with the Hippocratic notion of 'critical days'. Thus, the Hippocratic *Crisis* explained that 'by the fourth day many fevers will have resolved or will have killed their victims' (Christopher Hamlin, *More than Hot: A Short History of Fever* [Baltimore: Johns Hopkins University Press, 2014], p. 41).

46. Day, *Govinda*, p. 251.

47. Day, *Govinda*, pp. 369–71.

48. Day, *Govinda*, p. 369.

49. John Elliot, *Report on Epidemic Remittent and Intermittent Fever Occurring in Parts of Burdwan and Nuddea Divisions* (Printed at the Bengal Secretariat Office, 1863), p. 1.

50. Day, *Govinda*, pp. 361–2.

51. Day, *Govinda*, p. 362.

52. Day, *Govinda*, p. 363.

53. Day, *Govinda*, p. 362.

54. Day, *Govinda*, pp. 364–8.

55. Day, *Govinda*, p. 368.

56. Day, *Govinda*, p. 370.

57. Day, *Govinda*, p. 376.

58. Day, *Govinda*, pp. 361–2.

59. Elliot, *Report*; John Gay French, *Epidemic Fever in Lower Bengal Commonly Called Burdwan Fever* (Calcutta: Thacker, Spink & Co., 1875).

60. Baron, 'Reforming the Raj', pp. 177–216.

61. Leela Sami, 'Starvation, Disease and Death: Explaining Famine Mortality in Madras, 1876–1878', *Social History of Medicine* 24, no. 3 (2011): 700–19.

62. See, for instance, WR Cornish, 'The Sanitary and Medical Aspects of the Famine of 1876–77', in *Fourteenth Annual Report of the Sanitary Commissioner for Madras 1877*, edited by WR Cornish (Madras: Government Press, 1878), pp. i–li.

63. Baron, 'Reforming the Raj', p. 210.

64. For the colonial computations of adequate diets, see David Arnold, *Colonizing the Body: State Medicine and Epidemic Disease* (Berkeley: University of California, 1993), pp. 110–13 and David Arnold, 'The "Discovery" of Malnutrition and Diet in Colonial India', *The Indian Economic and Social History Review*, 31, no. 1 (1994): 1–26.

65. B.D. Basu, 'Indian Medical Celebrities', *The Medical Reporter*, 4 (1895), pp. 139–40, citation on p. 140. Roy was to finally succumb to this illness on 7 February 1887 at his family home in Burdwan.

66. Elliot, *Report*, p. 17.

67. Day, *Gobinda*, p. 376.

68. John Clark Marshman, *The Life and Times of Carey, Marshman and Ward: Embracing the History of the Serampore Mission*, vol. 2 (London: Longman, Brown, Green, Longmans and Roberts, 1858), p. 473.

69. Hepworth Dixon, *Robert Blake: Admiral and General at Sea* (London: Chapman & Hall, 1856), p. 12.

70. Dugald Stewart, Sir James Mackintosh, James Playfair, and Sir John Leslie, *Dissertations on the History of Metaphysical and Ethical and Mathematical and Physical Sciences* (Edinburgh: Adam & Charles Black: 1835), p. 586.

71. Stewart et al, *Dissertations*, p. 622.

72. See entry under 'spirit, n.' in Oxford English Dictionary, available at https://en.oxforddictionaries.com/definition/spirit, last accessed 18 August 2017.

73. Day, *Gobinda*, pp. 89, 100, 137.

74. Day, *Gobinda*, pp. 80, 104–7, 110, 261.

75. Day, *Gobinda*, p. 251.

76. Day, *Gobinda*, pp. 279, 280, 307, 311, 327, 329, 364.

77. Simon Schaffer, 'Godly Men and Mechanical Philosophers: Souls and Spirits in Restoration Natural Philosophy', *Science in Context* 1, no. 1 (1987): 53–85.

78. Day, *Gobinda*, pp. 19, 123, 296–7.

79. Hamlin, 'The "Necessaries of Life"', p. 375.

80. Anon., 'Review of *The Causes, Symptoms and Treatment of Burdwan Fever*', *The Medical Times and Gazette*, 1, 13 April 1876, p. 426.

81. Anon., 'Review of *The Causes, Symptoms and Treatment of Burdwan Fever*', *Journal of the National Indian Association* 73 (1877): 70–4.

82. Anon., 'Review of *The Causes, Symptoms and Treatment of Burdwan Fever*', *The Doctor* 6 (1 March 1876): 55.

83. Basu, *The Bengal Peasant*.

84. For a recent example, see Sarkar, 'Malaria and Medical Intervention'.

85. Basu, *The Bengal Peasant*, pp. 190–1.

86. Basu, *The Bengal Peasant*, p. 177.

87. Samir Dasgupta, 'Life in a Bengal Village', *Economic Development and Cultural Change* 13, no. 1 (1964): 115–17.

88. The 'fostering of life' or 'disallowing it to the point of death' are, of course, characteristic objectives of the new mode of power—biopower—that Michel Foucault identified as emerging gradually since the seventeenth century. But what I want to emphasize is that while Foucault is enormously helpful in documenting the transformation of 'life' into an administrative object, his analysis is mainly concerned with the progressive biologization of life. I do not think this purely biological idea of life ever completely banishes 'fluffier' notions of life. While death does signal the absolute limit of biological life, it is hardly any indicator of the quality of life lived, leave alone spiritual life. For a crisp statement of Foucault's thinking on biopower, see Michel Foucault, 'Right of Death and Power over Life', in *The Foucault Reader*, edited by Paul Rabinow (New York: Pantheon Books, 1984), pp. 258–72.

11

TECHNOLOGY AND HEALTH IN LATE COLONIAL INDIA

DAVID ARNOLD

The history of medicine in India is by now a well-established field. The past thirty years have produced a rich and extensive scholarly literature, mainly centred around what one might call the epidemic–institutional nexus of medical history. Such topics include the nature and impact of epidemic diseases, the rise of the medical professions, and the emergence of public health, the changing relationship between Western and indigenous medical practices, the growth of Christian medical missions and women's medical organizations, and the role played by critical sites of medical regulation and intervention from the army and the prison to the dispensary and the hospital.[1] At the same time, the medical archive has been extended to embrace a great diversity of English and vernacular sources. Yet, even so, there remain ways in which the empirical scope, analytical range and archival underpinning of the study of disease, health, and medicine in India can continue to be developed, and it is argued in this chapter that one of the most promising ways of doing so is through greater engagement with issues of technology. Technology in this context might signify a number of different things. It could refer to the techniques that physicians and a broad range of medical specialists employ in their work—in gynaecology, for instance, or ophthalmology. Or it could relate to mechanical devices that had a specific relationship with medicine and the body—from simple instruments like vaccination needles, stethoscopes, and syringes to more complicated objects like X-ray machines and ophthalmoscopes or the technologies surrounding contraception and reproduction.[2] But this chapter pursues technology in a rather different direction: I want to move into a largely doctor-less domain of health and argue for the importance of a set of 'everyday technologies' that in themselves had no direct and functional relationship with bodily health but which in the period from the 1890s to the 1940s began to impinge directly and indirectly on the lives and livelihoods, and hence on the physical well-being, of a large number of people in India. In other words, this chapter seeks to align considerations of health more closely with everyday experience and technological change.[3] Rather than look to the hospital, the prison, the laboratory, and the lock hospital as a site of enquiry, this discussion turns to less familiar medical locations, the street, the factory, and the home. It thereby seeks to address a range of sources—from newspapers to the reports of the police, the municipal authorities, and factory inspectors—and to move closer to a consideration of the people's health. Taking the city as its primary locus, the chapter seeks to expand subaltern readings of the determinants of health and its multiple conditions and subjectivities. It is not claimed that there was a single relationship here to be uncovered so much as a range of contexts and experiences that collectively illuminate the insistent framing of health by modern technology and the concurrent expectation that modern minds and, still more, modern bodies should accommodate themselves to the requirements of machines, or suffer the consequences for failing to do so. This might be read as a universal story of health and modern technology, but it also reflects on the social and cultural specificities of India and the changing nature of colonial governance.

On the Street

The street has been largely ignored in medical histories of South Asia, and yet much of what concerned modern health and medicine happened, and still happens, on or in close proximity to the street. Any revisionist attempt to 'locate the medical', at least within an urban context, must address the street as a critical site of medical display, practice, intervention, and reaction. In the past, as in any Indian town or city today, clinics and dispensaries, pharmacists, and bonesetters opened directly onto the street, advertising through words, signs, and images their varied medical offerings. Druggists sold their wares from roadside stalls or on city pavements, and, amidst the clutter of posters and advertising hoardings, patent medicines and miracle cures clamoured for attention. Indigenous oculists plied their trade on the street, drawing crowds by their claims to remove cataracts instantly, safely, painlessly.[4] Sidewalk shrines, as to the goddess Sitala, reminded passers-by of their need to propitiate deities that had the power to cause or moderate smallpox and other ailments. The victims of deforming diseases such as leprosy and of incapacitating injuries displayed their afflictions in hope of alms, and, as if to remind the living of their mortality, the dead were borne through the streets on their way to burial sites and cremation grounds. In an age of emergent public health, the street was a critical site of state intervention (as evident in the bubonic plague epidemic from 1896 onwards) but also of demonstrations against compulsory inoculation and hospitalization.[5] As persuasion rather than coercion came to the fore in colonial health policy, so, by the 1930s mobile dispensaries travelled the streets or vans displayed hoardings warning of the dangers of tuberculosis or urging smallpox vaccination. Disease, like medicine, lived—still lives—a very public life in India.

Over the past century, too, the street has become a theatre of death, not through disease as such but as a consequence of the rise of modern traffic, as vehicles collide or pedestrians, cyclists, street vendors, and labourers are knocked over, injured, or killed. Returning to India in the early 1980s after several years abroad, Prafulla Mohanti described how cities, towns, even villages, in his native Odisha had become choked with traffic. The chaotic, cacophonous traffic spilled over from congested city streets onto adjacent highways, with bellowing trucks and overcrowded buses competing for road-room with bullock carts, bicycles, cars, and jeeps. In the past, Mohanti observed, people used to be worried about epidemics like smallpox and cholera. Now, traffic accidents 'are regarded as a part of life. The fear of smallpox and cholera has been replaced by the fear of accidents. Before starting a journey by road, the villagers worship the goddess Durga for protection'.[6] Even if there is a degree of literary licence in Mohanti's elision of traffic with disease and the propitiation of disease deities with the invocation of Durga's protection against road accidents, one can still accept that in popular perception traffic has become a kind of life-threatening disorder and that earlier understandings of disease and its dangers have in part been transposed onto modern traffic. Certainly, behind Mohanti's personal observation lie a host of grim statistics. In 2010 alone traffic accidents cost an estimated 134,000 lives in India, up from 92,618 only six years earlier.[7]

Behind such statistics lies a long history. Across British India in 1933 there were 954 reported deaths from road accidents and 6,611 serious injuries, a seemingly miniscule figure by today's standards but a tally that was already beginning to rise year on year: even by 1935 road deaths had jumped to 1,309 and major injuries to 9,621. In relation to the number of motor vehicles on the road, this was three times the accident rate in England and Wales and twice that in Germany, though the actual number of deaths and injuries was far below the United States, where 23,000 automobile-related deaths were recorded in 1924 alone.[8] The sum of India's road deaths in the 1920s and 1930s appears small when compared to such headline causes of mortality as malaria and cholera, which in any one year might record in excess of half a million deaths, but they underscore the growing impact of industrial technology on human health and represent the start of what has grown to become a major epidemic of injury and death on India's streets and highways.

Accidents took many forms. City trams were one major cause as tramcars collided with other vehicles, as cyclists became trapped in tram tracks, or alighting passengers stepped into the paths of oncoming cars and taxis.[9] There was even an instance of a man sleeping outside a tram depot at night whose legs were crushed when the trams resumed work in the morning (those who slept on the streets were in constant danger): he died later in hospital.[10] Individuals who worked on the street, such as rickshaw-pullers and cart-haulers, were at risk both from the arduous physical nature of their labour and the dangers posed by other road users.[11] Contemporary newspapers (which, along with police reports, provide the main source of information) were full of episodes like the 'Serious Smash in Chowringhee' in June 1922, when two speeding taxi drivers in Calcutta struck a cyclist before colliding with a Tollygunge tram.[12] Car, taxi, truck, and bus drivers further added to the toll, as they drove carelessly, drunk, or at high speeds, or, in the case of trucks and buses, in vehicles that were overloaded and poorly maintained. Children playing at the roadside, old people slow to cross the road, and those who were hearing or visually impaired, cyclists, or pedestrians avoiding other street hazards were among the many victims. Transported by taxis and private cars, many of these casualties ended up in city hospitals, like Bombay's JJ Hospital, but usually too late to save their lives.[13]

Apart from defective and badly driven vehicles, in the eyes of the police and officials a general lack of 'road sense' among Indians was a fundamental cause of many accidents, especially where pedestrians and cyclists were involved; but there was also a growing European and Indian middle-class consensus that the poor, as uneducated and undisciplined city-dwellers, were often responsible for their own misfortune. They had yet to learn to respect, anticipate, and, where necessary, avoid the modern machine.[14] This, then, was a history of suffering and death in which the medical and public health professions played little part, until perhaps the victims became hospitalized. Laws were passed and municipal regulations introduced to try to maintain order and discipline on the streets and to protect the road-using public. It was left to the police and magistracy to try to educate, punish, and chastise the reckless, the hapless, and the vulnerable. Traffic police patrols were set up to catch offenders, policemen stood for hours on point-duty, and attempts were even made to control escalating urban noise pollution by banning the use of claxon horns at night or in inner-city locations.[15] Safety-first campaigns were instituted to warn schoolchildren of the dangers traffic posed.[16] On the other hand, those who found themselves repeatedly classed in official discourse as victims were not entirely supine, and there were not infrequent instances, as in Calcutta in April 1946, when, after a long spate of accidents caused by 'military-type vehicles', local residents responded with their own rough justice by attacking truck drivers and stoning or setting fire to their vehicles.[17]

Of course, it is possible to take too hostile a view of modern technology, on the streets or elsewhere. New modes of transport could be conducive to health as well as being its nemesis. Bicycles, vans and trucks could be used as vehicles to conduct health propaganda or to facilitate and extend the operations of vaccination squads, anti-malarial brigades, and mobile clinics. Motorized ambulances began to appear on city streets just as trucks (partly) replaced bullock-drawn conservancy carts. When bicycles were first introduced to India they were often, as in Europe and North America, lauded for their health-conferring benefits: the association between cycling and health had a particular appeal to many middle-class groups in India, such as the Parsis in Bombay and the bhadralok of Bengal.[18] But as the roads became more congested and as the affluent took to the greater comfort of their motor cars, the idea of cycling for health steadily diminished. Competitive cycling continued but mostly within stadia and other enclosed spaces. As the celebrated Parsi cyclist F.J. Davar complained in 1938, it was no longer safe to hold cycle races on public roads as the competitors were 'greatly obstructed by stray cattle, pigs and sheep, which very often caused accidents'.[19]

In the Factory

In moving from the open-air environment of the street to the enclosed or semi-enclosed world of the factory, we enter a different kind of physical space but one in which a number of comparable factors apply. In fact, the relationship between technology and health in Indian factories was twofold. On the one hand, external influences impacted the factory, most evidently when epidemics of cholera, plague, and influenza struck the cities: workers died or fled for their own safety, bringing industrial production to a standstill or rendering the weakened workforce incapable of sustained labour.[20] On the other hand, with poor ventilation, unfenced machines, defective latrines, and overworked, undernourished operatives, the factory was itself a site of disease, insanitary conditions, and industrial accidents that echoed or even exceeded those occurring on the streets outside.[21] Studies of factory labour in India have mostly focused on the larger, more organized industries, such as jute in Calcutta and cotton in Bombay, only marginally touching on the impact of industrial employment on workers' health.[22] Far less attention has been given to the multitude of smaller workshops, mills, and factories that sprang up all over India in the early twentieth century and the health conditions of their often casual or seasonal workers. In part this neglect reflects the small scale and dispersed nature of these enterprises and the consequent inability of state agencies to observe them as closely as they could larger factories in the metropolitan cities of Calcutta, Bombay, and Madras. But it also suggests relative unconcern on the part of the Indian public and emerging trade unions: few among these workers were unionized before the 1940s and their conditions rarely attracted high-profile attention.[23]

One indication of the violent career of the machine and its consequences for workers' health can be given through the example of Indian rice mills as documented not through health and sanitation returns but through the reports of the provincial factory inspectors.[24] Although India's factory legislation dates from1881, the first act was confined to factories with at least 100 employees, whereas most rice mills in India were far too small to fall within this remit. This figure was gradually reduced—to fifty employees in 1891 and twenty in 1911—at the same time as mechanized rice milling began to flourish across Madras, Bengal, and other major rice-consuming provinces. By 1937–8 there were 1,135 perennial rice mills in India (plus 175 operating only seasonally) with a combined workforce of 47,289 or, on average, roughly 36 workers for each registered rice mill (some remained too small to be registered at all).[25] But this statistic fails to capture the transitory nature of many rice mills (especially in the depression years of the 1930s), the casual and seasonal nature of their employment practices, the large number of women and juvenile employees, and the wide dispersal of the mills in towns and villages across India. The insufficient number of factory inspectors, men who were by profession engineers and not trained in medicine and public health, and the evasive practices of mill owners and managers made the task of routine inspection still more problematic.[26]

Nevertheless, the inspectors' reports give clear evidence of the health hazards rice-mill workers encountered. Given the cheap and flimsy materials used in the mills' construction, internal walls and grain stores were prone to collapse, killing labourers or causing broken ribs and fractured limbs. Men, women, and juveniles were required to carry excessively heavy loads of grain, itself a cause of strains and injuries but also a factor in causing them to trip and fall into vats of boiling paddy. Boilers overheated and burst, scalding nearby workers. In trying to repair or clean machines, or to remove husks from under moving parts, workers lost fingers, arms and legs, or developed tetanus and died in hospital a few days later.[27] Due to faulty wiring, workers were electrocuted as they handled machine parts and light fittings or as electric wires touched water.[28] With stacks of dry grain, husks, and sacks lying around, fires were frequent.[29] There was long-term harm to workers' health from the constant noise of machinery and the prevailing 'dust evil'. Like tanning works and cotton gins, the air in rice mills was full of irritating dust particles, which filled workers' eyes and choked their throats and lungs. Although some attempts were made at the factory inspectors' behest to improve ventilation in the mills, such remedial measures were in general too expensive for such small enterprises as rice mills and cotton gins to afford and so, in effect, were deemed impractical.[30] Although by the late 1930s, some rice mills (and similar small-scale industrial establishments) could boast of having an at least part-time medical officer, these appear to have had little impact on overall health conditions and may have been little more than a sop to the authorities.[31] As with the policing of road traffic, the expectations of late colonial factory governance far exceeded its capacity to deliver.

A further hazard to workers' health came from the unregulated use of corrosive and toxic substances, such as lime in tanneries, in which young Dalit labourers might be semi-immersed for several hours a day.[32] What happened to harm health inside the factory, in terms of dust, noise, and pollution, also connected to what happened adversely outside it. Rice and flour mills, dal-grinding machines, jute mills, tanneries, brickyards, and cement works spread a pall of pollution over adjacent residential areas, adding to the incidence of respiratory disease, contaminating water sources, and fouling food supplies. Some attempts were made, as in Calcutta in the 1900s, to try to restrict smoke pollution from factory chimneys or to relocate tanneries and workshops to the suburbs but to only limited effect.[33] India's historians have barely begun to examine the deleterious nature and adverse health consequences of urban and industrial growth, or the complex relationship between ideas of environmental and ritual pollution, but potentially this is a highly significant area for social and environmental history research.[34]

One of the alleged causes of accidents in rice mills and similar industries was the so-called 'carelessness of operatives'.[35] Apart from neglecting to turn off machines they were cleaning or to keep clear of moving parts, this was commonly attributed to the 'loose clothing' Indian workers wore—the dhotis, saris, turbans, and shawls—which became entangled in whirling machinery and dragged wearers to their deaths. Women's hair, too, became fatally trapped in conveyor belts and flywheels.[36] Given that workers often refused to wear the protective clothing supplied to them (again, at the inspectors' insistence) or to use the guardrails on their machines, this apparent rejection of even elementary safety measures reinforced the colonial (but also managerial) belief that these were premodern minds and premodern bodies, which like the undisciplined pedestrians and cyclists on the city streets, were the proximate cause, and not just the innocent victims, of industrial accidents. Under India's increasingly comprehensive factory acts, fines were sometimes levied on owners and managers for serious health and safety violations, but the penalties imposed were seldom sufficiently severe to change the way in which their works were run. Often a belief in instruction and education for the wayward and illiterate worker was seen to be the only practical long-term solution.[37]

While lax management practices received some share of the blame, it is striking how often in these factory inspection narratives workers were blamed for their own injuries and fatalities. If one of the expectations of the modern machine was that those who used it—whether in the home, the street or the factory—should obey the discipline of modern mechanized life, then a criticism repeatedly levied against working Indians was that they failed, even at the cost of their own lives, to meet those corporeal requirements and behavioural norms. The Madras Labour Commissioner, George Paddison, remarked in 1920, following a year in which 7 deaths, 6 serious injuries, and 656 minor injuries had occurred in provincial rice mills alone, that the majority of accidents were not the managers' fault. Rather, they were

> entirely due to the carelessness and stupidity of the operatives. They may almost be said to go out of their way to court disaster and this is undoubtedly due to their lack of intelligence or common-sense and at times even to inquisitiveness as to the mechanism of certain machinery which fascinates them. Month after month, year after year, the doctrine of care and self-preservation is propounded to the workmen but results are far from satisfactory.[38]

That much of the work in rice mills was performed by casual, unskilled, often seasonal labour, and was carried out in small, generally unregulated premises, some of which were 'totally unsuitable' for industrial use, added to the hazards of the workplace.[39] The quest for quick profits and the ready availability of cheap labour made factory owners and managers still more inattentive to workers' well-being. Considering the size of the workforce and the nature of the conditions involved, it is perhaps surprising that there were not even more serious injuries and deaths. In the decade 1922–31 there were 35 deaths and 32 serious injuries recorded in rice mills in the Madras Presidency. In the following decade (1932–41) 10 deaths and 64 serious injuries were reported.[40] As with all statistics relating to industrial accidents in India, the actual scale of mortality (and more especially of injury) is difficult to determine. Inspection was erratic and mill managers had every incentive to conceal the extent of workplace injuries for fear of prosecutions and fines. Rice mill workers seldom protested to the authorities about their conditions for fear of losing their jobs and even failed to claim benefits (such as maternity welfare payments) to which they were technically entitled but of which they may have been unaware or were discouraged by mill managers from requesting. Many ill or injured workers simply dropped out of employment and returned to their villages, or, distrusting Western medicine, sought the assistance of local *vaids* (indigenous doctors) and hakims.[41] In other words, the coming of the machine age and the rise of industrial labour in India had not been matched by a corresponding growth in the medicalization of the poorer classes.

In the Home

It could be argued that, like the street and the factory, the home saw a redefinition of what constituted health and ill health in the late colonial period. Certainly, the Indian home as a site of ill health and poor sanitary practice had often been highlighted in the medical and sanitary discourse of the early colonial period—as in complaints about the deplorable conditions in which Indian women gave birth at home or, conversely, about the ways in which the bodies of certain categories of the dead might be disposed of within the home rather than in approved burial grounds.[42] The home was further presented in sanitary discourse as a site of gender inequality and hence of adverse health conditions for women and their infant children, as through the seclusion of purdah and through the neglect of female well-being, factors that might, for instance, be conducive to a higher incidence of tuberculosis than among the adult male population.[43]

But, in part due to the changing nature of technology, the home acquired a new social and sanitary significance around the close of the nineteenth century. Many Indians turned to forms of self-medication rather than seeking formal doctoring, a process aided by the rise of self-help homoeopathy and the availability of pre-packed allopathic and Ayurvedic medicines, widely advertised through the technology of the printing press and made available through the Indian postal service. Indeed, one could argue that the printing press, and the rise of commercial advertising that accompanied it, played a major role in transforming medical practices in India, especially through the use of home remedies.[44] Newspaper advertising was similarly an important vehicle for the projection of a positive image of machines, with advertisements for typewriters, bicycles, gramophones, radios, electric fans, and sewing machines all projecting the idea of modern machines as being conducive to good health and human well-being or as themselves being the embodiment of health and happiness.[45] And yet the arrival of new machines in Indian (mostly middle-class) households could constitute a new source of danger to health as well as a means to protect or improve it. To take a trivial but suggestive example, the advent of sewing machines might occasion minor mishaps, in which children playing with their mother's sewing machine got their fingers caught and needed a doctor to free them from being trapped under the needle.[46] More alarmingly, the increased use of primus stoves in domestic kitchens by the 1920s led to a number of accidents (one assumes them to have been accidents rather than precursors of more recent 'dowry killings') in which stoves exploded or saris and other items of women's clothing caught light, resulting in death or serious injury—once again Indian clothing appeared as a common culprit.[47]

But let us turn again to the example of rice milling. There were many different forms of traditional rice husking in India—the two principal methods involved ramming a large, hand-held pestle into a wooden mortar to separate the outer husks from the inner grain or using a foot-operated treadle and mortar device (a *dhenki*), usually operated by two women. Traditionally, this was mostly women's work, whether done by the females of the household as part of their daily work or by low-caste women from outside the home. The advent of mechanized rice mills from the 1880s onwards began to undermine traditional rice preparation methods and to remove husking from the ambit of the home. There were 313 rice mills operating in India and

Burma by 1912: by the late 1930s this figure had risen fourfold for India alone and by then nearly 70 per cent of rice consumed in the Madras Presidency was machine-husked—a remarkable revolution in the mechanization of food preparation.[48] The expansion of mechanical milling clearly wasn't driven by health considerations. However, it helped make rice, a high-status food, more widely available to (and affordable by) urban dwellers, to industrial workers in the cities as to plantation labourers in the countryside, and to replace more nutritious or energizing grains such as the millets *ragi* and *cholum*, hitherto widely consumed in south India. Milling produced attractively clean and polished white rice and it freed women from the daily drudgery of cleaning and pounding rice at home. Rice milling was also a significant vehicle for local entrepreneurship, for it required little capital or prior expertise to set up a small rice mill, but, like other forms of increasingly mechanized food processing (such as flour milling, sugarcane crushing or groundnut decortication), it could yield significant profits for the owners.

But, in common with many other items of food now subject to mechanization, there were potential health risks involved—including adulteration, contamination, and the loss of nutritional content.[49] By the 1920s and 1930s rice milling in India (and across large parts of monsoon Asia) was coming under sustained attack on health grounds. Part of this critique came from colonial medical and public health experts. Although the incidence of beriberi in India was relatively low by the standards of many Southeast Asian countries (in part because of the widespread practice of parboiling in India which preserved part of the grain's vitamin B1, or thiamine, content) and was largely confined to one region (the Andhra delta), nutritional researchers led by Robert McCarrison and Wallace Aykroyd identified milled rice as a significant illustration of the wider problem of nutrition deficiency in India. They supported calls for the government to intervene to restrict intensive milling or sought to encourage the use of more varied diets, even for the poor, which would offset the thiamine deficiency attributed to heavily milled rice.[50] The critique of rice mills and the polished grain they produced also found echoes, for somewhat different reasons, in the nationalist camp. The Bengali patriot and industrialist Prafulla Chandra Ray seized on rice milling as a demonstration of how modern technology adversely affected health and employment. 'Hitherto', he wrote in 1932, 'husking of paddy was the only home industry in Bengal by means of which poor widows with infants in arms could eke out a miserable living.' At one time almost every home had had a dhenki. Now, he continued, thanks to the 'march of civilization', rice mills were springing up all over Bengal and depriving poor women of their scant income: 'A single rice mill snatches away morsels of bread from the mouths of hundreds of the destitute. A few capitalists are lining their pockets at the expense of thousands of their helpless sisters.'[51] Gandhi, too, took up McCarrison and Aykroyd's 'instructive' findings to inform his own critique of the perils of technological modernity and the unhealthy—and, to his eyes, unpatriotic—nature of modern consumption practices. Complementing his campaign to revive hand-spinning and the use of the *charkha* (spinning wheel), Gandhi's condemnation extended beyond rice milling to other dying rural crafts such as the making of *gur* (raw sugar) or the extraction of oil from oilseeds by means of bullock mills. Like Ray, he lamented the decline of what he saw as the self-sufficiency of the village and the employment rice husking gave to needy women.[52]

Despite the swadeshi sentiments and scientific objections, little was done under a still largely non-interventionist laissez-faire regime to halt the proliferation of rice mills or to revive hand-husking. But what the beriberi scare did do was enhance awareness of the dangers of nutritional disorders in general and to fuel the growing middle-class preoccupation with vitamins, tonics, and 'the horrors of malnutrition'.[53] An article in Bombay's *Illustrated Weekly* in 1939 observed that it was now hard to find rice that had not been 'robbed of its vitamins by milling. Few indeed are the places throughout the length and breadth of India to which the rice mill has not penetrated'.[54] But, conversely, by the late 1930s it was being proclaimed in the Indian press that 'beri-beri can now be cured',[55] and a wide market was emerging for drugs and dietary supplements that promised freedom from beriberi and kindred diseases. In other words, the sustained criticism of rice mills did not stop people from consuming polished rice. Rather, the problem was translated into one of how individual households could compensate for the problem that mechanized milling created by finding new ways of protecting their health and nutritional intake. But since only relatively well-to-do and educated families were able to respond in this way, the

burden of ill health in general, and poor nutrition in particular, shifted
still more emphatically to the labouring classes.

* * *

The history of health and disease in India has understandably been
dominated by the history of diseases (especially epidemics like smallpox, cholera, plague, and malaria), by the growth of medical services
and institutions, and by the rise of new sanitary regimes and competing
medical systems. It has been argued here, however, that one of the ways
in which we can seek to expand the empirical scope and analytical
ambitions of the academic study of health in South Asia is by looking
more closely at the problems and issues generated by the growth of
modern technologies and especially those 'everyday technologies' that
impinged directly or indirectly on the lives of the people at large and of
the poorer classes in particular.

The understanding of disease in modern India was always located in
something more than the body itself—in climate and the physical environment, in social practice and gender differentiation, in poverty and
caste hierarchies. But, from about the 1890s, the rise of urbanization,
industrial capitalism, and the modern machine endowed ill health and
disease with a whole new range of meanings and contexts above and
beyond those instituted by the bacteriological revolution and a more
intensive public health regime. The location for these technological
encounters was necessarily very varied. It might be the home, street, or
factory, as suggested here, but it might also be the school, the plantation, or the paddy field. The increasing ubiquity of the modern machine
helped create a new kind of health regime, in which the dangers, the
risks of accident, and injury arguably outweighed (especially for subaltern subjects) many of the discernible benefits. As the mortality from
once-feared epidemics, such as smallpox and cholera, declined, other
man-made epidemics—of urban traffic or industrial pollution—began
to take their place.

The nature of these modern technological encounters suggests two
further thematics. One is the way in which many of the accidents and
injuries associated with modern machines—in the home, at work,
on the street—were blamed on those who, viewed in a different
light, appeared to be their victims. The ignorance and inexperience

of workers and road users, the wearing of inappropriate or 'loose' clothing, the failure to obey traffic rules, to make use of protective guards on moving machines, or simply to anticipate what a machine might do next—these were causes repeatedly invoked to explain casualties and fatalities. To some extent this repeated condemnation of un-modern behaviour and un-modern bodies served merely to mask the greed and negligence of factory owners and managers and the ruinous state of poorly maintained and recklessly driven trucks and buses, and hence the ruthless, irresponsible, and exploitative nature of a relatively unconstrained capitalism. To a degree, too, it demonstrates the unwillingness or incapacity of the late colonial state to curb industrial excesses or to establish effective order on the streets, and the frustrations of governance this repeatedly entailed. But the un-modern critique also raises teasing questions about why rice mill and tannery workers, city cyclists and rickshaw-pullers did not do more to defend and protect their own health. Was ignorance really to blame or was it the destitution that forced them to toil, work-weary and underfed, in such hazardous and insalubrious conditions? This is a question that calls for further enquiry.

Again, the relationship posited in this chapter between modern health and modern technology encourages us to think of health less in terms of what doctors, surgeons, clinics, and hospitals might provide and more of the circumstances in which individuals and households encountered ill health and injury in the course of their daily lives. It prompts us to think of diseases—of eyes, lungs, and limbs in particular—in terms of the occupations of those who suffered from them and hence what normative ideas of health and ill health were for the average urban worker or middle-class householder. This in turn leads us to consider the kinds of historical source materials, hitherto under-explored, that might reveal more about these modern conditions. The health–technology nexus encourages us, too, to think further about the ways in which, in a modern society, the perceived responsibility for health and ill health might have shifted or been transferred to new objects and agencies. There might be, as Prafulla Mohanti suggests in the passage quoted earlier in this chapter, a kind of lateral shift in which established deities (and the rituals surrounding them) assume in modern times responsibility for preventing traffic accidents just as formerly they stood as guardians against the onset of smallpox, whooping-cough, and measles. But there is also a sense in which responsibility for health has extended far beyond the medical professions to become a wider central concern of the state—in which the police, the magistracy, and the factory inspector might play a significant role—as well as becoming primary expressions of public opinion and part of the widening domain of civil society institutions. That technological change has profound implications for how we think about modern health cannot be doubted. Perhaps it is time for historians of India to address these issues more centrally than they have done hitherto.

Notes

1. Examples include: Poonam Bala, *Imperialism and Medicine in Bengal: A Socio-Historical Perspective* (New Delhi: Sage, 1991); David Arnold, *Colonizing the Body: State Medicine and Epidemic Disease in Nineteenth-Century India* (Berkeley: University of California Press, 1993); Mark Harrison, *Public Health in British India: Anglo-Indian Preventive Medicine, 1859–1914* (Cambridge: Cambridge University Press, 1994); Anil Kumar, *Medicine and the Raj: British Medical Policy in India, 1835–1911* (New Delhi: Sage, 1998); Biswamoy Pati and Mark Harrison, eds, *Health, Medicine and Empire: Perspectives on Colonial India* (London: Sangam Books, 2001); Jane Buckingham, *Leprosy in Colonial South India: Medicine and Confinement* (Basingstoke: Palgrave, 2002); Guy N.A. Attewell, *Refiguring Unani Tibb: Plural Healing in Late Colonial India* (Hyderabad: Orient Longman, 2007); Biswamoy Pati and Mark Harrison, eds, *The Social History of Health and Medicine in Colonial India* (Hyderabad: Orient Longman, 2008); Projit Bihari Mukharji, *Nationalizing the Body: The Medical Market, Print, and Daktari Medicine* (London: Anthem Press, 2009); Pratik Chakrabarti, *Bacteriology in British India: Laboratory Medicine and the Tropics* (Rochester: University of Rochester Press, 2012); Rachel Berger, *Ayurveda Made Modern: Political Histories of Indigenous Medicine in North India, 1900–1955* (Basingstoke: Palgrave Macmillan, 2013). There has also been a very considerable journal literature, too extensive to acknowledge here.
2. For the importance of one of these investigative and diagnostic devices, the ophthalmoscope, and its proper use, see Henry Kirkpatrick, *Diseases of the Eye: A Manual for the Practitioner* (Calcutta: Butterworth, 1925), chapter 7.
3. Material for this chapter is partly drawn from a research project on 'Everyday Technology' funded by the ESRC from 2007 to 2010: see David

Arnold, *Everyday Technology: Machines and the Making of India's Modernity* (Chicago: University of Chicago Press, 2013).

4. For a vivid account, see R.P. Ratnakar, presidential address, 7th Conference of the All-India Ophthalmological Society, 20 June 1940, *Indian Journal of Ophthalmology* 2, no. 1 (1941): 28–9.

5. On the street as a site of sanitary intervention and public response during the Bombay plague, see the report of the city health officer, T.S. Weir, in *Administration Report of the Municipal Commissioner for the City of Bombay, 1896–97* (Bombay: 'Times of India' Steam Press, 1897), pp. 656–717.

6. Prafulla Mohanti, *Changing Village, Changing Life* (London: Viking, 1990), p. 24.

7. *Times of India* (Jaipur), 21 February 2012, p. 6. The World Health Organization reported 207,551 roads deaths in India in 2013, equivalent to 16.6 deaths per 100,000 of the population, a far higher figure than the 137,572 deaths recorded locally. Available at www.who./int/gho/road_safety/mortality/en, accessed 24 April 2016.

8. *Report of the Motor Vehicles Insurance Committee, 1936–37* (Delhi: Government of India, Manager of Publications, 1937), pp. 11, 14–15, 53; Ruth Schwartz Cowan, *A Social History of American Technology* (New York: Oxford University Press, 1997), p. 235.

9. For examples, see *Bombay Chronicle*, 9 December 1926, p. 4; *Bombay Chronicle*, 17 December 1933, p. 5.

10. Madras, Judicial, Government Order [GO] 1099, 4 July 1911, India Office Records [IOR], British Library, London. For the case of a taxi that drove over three sleeping people at night, see *Annual Report on the Police of the City of Bombay, 1935* (Bombay: Government Central Press, 1936), p. 34.

11. On Indian rickshaw-pullers, see Ahmad Mukhtar, *Report on Rickshaw Pullers* (Delhi: Manager of Publications, 1946). The hazardous life of the rickshaw-puller has been more fully described elsewhere: see David Strand, *Rickshaw Beijing: City People and Politics in the 1920s* (Berkeley: University of California Press, 1989), and James Francis Warren, *Rickshaw Coolie: A People's History of Singapore (1880–1940)* (Singapore: Oxford University Press, 1986), with its exemplary use of coroners' reports to document the hardships of rickshaw-pullers' lives.

12. *Statesman* (Calcutta), 25 June 1922, p. 9.

13. *Bombay Chronicle*, 4 January 1927, p. 5; *Bombay Chronicle*, 23 December 1933, p. 6; *Bombay Chronicle*, 1 January 1934, p. 1; *Bombay Chronicle*, 6 June 1938, p. 5.

14. *Report of the Motor Vehicles Insurance Committee*, p. 17; *Annual Report on the Police of the City of Bombay, 1935* (Bombay: Government Central Press, 1936), p. 41; *Bombay Chronicle*, editorial, 2 July 1938, p. 6.

15. As in Calcutta: *Statesman*, 22 January 1922, p. 4, and Bombay: *Illustrated Weekly of India*, 23 August 1936, late news supplement.

16. *Illustrated Weekly of India* (Bombay), 9 August 1936, pp. 45–6; *Illustrated Weekly of India* (Bombay), 2 January 1938, p. 17.

17. *Bombay Chronicle*, 1 April 1946, p. 5. For related incidents, see *Statesman*, 3 January 1946, p. 3; *Statesman*, 5 January 1946, p. 7.

18. Oscar Jennings, *Cycling and Health*, 2nd ed. (London: Iliffe and Sons, 1893). On the association of Parsis with cycling and health, see H.D. Darukhanawala, *Parsis and Sports and Kindred Subjects* (Bombay: H.D. Darukhanawala, 1935), pp. 43, 372–81.

19. *Bombay Chronicle*, 30 June 1938, p. 10.

20. As, for instance, when plague struck factories in Cawnpore (Kanpur) in 1902 and 1904 (annual reports of the U.P. inspector of factories for these years, in V/24/1633 [IOR]).

21. It is worth putting street and factory deaths in context: in Bombay in 1908, 59 deaths were attributed to accidents involving machinery and 36 to moving vehicles, while many more (262) were caused by 'privation and starvation' and drowning (192) (*Administration Report of the Municipal Commissioner for the City of Bombay, 1908–09* [Bombay: Bombay Gazette Electric Printing Works, 1909], p. 72).

22. Dipesh Chakrabarty, *Rethinking Working-Class History: Bengal, 1890–1940* (Princeton: Princeton University Press, 1989); Samita Sen, *Women and Labour in Late Colonial India: The Bengal Jute Industry* (Cambridge: Cambridge University Press, 1999). But see Ahmad Mukhtar, *Factory Labour in India* (Madras: Annamalai University, 1930).

23. For a further consideration of factory health, see David Arnold, *Toxic Histories: Poison and Pollution in Modern India* (Cambridge: Cambridge University Press, 2016), pp. 192–9.

24. Among other locations where accident rates and fatalities were high in India in this period were sawmills, mines, railway workshops, and marshalling yards, not surprisingly in view of the nature of the machinery and working conditions involved.

25. B.P. Adarkar, *Report on Labour Conditions in the Rice Mills* (Delhi: Manager of Publications, 1946), p. 1.

26. Mukhtar, *Factory Labour*, pp. 221–8. As late as 1945, it was complained that India had no equivalent of Britain's medical factory inspectors and that the role of surgeons was confined to certifying the age of juvenile workers (C.K. Lakshmanan, 'Desirability of Instituting a Medical Inspectorate of Factories and Mines in India', appendix 1 to *Indian Industrial Health Advisory Committee, 1945–6* [IOR], pp. 5–8).

27. For example, Madras, Judicial, GO 1248, 7 August 1912 (IOR); Madras, Judicial, GO 1608, 24 July 1914 (IOR); Madras, Development, GO 940,

3 June 1923 (IOR); Madras, Development, GO 838, 10 June 1926 (IOR); *Report on the Working of the Indian Factories Act in the Madras Presidency, 1934* (Madras: Government Press, 1935), p. 22.

28. *Report of the Working of the Factories Act, Madras, 1915* (Madras: Government Press, 1916), p. 14; *Report of the Working of the Factories Act, Madras, 1941* (Madras Government Press, 1942), p. 51.

29. For example, Madras, Judicial, GO 1683, 19 July 1915 (IOR); Madras, Development, GO 1282, 14 July 1924, (IOR).

30. *Report of the Indian Factory Labour Commission, 1908*, vol. 2, *Evidence* (Simla: Government Central Branch Press, 1908), p. 297; *Annual Report on the Working of the Indian Factories Act in the Punjab, 1922* (Lahore: Government Press, 1923), pp. 2–3; *Annual Report on the Administration of the Factories Act in Bengal, 1938* (Calcutta: Government Press, 1939), pp. 11–12.

31. For example, *Report on the Working of the Indian Factories Act in the Madras Presidency, 1938* (Madras: Government Press, 1939), p. 30.

32. Margaret Bourke-White, *Halfway to Freedom* (New York: Simon and Schuster, 1949), pp. 131–9.

33. *Calcutta Municipal Gazette*, 2 May 1925, p. 991; *Statesman*, 7 February 1933, p. 4; Michael R. Anderson, 'Public Nuisance and Private Purpose: Policed Environments in British India, 1860–1947', SOAS Law Department Working Papers, no. 1, 1992.

34. But see Kelly D. Alley, *On the Banks of the Ganga: When Wastewater Meets a Sacred River* (Ann Arbor: University of Michigan Press, 2002); Awadhendra Sharan, *In the City, Out of Place: Nuisance, Pollution, and Dwelling in Delhi, c. 1850–2000* (New Delhi: Oxford University Press, 2014).

35. A.G. Clow, 'Indian Factory Law Administration', *Bulletin of Indian Industries and Labour*, no. 8 (Calcutta: Superintendent of Government Printing, India, 1921): 26.

36. Madras, Judicial, GO 1248, 7 August 1912 (IOR); Madras, Development, GO 940, 3 June 1923 (IOR); Madras, Development, GO 940, 25 June 1931 (IOR). 'Loose clothing' was also identified as a cause of accidents in cotton-ginning factories (*Annual Report on the Working of the Indian Factories Act in the Punjab, 1925* [Lahore: Government Press, 1926], p. 6; *Annual Report on the Working of the Indian Factories Act in the Punjab, 1929* [Lahore: Government Press, 1930], p. 11). A plea that tight-fighting clothing would save workers' lives was made as early as 1897 by the factory inspector for the North-Western Provinces, but with the oft-repeated reservation that this would be almost impossible to enforce (C.A. Walsh to Chief Secretary, NWP, 16 May 1898, V/24/1633 [IOR]).

37. Madras, Development, GO 880, 17 June 1925 (IOR).

38. Madras, Revenue (Special), GO 1206, 2 July 1920 (IOR). For a similar sentiment about the 'carelessness and ignorance' of uneducated workers

who 'generally are not of high intelligence', see Madras, Development, GO 1090, 30 June 1928 (IOR).

39. *Annual Report on the Administration of the Factories Act in Bengal, 1936* (Calcutta, 1937), pp. 20–1.

40. Figures calculated from the annual reports of the factory inspectors for Madras. 'Serious injuries' meant permanent disablement.

41. These issues are discussed in Mukhtar, *Factory Labour*.

42. On the latter, see *Correspondence Relating to a Proper Enactment for the Regulation of Places Used for the Disposal of Corpses in the Town and Island of Bombay* (Bombay: Bombay Education Society's Press, 1855).

43. Conditions in 'the home', in practice often a one-roomed tenement, were particularly held responsible for the high incidence of infant mortality in Bombay (*Administration Report of the Municipal Commissioner for the City of Bombay, 1915–16* [Bombay: Times Press, 1916], pp. 16–19). On purdah, see *Report of the Municipal Administration of Calcutta, 1919–20* (Calcutta: Corporation Press, 1920), vol. 1, pp. 62–3.

44. By the mid-twentieth century the promotion of drugs and medicines was of one of the leading sources of advertising revenue in India (*Report of the Press Commission* [New Delhi: Manager, Government of India Press, 1954], vol. 1, p. 80).

45. Arnold, *Everyday Technology*, chapter 5.

46. Such an episode occurs in Ikramulla's 'Le Gayi Pawan Urha' [The Wind Carried All Away] (1962), in *The Penguin Book of Classic Urdu Stories*, edited by M. Asaduddin (New Delhi: Penguin, 2006), pp. 255–6.

47. For example, *Bombay Chronicle*, 22 January 1927, p. 4.

48. K. Ramiah, *Rice in Madras: A Popular Handbook* (Madras: Superintendent, Government Press, 1937), chapter 8; W.R. Aykroyd, B.G. Krishnan, R. Passmore, and A.R. Sundarajan, *The Rice Problem in India*, Indian Medical Research Memoirs, no. 32 (Calcutta: Thacker, Spink & Co., 1940), p. 64.

49. As, for instance, with the contamination of mustard oil, widely used for cooking in eastern India, with the poisonous seeds of *Argemone mexicana* ('prickly poppy'), which resulted in fatal outbreaks of epidemic dropsy (Arnold, *Toxic Histories*, pp. 175–6).

50. David Arnold, 'British India and the "Beriberi Problem", 1798–1942', *Medical History* 54, no. 3 (2010): 295–314.

51. Prafulla Chandra Ray, *Life and Experiences of a Bengali Chemist*, vol. 1 (Calcutta: Chuckervertty, Chatterjee & Co., 1932), p. 367. These views on the negative impact of mechanized milling received convincing support from a detailed research study, Hashim Amir Ali, 'The Rice Industry in Lower Birbhum: A Survey', *Vishva-Bharati Rural Studies* 3 (1934) 35–45.

52. M.K. Gandhi, *Diet and Diet Reform*, 2nd ed. (Ahmedabad: Navajivan Press, 1940), p. 18; 'Swadeshi', 6 August 1934, *Collected Works of Mahatma Gandhi* vol. 58 (New Delhi: Publications Division, Ministry of Information and Broadcasting, 1974), pp. 293–4; 'Polished v. Unpolished', *Collected Works of Mahatma Gandhi*, vol. 59 (New Delhi: Publications Division, Ministry of Information and Broadcasting, 1974), p. 226.
53. *Bombay Chronicle*, 15 June 1938, p. 11.
54. *Illustrated Weekly of India*, 29 January 1939, p. 67.
55. *Illustrated Weekly of India*, 16 January 1938, p. 73.

AFTERWORD
Making 'the Medical'

MARK HARRISON

The chapters in this volume have clearly demonstrated the instability of 'the medical' as an analytical category. When examined closely, its boundaries become altogether less distinct and more porous than commonly imagined. Moreover, the authority of Western medicine, often regarded as a colonizing force in its own right, appears contingent and fragile. Challenges and adaptations to biomedicine—as the Western tradition came to be known—have taken many forms and have long fascinated scholars of 'colonial medicine', in particular.[1] But what is distinctive about this volume is that it has sought 'the medical' not only in hospitals, dispensaries, and other professionalized spaces but also in penal establishments, infrastructure, the workplace, and the home. In such contexts, 'the medical' lacked precise definition, its authority often being dependent on the whims of non-medical actors. And yet, there is no disguising the fact that the period covered by this volume was marked by the emergence of a relatively distinct domain that has come to be known as 'medical'. In this afterword, I shall therefore concentrate on the first part of what the editors—following Hacking—refer to as the 'historical ontology' of 'the medical'; the process by which it came into being.

At the end of the eighteenth century, the term 'medical' was used chiefly to denote those persons and practices specializing in 'physic' (as distinct from surgery or the apothecary's trade). Persons involved in this line of work normally held degrees in medicine but physic (or 'internal medicine') was also practised by a growing body of men whose work moved readily between medicine and surgery—prototype 'general practitioners'.[2] The many 'surgeons' of the European trading companies were among the more important populations constituting the latter category,[3] alongside those of the armed forces.[4] In the coming century, 'the medical' came to refer to a broader spectrum of activities, spanning the formerly distinct provinces of physic, surgery, and pharmacy. This reflects the emergence of a unified profession in mid-century, after which it is likely that the term had a boundary function, demarcating those areas which were, by law or convention, the preserve of qualified practitioners.[5] But even before the medical profession—in the modern sense of the term—came into being, the 'medical' was moving beyond the purely professional to encompass those aspects of everyday life and institutions which entailed the regulation of health. Medicine and its practitioners were becoming steadily more important as arbiters of health and well-being and played a much bigger role in non-medical institutions. This process accelerated in the years after 1900 and particularly after the First World War, at which point the objectives of the profession, the state, and industry became more closely intertwined.[6]

These trends may be seen clearly in the titles of publications during the two centuries covered by this volume. Google Ngrams viewer, for example, shows an exponential growth in publications bearing the title 'medical' during the nineteenth century, together with its application to a greater variety of subjects. In the eighteenth century, the bulk of 'medical' titles were professional journals, but by the middle of the nineteenth century a wider range of 'medical' subjects is reflected in publication titles, including those relating to insurance and law. By the twentieth century, there were also a greater number of 'medical' works dealing with issues affecting home, workplace, and civil society. If the *Times of India* database is a reliable guide, then this general Anglophone pattern was reflected in the particular case of India, showing a sharp increase in references to 'the medical' in the last four decades of the nineteenth century and continued growth thereafter. The establishment of medical departments in military and civil administrations during the 1860s accounts for many of these references, as does the growth of institutions such as hospitals and medical colleges and the number of practitioners associated with them. 'Medical' plants, women, and societies also figure prominently. Within a few decades, lawsuits and qualifications (the standard and applicability thereof) become more noticeable, as do references to 'the medical' as a domain contested between different types of practitioners and in relation to the welfare of the population.

Indeed, one of the most notable features of 'the medical' as reflected/constituted in *The Times* is the partial incorporation of non-Western forms of healing. Despite the critical standpoint of most of the newspaper's correspondents and readers, it is clear that certain forms of non-Western medicine were becoming politically important by the early twentieth century and could not easily be ignored. The same is true of unlicensed practice by persons claiming to be 'doctors', together with many other persons who seemed to make a living from selling or using what appeared to be Western pharmaceuticals. As I shall argue in this chapter, there is evidence that a commodity-based, pan-medical culture had come into being by the turn of the twentieth century. Although distinctions between different forms of healing and medicine persisted and in many respects became more rigid, their authority increasingly rested on their ability to produce, advertise, and distribute a range of material artefacts. In this unregulated marketplace, many new forms of medicine came into being, blurring boundaries between different 'traditions' and creating a distinctively Indian medical space.

In accounting for the rise of 'the medical', the most obvious starting point is the state. As several of the authors in this volume remind us, 'the medical' is sometimes visible only in those traces that are left in official records. This is problematic for historians, who have regularly to confront the problems of distortion and omission. But it is also indicative that the state had a powerful role in constituting the medical, just as medicine came increasingly to shape the state's institutions and practices. The parameters of 'the medical' developed in line with the modern nation state's desire to know and regulate its population. Though by no means co-terminus with 'biopower'—in the Foucauldian sense of the term—medicine served to subjugate the population and eventually to nurture it as an economic asset. Beginning in the Renaissance, this process accelerated in the eighteenth century, with the transition from regal power over distinct, semi-hereditary 'estates' to those in which monarchical power was removed or superseded. These states were simultaneously engaged in the rapid expansion of their armed forces, which were required to fight wars against rival states on an increasingly global scale. Medical practitioners began to carve out a niche for themselves within burgeoning military and naval bureaucracies and in the trading companies through which wealth flowed into the capitals of Europe. Their role as managers of health soon expanded into other sectors in which 'massification' was taking place, most obviously in the new industrial towns but also in prisons, workhouses and other institutions regarded as vital to the maintenance of order.[7]

Employment within state bureaucracies expanded the reach of medicine and the numbers of persons trained to practice it, but it also changed the nature of medicine. The armed forces were initially the most powerful engine of this change. As the number of practitioners employed to practice surgery and medicine increased, the boundaries between these old 'estates' became blurred. The East India Company followed suit, as it began its transition from trading company to territorial power. Practitioners employed in these bureaucracies played a major part in the drive for the reform of medical learning, professional unification, and state recognition. This new breed of medical practitioner—adept at managing populations—subsequently became essential in the management of other institutions. Having demonstrated their worth to the state, medical practitioners were able to acquire legal recognition and protection of their new professional monopoly. This eventually increased their prestige but initially created suspicion because hitherto diverse groups of practitioners, with historic ties to a range of institutions, became self-referential. The tension created by professionalization was probably most evident within the armed forces, where the new outlook of medical practitioners created tensions with combatants. Doctors came to be looked upon as little more than civilians in uniform.[8]

The importance of the military in the formation of a distinctively medical space has often been overlooked, even by Foucault.[9] Philanthropic institutions for the care of the poor and infirm were—as Foucault and numerous historians have noted—important in the expansion of medicine and in the medicalization of certain areas of life.[10] But these developments were less noticeable in civilian than in military and naval contexts and it was in the latter that the operation of 'biopower' first became evident—in codes of behaviour ('discipline') and in the management of health ('biopolitics').[11] However, in the context of colonial India, the military origins of the medical are difficult to avoid and have been remarked upon by numerous scholars who have examined the growth of the colonial government's medical functions and institutions.[12] It is well known that civilian medical bureaucracies grew out of and continued to overlap with military ones, their most senior personnel, officers of the Indian Medical Service, serving two years in the military before being able to take up civilian employment.[13] However, by the middle of the century, other branches of government, such as police, and bodies at local and municipal levels also began to employ medical-sanitary workers, the most senior of which held qualifications in medicine or public health. Around this professional core were assembled a vast number of subordinate staff in the form of assistant surgeons, hospital assistants, vaccinators, and an even greater number of non-medical workers who sometimes performed functions such as sanitary work.

It is seldom easy to delineate a strictly medical sphere of influence in such cases but these medical and quasi-medical occupations were organized and enabled by the growth of the colonial state, its object being to know and manage the populations over which it ruled.[14] As the essays collected here show, 'the medical' also figured—albeit sometimes indistinctly—in other realms of state activity; juridical, penal, and so forth. In these areas, 'medical' knowledge was often difficult to distinguish from other forms, such as the ethnographic and sociological. Nevertheless, it is clear that medical considerations began to shape the regulation and conduct of non-medical institutions. As in the armed forces, the professionalization of medicine made its practitioners more confident and assertive. Over time, it therefore becomes easier to identify 'the medical' within state institutions, especially when professional agendas came into conflict with political realities. In British India, we can see this at various levels of state administration, as medical officers formed different views about policy from senior officials. Some pressed the government much further than it was prepared to go in the funding of public and medical research or the regulation of social and personal life.[15] The same was true at municipal level, where there were clashes between health officers and Indian municipal commissioners about funding and the scale and pace of sanitary reform.[16] Behind these conflicts lay not only the realities of colonial economics but a conception

of medicine as central to human life.[17] Medicine had become synonymous with civilization and the expansion of its remit a kind of a moral
crusade.[18] As more Indians began to be trained in Western medicine,
these demands acquired a political edge, highlighting aspects of health
and medicine that had been ignored by the colonial administration.[19]

In India, 'the medical' originated primarily within state bureaucracies and grew in line with their expansion. As in other countries, this
fostered a mutually dependent relationship between governance and
medical expertise.[20] However, government growth is not a sufficient
explanation for the creation of what came to be understood as 'the
medical', as it was never confined solely to those aspects of medicine
fostered or dispensed by the government. Other domains of medical
practice such as Christian missions must also be considered, although
they were probably much less important in shaping the medical realm
in India than in some other colonies.[21] Their influence was most keenly
felt in places in which the state was most distant from the lives of the
people, such as in 'tribal' areas or on the frontier.[22] Far more important in constituting 'the medical' were the diverse array of practices
and practitioners often (misleadingly) referred to as Indian medical
'systems'. Despite wilful indifference on the part of the state and most
Western doctors, non-Western medical practices continued to flourish
and diversify. They adapted in ingenious ways to the challenges posed
by Western medicine, which had gained a hold on Indian society
primarily as a result of state sponsorship and the mass manufacture of
pharmaceutical products. The wide distribution of medicines across the
subcontinent (increasingly connected by roads, railways, and canals)
and their advertisement in English language and vernacular publications meant that Western medicine could make its presence felt despite
the lack of medical institutions outside the larger towns and cities.
Practitioners of 'Indian' medicine began to adopt these techniques,
advertising their products and services in similar ways to Western
practitioners, in the pages of vernacular newspapers and journals.[23]
Some even employed 'Western' and 'Indian' remedies together in their
practice.[24] These tactics enabled Indian medical 'traditions' to prosper
despite the institutionalization of Western medicine and the cultural
authority this bestowed.[25]

At the end of the nineteenth century and in the early twentieth
century, a commodity-based medical culture had come into being,

spawning myriad forms of medical practice, not readily identifiable as either Indian or Western.[26] It was evident not only in the marketplace but in the care of the self and in areas such as sexuality, reproduction, and physical regeneration, in which various pills and elixirs played an important part.[27] The increasing export of 'Indian' medical commodities also presented a certain version of this culture to the rest of the world.[28] After Independence, the export of 'Ayurvedic' and other such products was accompanied by the export of generic Western drugs and medical technologies. A favourable legislative environment and India's non-aligned status allowed the new nation to become one of the principal suppliers of medicines and medical technologies to the developing world.[29] Within India, too, the unregulated nature of the pharmaceutical market enabled a pluralistic medical culture to persist, for good or ill. These several factors have perpetuated a version of 'the medical' which is synonymous with material artefacts.

The growth of India's medical commodity culture was to some degree dependent on the state, which dispensed increasing quantities of popular drugs and assisted in the development of medical technologies after Independence. But much also depended on the entrepreneurship of medical practitioners outside the state sector, who fashioned exclusive professional domains through journals, professional societies, and clubs, as well as founding private hospitals, sometimes in conjunction with Indian philanthropists.[30] Their aim was simultaneously to expand professional opportunities, while closing down competition through regulation of the medical market. Demands for the control of 'quacks' began to appear with increasing frequency from the 1890s, as Indian practitioners became more assertive in pressing their claims,[31] but legislation to regulate medical practice along British lines was not passed until 1912.[32]

From the early twentieth century, the expansion of 'the medical' was, therefore, propelled through the activities of practitioners in private employment. Despite the growth of government hospitals and dispensaries in urban areas,[33] most rural areas and small towns still had none. Even where they did exist, Indians tended to use them selectively and sometimes as a last resort.[34] Indeed, in 1910, the Government of India admitted that it would never allocate sufficient resources to remedy this situation and decided instead to foster the growth of the 'independent' profession, that is, those persons qualified in Western

medicine but working outside the state sector.[35] Its primary intention
was to boost the number of private practitioners in the smaller towns,
but this also gave more power to Indians employed in state medical
institutions. In order to incentivize the independent profession, it
was thought desirable to accede to the demands of bodies such as
the Bombay Medical Union, which sought greater representation in
senior posts at government hospitals, for example, as part-time hospital
consultants. These new medical career paths, outside the military or
quasi-military services, came to be regarded as desirable among the
Indian elite.[36]

The growing assertiveness of Indian doctors, and their involvement in nationalist politics, facilitated the passage of medicine into
the political arena. After 1919, when Indians began to take charge
of provincial government departments, health and medicine figured
more prominently as political concerns, not only in demands for
greater recognition of Indian medicine or more Indian representation in government jobs, but also in comparisons of India with other
states. In the eyes of many nationalists, the British administration had
neglected the health of Indians, some of whom looked, like other
progressives around the world, to the health care systems of the
Soviet Union.[37] International comparisons were made possible by the
global reporting of 'medical' issues, sometimes in sections of newspapers entitled 'Medical News'. These included disasters such as the
malaria epidemic which struck the Punjab and the United Provinces
in 1908 and the influenza of 1918–19, but also more mundane professional matters and the development of medical science and institutions. The formation of international bodies such as the League of
Nations Health Organization in 1919 (a repository of health statistics
and an active investigator of health conditions) and intervention by
bodies such as the Rockefeller Foundation also meant that progress
in medicine and health was seen in relation to other countries and
colonies.[38] The 'medical' in India thus began to be shaped by international standards and expectations, and this process continued apace
after Independence, with the involvement of other nations—under
the auspices of the World Health Organization—in campaigns to
eradicate smallpox and malaria.[39]

In the nineteenth and twentieth centuries, the trends described
here worked together to fashion a relatively distinctive domain which

we have come to know as 'medical', even though, in contexts such as the Andaman forests, it may still be difficult to locate. What is or is not 'medical' remains contentious but such disputes ought not to detract from the fact that numerous aspects of human experience have been extricated from wider categories of understanding and have come to be regulated in accordance with medical expertise; in other words, 'medicalized'. That we feel the need to interrogate or deconstruct 'the medical' is in itself an admission that it has shaped our social institutions and subjectivities. Although it originated—like 'the economy,' 'society,' and other categories through which we have come to understand the modern world—from amidst the structural transformations of the last few centuries, it is imagined and renewed through every-day practices. 'The medical' is more than a category of analysis; it is a state of mind.

Notes

1. David Arnold, *Colonizing the Body: State Medicine and Epidemic Disease in Nineteenth-Century India* (Berkeley: University of California Press, 1993). See also, P. Bala, ed., *Biomedicine as a Contested Site: Some Revelations in Imperial Contexts* (Lanham, etc.: Lexington Books, 2009); A. Cunningham and B. Andrews, eds, *Western Medicine as Contested Knowledge* (Manchester: Manchester University Press, 1997); D. Arnold, ed., *Imperial Medicine and Indigenous Societies* (Manchester: Manchester University Press, 1988).

2. Anne Digby, *Making a Medical Living: Doctors and Patients in the English Market for Medicine, 1720–1911* (Cambridge: Cambridge University Press, 1994); Irvine Loudon, *Medical Care and the General Practitioner, 1750–1850* (Oxford: Clarendon Press, 1986).

3. Mark Harrison, *Medicine in an Age of Commerce and Empire: Britain and Its Tropical Colonies 1660–1830* (Oxford: Oxford University Press, 2010); Iris Bruijn, *Ship's Surgeons of the Dutch East India Company: Commerce and the Progress of Medicine in the Eighteenth Century* (Leiden: Leiden University Press, 2009).

4. M. Ackroyd, L. Brockliss, M. Moss, K. Retford, and J. Stevenson, *Advancing with the Army: Medicine, the Professions, and Social Mobility in the British Isles, 1790–1850* (Oxford: Oxford University Press, 2006).

5. Penelope J. Corfield, *Power and the Professions in Britain 1700–1850* (London and New York: Routledge, 1995), chapter 6; J. Parry and N. Parry, *The Rise of the Medical Profession: A Study of Collective Social Mobility* (London: Croom Helm, 1976).

6. John Pickstone, 'Production, Community, and Consumption: The Political Economy of Twentieth-Century Medicine', in *Medicine in the Twentieth Century*, edited by R. Cooter and J. Pickstone (London: Harwood, 2000), pp. 1–19.

7. Christopher Lawrence, *Medicine in the Making of Modern Britain 1700–1920* (London: Routledge, 1994).

8. Mark Harrison, 'Medicine and the Management of Modern Warfare', *History of Science* 34 (1996): 386.

9. Michel Foucault, 'The Politics of Health in the Eighteenth Century', in *Power/Knowledge: Selected Interviews and Other Writings 1972–1977*, edited by C. Gordon (Brighton: Harvester Press, 1980), pp. 166–82.

10. See, for example, A. Borsay and P. Shapely, eds, *Medicine, Charity and Mutual Aid: The Consumption of Health and Welfare in Britain, c.1550–1950* (Aldershot: Ashgate, 2007); L. Granshaw and R. Porter, eds, *The Hospital in History* (London: Routledge, 1989).

11. See, for example, Erica Charters, *Disease, War, and the Imperial State: The Welfare of the British Armed Forces during the Seven Years' War* (Chicago: University of Chicago Press, 2014); G. Hudson, ed., *British Military and Naval Medicine, 1600–1830* (Amsterdam and New York: Rodopi, 2007).

12. For example, David Arnold, 'Medical Priorities and Practice in Nineteenth-Century British India', *South Asia Research* 5 (1985): 167–83; Radhika Ramasubban, 'Imperial Health in British India', in *Disease, Medicine, and Empire*, edited by R. MacLeod and M. Lewis (London: Routledge, 1988), pp. 38–60.

13. Mark Harrison, *Public Health in British India: Anglo-Indian Preventive Medicine 1859–1914* (Cambridge: Cambridge University Press, 1994).

14. Harrison, *Public Health*, chapters 7–8; Amna Khalid, '"Unscientific and Insanitary": Hereditary Sweepers and Customary Rights in the United Provinces', in *Public Health in the British Empire: Intermediaries, Subordinates, and the Practice of Health, 1850–1960*, edited by R. Johnson and A. Khalid (Abingdon: Routledge, 2012), pp. 51–70; Amna Khalid, '"Subordinate" Negotiations: Indigenous Staff, the Colonial State and Public Health', in *The Social History of Health and Medicine in Colonial India*, edited by B. Pati and M. Harrison (Abingdon: Routledge, 2009), pp. 45–73; S. Bhattacharya, M. Harrison, and M. Worboys, *Fractured States: Smallpox, Public Health and Vaccination Policy in British India 1800–1947* (Hyderabad: Orient Longman, 2005).

15. Mark Harrison, 'Towards a Sanitary Utopia? Professional Visions and Public Health in India, 1880–1914', *South Asia Research* 10 (1990): 19–40.

16. Partho Datta, *Planning the City: Urbanization and Reform in Calcutta c.1800–c.1940* (New Delhi: Tulika Books, 2012); Sandip Hazareesingh,

The Colonial City and the Challenge of Modernity: Urban Hegemonies and Civic Contestations in Bombay (1900–1925) (Hyderabad: Orient Longman, 2005); Harrison, *Public Health*, chapters 7–8.

17. Arnold, *Colonizing the Body*.

18. See, for example, Pratik Chakrabarti, *Bacteriology in British India: Laboratory Medicine and the Tropics* (Rochester, New York: University of Rochester Press, 2012).

19. For example, Arabinda Samanta, 'Negotiating Subalternity in Everyday Life: Social Construction of Tuberculosis in Colonial and Post-colonial India', in *Medical Encounters in British India*, edited by D. Kumar and R. Sekhar Basu (Delhi: Oxford University Press, 2013), pp. 253–74; Mridula Ramanna, *Western Medicine and Public Health in Colonial Bombay 1845–1895* (London: Sangam Books, 2002).

20. Roy MacLeod, ed., *Government and Expertise: Specialists, Administrators and Professionals, 1860–1919* (Cambridge: Cambridge University Press, 2003).

21. Most notably in Africa, see D. Hardiman, ed., *Healing Bodies, Saving Souls: Medical Missions in Asia and Atlanta* (Amsterdam: Rodopi, 2006).

22. For example, David Hardiman, *Missionaries and Their Medicine: A Christian Modernity for Tribal India* (Manchester: Manchester University Press, 2008); '"Clinical Christianity": The Emergence of Medical Work as a Missionary Strategy in Colonial India, 1800–1914', in *Health, Medicine and Empire: Perspectives on Colonial India*, edited by B. Pati and M. Harrison (Hyderabad: Orient Longman, 2001), pp. 88–136.

23. See, for example, Madhuri Sharma, *Indigenous and Western Medicine in Colonial India* (New Delhi: Foundation Books, 2012); Guy Attewell, *Refiguring Unani Tibb: Plural Healing in Late Colonial India* (Hyderabad: Orient Longman, 2007); Kavita Sivaramakrishnan, *Old Potions, New Bottles: Recasting Indigenous Medicine in Colonial Punjab 1850–1945* (Hyderabad: Orient Longman, 2006).

24. Anil Kumar, 'The Indian Drug Industry under the Raj, 1860–1920', in Pati and Harrison, *Health, Medicine and Empire*, pp. 356–85; J.H. Hume, 'Medicine in the Punjab, 1849–1911' (unpublished Ph.D. diss., Duke University, 1977).

25. K.N. Panikkar, 'Indigenous Medicine and Cultural Hegemony', in K.N. Panikkar, *Culture, Ideology, Hegemony: Intellectuals and Social Consciousness in Colonial India* (New Delhi: Tulika Books, 1995), pp. 145–75.

26. D. Hardiman and P.B. Mukharji, eds, *Medical Marginality in South Asia: Situating Subaltern Therapeutics* (Abingdon: Routledge, 2012); Projit Bihari Mukharji, *Nationalizing the Body: The Market, Print and Healing in Colonial Bengal, 1860–1930* (London: Anthem Press, 2009).

27. For example, S. Hodges, ed., *Reproductive Health in India: History, Politics, and Controversies* (New Delhi: Orient Longman, 2006).

28. Madhulika Banerjee, *Power, Knowledge, Medicine: Ayurvedic Pharmaceuticals at Home and in the World* (Hyderabad: Orient BlackSwan, 2009); Maarten Bode, *Taking Traditional Knowledge to the Market: The Modern Image of the Ayurvedic and Unani Industry 1980–2000* (Hyderabad: Orient BlackSwan, 2008).

29. Stanislaw Kachnowski, 'A History of Medical Technology in Post-Colonial India: The Development of Technology in Medicine from 1947 to 1991' (unpublished D.Phil. diss., University of Oxford, 2016).

30. For example, 'The Rajkumari Leper Asylum', *Indian Medical Reporter*, 16 October 1895, p. 275.

31. For example, Letter to the Editor from 'A civil-hospital assistant', *Indian Medical Reporter*, 26 July 1895, p. 125.

32. Harrison, *Public Health*, p. 12.

33. Samiksha Sehrawat, *Colonial Medical Care in North India: Gender, State, and Society, c.1840–1920* (New Delhi: Oxford University Press, 2013).

34. Moizuddin, Deputy Collector, Nara Valley, to Deputy Commissioner, Thar and Parkar, 26 November 1910, General Dept., vol. 73, 1913, Maharashtra State Archives, Mumbai.

35. A. Earle, Officiating Secretary to Government of India, Home Department (Medical) to Secretary to General Department, Government of Bombay, 22 February 1911, General Department, vol. 73, 1913, Maharashtra State Archives, Mumbai.

36. Mark Harrison, 'Introduction', in *From Western Medicine to Global Medicine: The Hospital beyond the West*, edited by M. Harrison, M. Jones, and H. Sweet (Hyderabad: Orient BlackSwan, 2009), p. 26.

37. Mark Harrison, 'A Global Perspective: Reframing the History of Health, Medicine, and Disease', *Bulletin of the History of Medicine* 89 (2015): pp. 671–2.

38. Shirish N. Kavadi, 'Rockefeller Public Health in Colonial India', in *Histories of Medicine and Healing in the Indian Ocean World*, vol. 2, edited by A. Winterbottom and F. Tesfaye (Basingstoke: Palgrave Macmillan, 2016), pp. 61–88; Sunil Amrith, *Decolonizing International Health: India and Southeast Asia, 1930–65* (Basingstoke: Palgrave, 2006).

39. Sanjoy Bhattacharya, *Expunging Variola: The Control and Eradication of Smallpox in British India 1947–1977* (Hyderabad: Orient Longman, 2006). Randall M. Packard, *The Making of a Tropical Disease* (Baltimore: Johns Hopkins Press, 2007); Randall M. Packard, 'Malaria Dreams: Postwar Visions of Health and Development in the Third World', *Medical Anthropology* 17 (1997): 279–96.

EDITORS AND CONTRIBUTORS

Editors

Rohan Deb Roy is Lecturer in South Asian History at the University of Reading. He received his PhD from University College London, UK, and has held postdoctoral fellowships at the Centre for Studies in Social Sciences' Calcutta, India, at the University of Cambridge, UK, and at the Max Planck Institute for the History of Science, Berlin, Germany. He has been a Barnard-Columbia Weiss International Visiting Scholar in New York, USA. He is the author of *Malarial Subjects: Empire, Medicine and Nonhumans in British India, 1820–1909* (2017).

Guy N.A. Attewell is an independent researcher, and divides his time between Tamil Nadu, India, and the UK. He was formerly a Researcher in the Department of Social Sciences at the French Institute of Pondicherry, India, and taught in University College London, Wellcome Trust Centre for the History of Medicine, UK. He has published on the history of late colonial medicine in India, Islam and medicine, the circulation of medicinal plant knowledge between Europe and India, and bone-setting practices in contemporary India. Among other things, he currently devotes himself to experiments in non-conventional education for secondary school students in Auroville, Tamil Nadu.

Contributors

Clare Anderson is Professor of History at the University of Leicester, UK. Her research centres around the history of incarceration and penal colonies, and their intersections with other modes of confinement and coerced labour, with a focus on South and Southeast Asia, the Indian Ocean, and Australia. Her publications include *Convicts in the Indian Ocean: Transportation from South Asia to Mauritius, 1815–53* (2000), *Legible Bodies: Race, Criminality and Colonialism in South Asia* (2004), *Subaltern Lives: Biographies of Colonialism in the Indian Ocean World, 1790–1920* (2012) and, with Madhumita Mazumdar and Vishvajit Pandya, *New Histories of the Andaman Islands: Landscape, Place and Identity in the Bay of Bengal, 1790–2012* (2016).

David Arnold, Emeritus Professor of History at the University of Warwick, UK, was previously Professor of South Asian History at the School of Oriental and African Studies, London, UK. His published work has addressed various aspects of modern Indian history, with particular reference to science, technology, and medicine. His published work includes *Colonizing the Body: State Medicine and Epidemic Disease in Nineteenth-Century India* (1993), *Science, Technology and Medicine in Colonial India* (2000); *The Tropics and the Traveling Gaze: India, Landscape, and Science, 1800–1856* (2006), *Everyday Technology: Machines and the Making of India's Modernity* (2013), and *Toxic Histories: Poison and Pollution in Modern India* (2016).

Calum Blaikie is a Postdoctoral Researcher in the European Research Council-funded 'Reassembling Tibetan Medicine' (Ratimed) project, based at the Institute for Social Anthropology, Austrian Academy of Sciences, Vienna, Austria. He holds a PhD in Social Anthropology from the University of Kent, UK, and has over fifteen years of experience in research and applied work concerning Sowa Rigpa (Tibetan medicine) in Himalayan India, Nepal, and Bhutan. His research focuses on social networks and flows of medicinal raw materials, the production and circulation of Tibetan medicines, and the integration of traditional medicine into public health care.

Mark Harrison is Professor of the History of Medicine at the University of Oxford, UK, where he is Director of the Wellcome Unit for the History of Medicine and co-Director of the Wellcome Centre for Ethics and Humanities and the Oxford Martin Programme on Collective Responsibility for Infectious Disease. He has written widely on the history of medicine and health in India and on global themes. He is currently working on the history of malaria in British India.

Madhumita Mazumdar is Associate Professor at the Dhirubhai Ambani Institute of Information Communication Technology, Gandhinagar, Gujarat, India. She has a specialized interest in the social and cultural history of science and technology in India. She is presently involved in research on the historical legacies of colonial science in the shaping of contemporary developmentalist agendas and tribal welfare policies in the Andaman Islands. She has recently co-authored a book, with Clare Anderson and Vishvajit Pandya, titled *New Histories of the Andaman Islands: Landscape, Place and Identity in the Bay of Bengal, 1790–2012*.

James H. Mills researches the social history of drugs and narcotics, and the history of health and medicine in the British empire. His publications include *Cannabis Britannica: Empire, Trade, and Prohibition, 1800–1928* (2003) and *Cannabis Nation: Control and Consumption in Britain, 1928–2008* (2012). He has also co-edited (with Patricia Barton) *Essays in Modern Imperialism and Intoxication 1500–1930* (2007). He is currently the Principal Investigator on the Wellcome Trust Investigator Award-funded project 'The Asian Cocaine Crisis: Pharmaceuticals, Consumers and Control in South and East Asia, c. 1900–1945'.

Durba Mitra is Assistant Professor of Studies in Women, Gender, and Sexuality, and Carol K. Pforzheimer Assistant Professor at the Radcliffe Institute at Harvard University, USA.

Projit Bihari Mukharji is Associate Professor in History and Sociology of Science at the University of Pennsylvania, USA. His work has focused largely on the vernacularization of 'Western' medicine (*Nationalizing the Body*, 2009), subaltern therapeutics (*Medical Marginality in South Asia*, 2012), and the modernization of Ayurveda (*Doctoring Traditions*,

2016). Currently he is working on a history of genetics, race, and human difference in South Asia.

Vishvajit Pandya is Professor of Anthropology at the Dhirubhai Ambani Institute of Information Communication Technology, Gandhinagar, Gujarat, India. He completed his PhD from the University of Chicago, USA, and has worked among the indigenous communities of the Andaman and Nicobar Islands since 1982. He has held teaching positions in the United States and New Zealand. He has published widely on the Andamanese indigenous groups and has had a particular interest in the anthropology of medicine. He is the author of *Above the Forest: A Study of Andamanese Ethnoanemology, Cosmology, and the Power of Ritual* (1993), *In the Forest: Visual and Material Worlds of Andamanese History (1858–2006)* (2009) and co-author, with Clare Anderson and Madhumita Mazumdar, of *New Histories of the Andaman Islands: Landscape, Place and Identity in the Bay of Bengal, 1790–2012* (2016). He is also the founder and Honorary Director of the Andaman and Nicobar Tribal Research Institute at Port Blair, India.

Shubha Ranganathan is Assistant Professor in the Department of Liberal Arts, Indian Institute of Technology Hyderabad, India. Her work is broadly located at the interface of culture and mental health, particularly with reference to women's health and illness. Her doctoral research explored women's experiences of spirit possession, trance, and healing while residing in Mahanubhav temples in Maharashtra. Her current work engages with issues surrounding the politics of mental health and healing, and contemporary debates around the legitimacy and credibility of indigenous healing practices. She is also involved in ethnographic studies of the practices of biomedical psychiatry and indigenous healing shrines.

Jonathan Saha completed his PhD at the School of Oriental and African Studies, London, UK, in 2010. Jonathan is currently Associate Professor of Southeast Asian History at the University of Leeds, UK. He has published on the history of corruption in British Burma, notably in his 2013 monograph *Law, Disorder and the Colonial State: Corruption in Burma c.1900*. He has also written widely on the subjects of crime, justice, psychiatry, and animals in the colony in a range of journals, including *Modern Asian Studies, Past and Present,* and *The American Historical Review.*

Sudipta Sen is Professor of History, University of California, Davis, USA. His work has largely focused on the early history of British India. He is the author of *Empire of Free Trade: The English East India Company and the Making of the Colonial Marketplace* (1998), and *Distant Sovereignty: National Imperialism and the Origins of British India* (2002). His current book projects include *Ganga: Many Pasts of an Indian River* (forthcoming) and *Imperial Law and Order: Crime, Punishment and Justice in Early British India, 1770–1830* (forthcoming).

Chandak Sengoopta is Professor of History at Birkbeck College, University of London, UK. Educated in India and the USA, he works on the history of medicine and the cultural history of modern India. He is the author of many papers and several books, of which *The Rays before Satyajit: Creativity and Modernity in Colonial India* (2016) is the latest.

INDEX